W9-AEL-421

Professional Nursing

Concepts, Issues, and Challenges

John Daly, PhD, RN, FRCNA, FINE, FCN, is Professor of Nursing and Foundation Head of the School of Nursing, Family & Community Health, University of Western Sydney. He is one of Australia's leading scholars in Nursing. Dr. Daly's research focuses on cardiovascular nursing, the experience of illness and transcultural nursing. He is active in international publications projects in nursing scholarship and is well published in textbooks and refereed journals.

Sandra Speedy, EdD, MURP, BA (Hons), Dip. Ed., RN, is currently Executive Dean, Faculty of Law, Business and the Creative Arts, at James Cook University and Professor Emeritus. She has an extensive history in nursing education at all levels, working across the range of administrative, academic and service areas. Her areas of research interest include gender issues in management, dysfunctional organizations and cultural challenges in organizations. She has published in a wide range of areas in nursing, health, sociology and management. She is a consultant clinical psychologist and conducts a psychotherapy practice.

Debra Jackson, PhD, RN, MCN, is Associate Professor of Nursing at the School of Nursing, Family & Community Health, University of Western Sydney. Dr. Jackson's research focuses on women's and family health nursing, family support, building resilience in individuals and families, nursing leadership, and nursing workforce issues. She is well published in refereed journals and textbooks.

Vickie A. Lambert, DNSc, RN, FAAN, is Dean and Professor Emerita, School of Nursing, Medical College of Georgia, and an international nursing consultant with Lambert & Lambert Nursing Consultants. She has held visiting professorships in Australia, China, Japan, South Korea and Thailand. Dr. Lambert's research focuses on role stress and coping skills among hospital nurses from America, Asia, and Oceania. She has numerous publications in textbooks and journals, as well as having served as Editor of an international nursing and health sciences journal.

Clinton E. Lambert, PhD, RN, CS, FAAN, is an international nursing consultant with Lambert & Lambert Nursing Consultants. He is a retired US Army psychiatric clinical nurse specialist and the former owner and counselor, Lambert Counseling Services, in rural Georgia. Dr. Lambert has held visiting professorships in Australia, China, Japan, South Korea, and Thailand. His research focuses on role stress and coping skills among hospital nurses from America, Asia, and Oceania. Dr. Lambert has published extensively in books and professional journals, as well as having served as Editor of an international nursing and health sciences journal.

Professional Nursing
Concepts, Issues, and Challenges

John Daly, PhD, RN, FRCNA, FINE, FCN
Sandra Speedy, EdD, MURP, BA (Hons), Dip. Ed., RN
Debra Jackson, PhD, RN, MCN
Vickie A. Lambert, DNSc, RN, FAAN
Clinton E. Lambert, PhD, RN, CS, FAAN

Editors

Springer Publishing Company

RT
82
.P757
2005

Copyright © 2005 by Springer Publishing Company, Inc.

All rights reserved

No part of this publication may be reproduced, stored in a retrieval system, or transmitted in any form or by any means, electronic, mechanical, photocopying, recording, or otherwise, without the prior permission of Springer Publishing Company, Inc.

Springer Publishing Company, Inc.
11 West 42nd Street, 15th Floor
New York, NY 10036-8002

Acquisitions Editor: Ruth Chasek
Production Editor: J. Hurkin-Torres
Cover design by Joanne Honigman

05 06 07 08 09 / 5 4 3 2 1

Library of Congress Cataloging-in-Publication Data

Professional nursing : concepts, issues, and challenges / edited by
   John Daly . . . [et al].
     p.; cm.
   ISBN 0-8261-2554-9
   1. Nursing.   2. Nursing—United States.
   [DNLM: 1. Nursing. WY 16 P96443 2005] I. Daly, John, 1958–
   RT82.P757 2005
   610.73—dc22

                                                                           2004027269

Printed in the United States of America by Maple-Vail.

Contents

Contributors

Robert L. Anders, DrPH, RN, APRN, CS, CNAA
Associate Dean, College of Health Sciences
Professor and Director of School of Nursing
University of Texas at El Paso, Texas, USA

Margaret M. Andrews, PhD, RN, CTN, FAAN
Professor and Director, School of Nursing
University of Northern Colorado, Greeley, Colorado, USA

Sally Borbasi, PhD, RN, MA(Ed), BEd(Nursing)
Associate Professor of Nursing
School of Nursing & Midwifery
Flinders University, Adelaide, South Australia, Australia

Debra A. Bournes, PhD, RN
Director of Nursing, New Knowledge and Innovation
University Health Network
Assistant Professor
University of Toronto, Toronto, Canada

Esther Chang, PhD, RN, CM, FCN(NSW)
Professor of Nursing and Director of Research
School of Nursing, Family & Community Health
University of Western Sydney, Sydney, New South Wales, Australia

William K. Cody, PhD, RN, BSN, BS, MSN
Professor and Chair, Department of Family and Community Nursing
Executive Director, Nursing Center for Health Promotion
University of North Carolina at Charlotte, Charlotte, North Carolina, USA

Jane Conway, RN, BHlth Sc, BN(Hons)
Graduate Diploma in Further Education and Training
Lecturer
Faculty of Nursing
University of Newcastle, Newcastle, New South Wales, Australia

Philip Darbyshire, PhD, RNMH, RSCN, DipN(Lond), RNT, MN
Professor of Nursing, Women's & Children's Hospital
University of South Australia and Flinders University,
Adelaide, South Australia, Australia

Doug Elliott, PhD, RN, BAppSc, MAppSc
Professor of Nursing (Critical Care)
Nursing Education and Research Unit, Prince of Wales Hospital, Randwick
& Department of Clinical Nursing,
Faculty of Nursing
The University of Sydney,
Sydney, New South Wales, Australia

Suzanne Gordon, BA
Adjunct Professor
McGill University, School of Nursing
Montreal, Quebec, Canada
Visiting Scholar
Boston College School of Nursing, Boston,
Massachusetts, USA

Pamela J. Haylock, RN, MA
Cancer Care Consultant, Medina, Texas
Doctoral Student, Medical Branch School of Nursing
University of Texas, Galveston, Texas, USA

Gladys L. Husted, MA, PhD, RN
Professor of Nursing
Duquesne University
Pittsburgh, PA

James H. Husted
Independent Scholar
Pittsburgh, PA

M. Katherine Maeve, PhD, RN
Research Associate Professor
Center for Health Promotion and Risk Reduction in Special Populations
College of Nursing
University of South Carolina,
Columbia, South Carolina, USA

Margaret McMillan, PhD, RN, FCN
Professor of Nursing and Deputy Executive Dean
Faculty of Health
University of Newcastle,
Newcastle, New South Wales, Australia

Gail J. Mitchell, PhD, RN
Assistant Professor
School of Nursing
York University, Toronto, Canada

Ellen Murphy, MS, JD, FAAN
Professor of Nursing
College of Nursing
University of Wisconsin,
Milwaukee, Wisconsin, USA

Kathleen M. Nokes, PhD, RN, FAAN
Professor of Nursing
Hunter-Bellevue School of Nursing
Hunter College
City University of New York, New York, USA

Akram Omeri, PhD, RN, CTN, MCN, FRCNA
Transcultural Nurse Consultant, Australia
Adjunct Associate Professor
School of Nursing, Family and Community Health University of Western Sydney
Sydney, Australia

Judith M. Parker, AM, PhD, RN, BA(Hons)
Visiting Professor
Department of Nursing Studies
The University of Hong Kong, Hong Kong

F. Beryl Pilkington, PhD, RN
Associate Professor
School of Nursing
York University, Toronto, Ontario, Canada

Catherine Reavis, EdD, APRN, BC
Family Nurse Practitioner and Associate Professor
Georgia Southern University, Statesboro, Georgia, USA

David R Thompson, BSc, MA, PhD, MBA, RN, FRCN, FESC
Professor of Clinical Nursing and Director
The Nethersole School of Nursing
The Chinese University of Hong Kong, Hong Kong, China

Jean Watson, PhD, RN, HNC, FAAN
Distinguished Professor of Nursing
Endowed Chair in Caring Science
College of Nursing
University of Colorado Health Sciences Center
Denver, Colorado, USA

Foreword

How is the nursing discipline defined? Who is a nurse? What is nursing? What are the major changes in nursing as a profession and a discipline? In what ways did the internal changes in the discipline of nursing affect the progress of knowledge that provides the base for nursing practice?

These are major questions that provided the impetus for the editors to design and produce this book. This book defines the discipline of nursing through its major components: theory, philosophy, ethics, art, science, image and identity. It is a book that also provides opportunities for readers to critically think about the nature of nursing and the issues that confront nurses.

There are many dialogues in the literature about the relationship between art and science, disciplinary and interdisciplinary, and history and contemporary issues in nursing. In this volume, the editors provide a reader-friendly, critical, and coherent summary of each of these issues, making this volume very significant reading for every nurse no matter what her/his level of education is. For those who think of nursing as a set of tasks, or believe that nursing could be defined through its activities, or that nurses are only doers, this volume of readings could quickly dismiss these myths, and will debunk stereotypes that have been attached to nurses and nursing.

Furthermore, the readings provided in this book challenge any claim that the discipline of nursing needs new definitions or the claim that progress in its art and science have been slow. It is an impressive volume by a number of international authors who are well published, whose writings are familiar to many, and whose arguments are cogent and well supported. They address many issues and questions facing the discipline of nursing. While some of these questions may not be new, the dialogue about them continues to be important to advance the discipline forward.

The discipline of nursing has evolved to reflect the complexities of human being's experiences with health and illness and the profound in-depth web of relationships in the health care systems, and the various chapters in this book highlight the progress made in the nature of the intellectual dialogue and discourse in nursing. It is a book that is a very significant reference for any nurse who is engaged in critical analysis of the history and the structure of the discipline as well as the nurse who wants to practice based on evidence. The editors and authors address the historical origins of the discipline and profession, and build on this history to frame discourses that are shaping the more contemporary issues in health care such as disparities in health care, gender and race inequities, and unsafe care for patients.

This is a comprehensive volume that provides the reader with a rounded view of the totality and complexity of the discipline of nursing. It provides an analysis of different components upon which nursing as a discipline and a profession can be understood, and without which nursing could be and usually is reduced to a set of skills and tasks. Anyone who doubts the global impact on nursing or the profound influence of image and gender stereotypes on progress made in nursing as a discipline or a profession, should review this text which provides intellectually compelling arguments. The history is daunting, the present is compelling, and the future is being shaped by the critical dialogues that this volume will create.

Afaf I. Meleis, PhD, DrPS (hon), FAAN
Professor of Nursing and Sociology
Margaret Bond Simon Dean of Nursing
University of Pennsylvania
Philadelphia, PA

Preface

This book has been written to facilitate consideration and understanding of key ideas that underpin nursing as a discipline in a global context. The book is, in a sense, groundbreaking, in that it is a collaboration between American, Canadian, British, and Australian nurses. The topics selected for inclusion represent a distillation of international nursing knowledge, and are drawn from an immense base of research and scholarly endeavor. They are highly relevant to nursing internationally, and correspond to many of the concerns and challenges confronting contemporary nursing. This edition was written especially for American nurses. British and Australian editions, each tailored to the special needs of nurses in those countries, have already been published.

Engagement with the text, and completion of the reflective exercises that follow each chapter, will assist beginning students of nursing to develop a solid theoretical foundation for nursing, including an understanding of the commonality of key ideas in nursing culture and scholarship. We trust that this text will enable readers to understand the global as well as the local nature of nursing knowledge, practice, and related health care issues. The unique concerns and challenges confronting nursing are clarified as the process of professionalization unfolds.

We acknowledge that a number of individuals provided assistance and advice to the editors as they planned and prepared this work. Special thanks go to Dr. May Wykle, RN, PhD, FAAN, Professor of Nursing at Case Western Reserve University, Cleveland, Ohio, and Ms. Nancy Dickenson-Hazard, RN, MSN, Chief Executive Officer of Sigma Theta Tau International, for encouragement and believing in the project. We also convey thanks to Vaughn Curtis of *Elsevier* in Australia, and to Ruth Chasek of *Springer Publishing* in New York, for supporting and guiding the project. Alison Sheppard and Patricia Corbett of the University of Western Sydney are acknowledged for their exceptional secretarial and administrative assistance.

John Daly
Sandra Speedy
Debra Jackson
Vickie Lambert
Clinton Lambert

So, You Want to Be a Nurse

Pamela J. Haylock

LEARNING OBJECTIVES

Upon completion of this chapter, readers should have gained:

- Knowledge of the history of nursing in the U.S.
- An understanding of the complexities engendered by variations in educational preparation for entryintopractice
- Insights into the development of nurse practice acts and licensure
- An ability to define and differentiate licensure, expert practice, certification, and advanced practice nursing
- An understanding of the relationship between nursing ethics and codes of conduct

KEY WORDS

Nursing, practice, regulation, specialization, licensure, codes of conduct

INTRODUCTION

So, you want to be a nurse? Hopefully, you've chosen well—and your decision-making process integrates a basic understanding of who nurses are, some appreciation of the career possibilities that nursing education can prepare an individual to pursue, and how nurses prepare for career choices. The U.S. Department of Labor Bureau of Labor Statistics

(2003) tells us that there are more than two million nursing jobs and that nursing is one of ten occupations projected to have the largest number of new jobs in the foreseeable future. Today's nurses have an amazing array of career opportunities including those found in the armed services, home care, public health, critical care and emergency settings, schools, long-term and rehabilitation facilities, community health clinics, corporations, governmental agencies, and offices of elected officials involved in health policy—just to name a few. Undoubtedly, many nursing roles are as yet undefined and unimagined. Earnings are "above average," particularly for advanced practice nurses (Bureau of Labor Statistics, 2003).

Nurses who are effective and successful in achieving career goals generally consider nursing more than just a job; instead, it is a career with entrée to a profession based in fundamental values, morals, and human service. Nursing is a relatively new profession built on a foundation of caring and attention to human needs—a "holistic" tradition that complements, coexists, contrasts, and sometimes clashes with the medical model of disease and cure that characterizes the U.S. health care system. Although nursing has never been purely women's work—there have always been men in nursing and there are growing numbers of men in nursing today—the influence of socially determined women's roles remains strong.

The nursing profession is a work in progress; nursing today is unlike nursing in the past and will most certainly be different from nursing five, ten, or twenty years hence. Nurses entering the profession now must embrace change and integrate emerging science, creativity, and passion with professional discipline.

NURSING DEFINED

Nursing is an evolving profession. Oberle and Allen (2001) write: "Nursing is a societally mandated, socially constructed practice profession existing to serve a public that has certain expectations of nurses and nursing actions" (p. 150). Nursing today is in many ways a far different vocation from what it was at its inception and from what it will be in the future. Nurses around the world share a common history and traditions arising from their beginnings. A basic understanding of the history and traditions can be useful to nurses as they approach the challenges that face the profession as well as individual nurses.

Florence Nightingale is widely recognized inside and outside of the nursing profession as its founder. Many nursing traditions have their basis in Nightingale's beliefs and her experiences as an extremely well-educated, brilliant, wealthy, and privileged woman (even by modern standards), and in the customs of the Victorian era during which she lived. Nightingale's vision for nursing was that it would be a noble calling for women. Some traditions have served nursing well, such as Nightingale's insistence that nurses be educated and exemplify high moral standards. Conversely, many of nursing's current dilemmas, particularly its domination by the medical profession and conflicts with the traditional medical model of health care, arose from Nightingale-era perceptions of women in general, and women's roles in particular (Ashley, 1976). Nightingale's influence inadvertently led to the perception of altruism and what Reverby (1987) referred to as a "caring profession in a society that does not value caring" (p. 1). Nevertheless, Nightingale left a timeless legacy of commitment to a profession that would serve humanity—and its practitioners—well. Contemporary nurses must adapt or change long-held traditions in order for nursing to successfully address modern societal needs.

Since the nineteenth century, American nursing evolved and coexisted with hospitals; nurses kept hospitals functioning, while hospitals provided nurses with employment (Lynaugh & Brush, 1996). This relationship has historically been problematic, but sweeping changes in the health care environment, beginning in 1965 with the introduction of Medicare, Medicaid, and prospective payment systems, have generated changes in nursing practice and practice settings, which are increasingly outside of acute care hospitals (O'Neil & Coffman, 1998). These changes have revolutionized health care delivery, and have transformed role expectations and educational preparation among the health care professions, particularly nursing. Growing recognition of the importance of work satisfaction to maintaining an adequate nursing work force necessitates attention to the creation and sustenance of healthy, healing work cultures as an imperative for all nurses (Porter-O'Grady, 2000; Wesorick, 2002). Data compiled by the American Nurses Credentialing Center's magnet hospital program clearly documents the relationship of nurses' work environment to positive patient outcomes (Aiken, Havens, & Sloane, 2000).

Despite different interests and areas of expertise, there is agreement on the fundamental responsibilities of nurses identified in the International Council of Nurses (ICN) Code of Ethics for Nurses: to promote health; to prevent illness; to restore health; and to alleviate suffering (ICN, 2000). Nursing leader Virginia Henderson, sometimes referred to as the twentieth century's Florence Nightingale (Halloran, 1995), was invited by the ICN to produce a document to describe nursing independent of technology and medicine (Styles, 1997; Halloran, 1995). *Basic Principles of Nursing Care,* first published in 1960 and now translated into some 30 languages, provides the globally recognized working definition of nursing:

> The unique function of the nurse is to assist the individual, sick or well, in the performance of those activities contributing to health or its recovery (or to peaceful death) that the person would perform unaided given the necessary strength, will or knowledge. And to do this in such a way as to help the individual gain independence as rapidly as possible. (Henderson, 1997, p. 22)

Henderson's argument for the distinct nature of nursing emphasizing nurses as "providing the strength, will and knowledge to help others be independent" (Halloran, 1995, p. xvi), remains an enduring perspective of professional nursing in the twenty-first century. Henderson recognized the human need for nursing and nurses' potential to meet human needs in their endless varieties, and articulated the importance of a scholarly and artistic approach to care of individual patients (Halloran, 1995, p. xvi). Henderson warned of the "danger of thinking that any one set of prerequisites, any one type of preparation, or any era has the final answer to the question of producing the creative nurse" (Halloran, 1995, p. 9), and in doing so, confirmed the importance of adaptability and creativity that promote professional nursing practice over time. Henderson's influence on contemporary nursing practice is readily evident. The American Nurses Association's *Code of Ethics for Nurses* (2001), its many scope of practice statements, and state nurse practice acts integrate the responsibilities identified by ICN and the functions delineated by Henderson.

NURSING EDUCATION

Unlike other professions, nursing in the United States has three entry levels, a situation leading to misunderstandings and misconceptions among the public, nurses, and other health care professions, and among nurses themselves, relating to who and what a nurse is (Christman, 1998). The entry-into-practice issue in the United States generally sparks passionate debate. In 1964 the American Nurses Association (ANA) proposed a goal of mandating BSN education as the basic entry level by 1985. More than forty years later, only one state (North Dakota) had enacted legislation limiting entry into registered nursing practice to a minimum baccalaureate degree. However, this legislation has been recently overturned in that state. Efforts to achieve a standard entry-into-practice have historically met with resistance from many groups, leading some to conclude that American society "saw nursing as a logical extension of women's work, not as a scientific profession" (Leighow, 1996, p. 3). Community college faculty and administrators oppose measures that would limit enrollment. Minority groups suggest that their constituents could not afford college preparation. And, despite evidence of decreased overhead expenses and the positive relationship between nurses' educational preparation and patient outcomes, hospitals continue to support diploma and community college programs because they produce RNs more quickly, a significant consideration in light of the current nursing shortage (Christman, 1998; McClure, 2003). Although Christman is the most vocal advocate of a single, advanced, entry-into-practice level, there is growing recognition of the negative consequences of stratified preparation and stratified levels of nursing care (Jacobs, DiMattio, Bishop, & Fields, 1998; McClure, 2003). Nursing leaders insist that the time has come to move the entry-into-practice issue forward but lack consensus—and some say, the courage—to achieve this goal (Cathcart, 2003; Long, 2003; McClure, 2003).

Despite the decades-long debate over entry-into-practice education, basic nursing educational preparation for registered nurses (RN) in the U.S. remains stratified: Community colleges grant the associate degree in nursing (ADN); the few remaining hospital-based schools of nursing offer diplomas; and collegiate programs award the bachelor of science in nursing (BSN) degree. Graduates of any of these programs are qualified to take the registration examination offered by state boards of nursing. Regardless of educational preparation, graduates of the various preparatory programs all hold the same RN licensure.

Requirements and basic competencies for individuals to enter the nursing profession typically include:

- Graduation from a recognized basic nursing education program
- Meeting specific requirements of a state board of nursing

Passing the National Council of State Boards of Nursing (NCSBN) National Council Licensure Examination (NCLEX-RN®) for registered nurses NCSBN data indicates that approximately 80% of individuals taking the NCLEX-RN exam for the first time achieve a passing score, with lower pass rates for those repeating the exam (40%) and those who are foreign-educated (40%) (NCSBN, 2003).

REGULATION OF PRACTICE

Nurses must recognize the political nature of the nursing discipline. Indeed, what we are allowed to do and where we do it are mandated through political processes that result in nurse practice acts. In the United States and its five territories, Boards of Nursing (BON) are the authorities over nursing practice, established to protect the public's health and safety by overseeing and ensuring safe nursing practice, and holding regulatory and disciplinary responsibility for the profession (NCSBN, 2003). North Carolina enacted the first state law regulating nursing practice in 1903, and in 1938, New York legally mandated licensing for nurses. A few states maintain two boards, one for registered nurses and one for licensed practical or vocational nurses, though increasingly, boards are merging to create one board governing nursing practice.

The composition of BON membership also differs from state to state. Professional nursing organization leaders, representatives of the public at large, governmental agencies, hospital administrators, physicians, and pharmacists are among state BON members. Most often, BON members are political appointees, offered board positions at the discretion of state and territorial governors.

Nurse practice acts define the scope of nursing practice in each state and territory (hereinafter, references to "states" assumes inclusion of territories as well). In some states, nurses have exclusive control over BON functions and, therefore, nursing practice in these states; in other states, multidisciplinary boards, commissions, and non-nursing review committees make recommendations or develop legislation relative to nursing practice. Although regulations vary from state to state, nurse practice acts typically:

- Define the authority, composition, and powers of the board of nursing
- Define nursing and boundaries of the scope of nursing practice
- Identify types of licenses and titles

- State requirements for licensure
- Protect titles
- Identify grounds for disciplinary action (National Council of State Boards of Nursing, 2003)

Because of state-to-state variations, knowledge of the defined scope of practice and the nurse practice act in the state in which she or he practices is essential to every nurse.

Recognizing realities of contemporary nursing practice, several state BONs and state nurses associations (SNAs) initiated steps toward multistate nurse licensure in 1999, using language proposed by the National Council of State Boards of Nursing (NCSBN, 2003). Under this "Nurse Licensure Compact," states agree to mutual recognition which would allow a nurse to obtain one state license that grants a multistate privilege to practice across state lines (Nurse Licensure Compact Administrators, 2003). States join the Compact by enacting adoptive legislation. The nurse assumes responsibility for knowing the laws governing practice in each state in which she or he practices. A final report, drafted in 2004, allows revisions to the Compact to be made in the 2005 legislative sessions of each state.

SPECIALIZATION AND CERTIFICATION

In the United States, there are now approximately eighty specialty nursing organizations, a reflection of the vision of Hildegarde Peplau, another important twentieth century nursing leader who recognized the necessity of specialty focus to the development of clinical expertise.

The catalyst for specialization in nursing involves "avante garde [nurses] who sense a need to move in a direction that interests them or toward which they have an opportunity" (Peplau, 2003, p. 3). After this initial movement, a particular specialty's survival depends on the degree of interest among nurses working in this arena and the nursing population's willingness to learn, and to create and support innovations in professional nursing. Government funding and financial support from nongovernmental sources—such as scholarships, support for re-educating faculty, and research incentives—aid these efforts, stimulate development of the specialty, and prepare experts within a practice specialty. Specialty practice areas are most often defined according to practice settings (e.g., schools, mental health facilities, in-flight care), organs and body systems (e.g., heart, kidney), age of the client or patient (e.g., infants, children, adults, elderly), degree of illness (e.g., chronic, acute, convalescent, intensive care), clinical services (e.g., infusion center, physician office, labor and delivery), and fields of knowledge (e.g., cancer, orthopedics).

The expert nurse clinician has a broader understanding of the context of his or her practice area than does a general practitioner. As scientific knowledge continues to grow at an astounding rate, nurse generalists find it increasingly difficult, if not impossible, to integrate new knowledge into clinical practice. Focusing on one area of knowledge is imperative for nurses to offer true clinical expertise (Clark, 1995). And who among us would want "inexpert" nursing care?

Along with the obvious benefits of specialization by individual nurses and the support for expert practice offered by specialty organizations, splintering nursing into many specialty and subspecialty organizations creates significant dilemmas among practitioners and health care delivery systems. Christman (1998) refers to this phenomenon as "tribalism" and warns of its inherent lack of cohesion and cooperation among personnel in work settings, in care delivery systems, and within the nursing profession. Lack of cohesion and cooperation is a major factor in professional nursing's inability to influence public policy to any significant degree.

Licensure is the legal mechanism for ensuring basic competence for entry into practice, and it is the minimum requirement for professional nursing. RN licensure, however, does not indicate acquired knowledge beyond the required minimum. Some states require continuing education for license renewal, but other states require only payment of renewal fees. The aim of certification, a voluntary process undertaken by qualifying individual nurses, is to validate competencies in designated practice areas, signifying the certified nurse has acquired knowledge beyond the entry level. Indeed, there is evidence that nursing education and nursing practice in clinical specialty areas are influenced by specialty certification processes (Esper, Lockhart, & Murphy, 2002). Certification processes are offered by nongovernmental organizations including specialty nursing organizations and the American Nurses Credentialing Center (ANCC). Qualifying criteria for certification generally includes:

- An active RN license
- Demonstrated educational preparation beyond the entry level
- Specified level of supervised experience in the specialty area
- Successful completion of the certification examination

The entry-into-practice issue also plays a role in certification processes; many certifying bodies require the baccalaureate as a minimum qualifying credential for certification. The ANCC model of credentialing makes certification accessible to all qualified registered nurses. ANCC examinations lead to *certification* for associate degree and diploma prepared registered nurses, and *board certification* designates nurses with baccalaureate and higher preparation (ANCC, 2003).

ADVANCED PRACTICE NURSING

Although the advanced practice nursing role originated in 1877 when nurses began to administer anaesthesia, the term "advanced practice nursing" first appeared in nursing literature in the 1980s (Oberle & Allen, 2001). Advanced practice nursing is distinguished from expert practice in that the advanced practice nurse (APN) combines experiential knowledge with greater theoretical knowledge acquired through graduate study, and increased communication and relational skills (Oberle & Allen, 2001). Today, the title *advanced practice nurse* designates a registered nurse who has met graduate degree educational requirements, has expert clinical knowledge, and provides direct patient care. Advanced practice is defined as:

the application of an extended range of practical, theoretical, and research-based therapeutics to the phenomena experienced by patients within a specialized clinical area of the larger discipline of nursing. (Hamric, 1996, p. 47)

Four groups of APNs are recognized: certified registered nurse anaesthetists; certified nurse midwives; clinical nurse specialists (CNS); and nurse practitioners (NP). Of these, the CNS role is probably the most nebulous and diverse, with complex variations in implementation, process, and outcomes according to specialty practice area. Advanced practice roles typically make certification a requirement for practice. NPs are generally required to hold a second license to practice in this advanced role because of their prescription-writing privileges. The lack of uniform standards for advanced practice nursing precluded its inclusion in the initial Compact draft, but Compact provisions will eventually address the various forms of advanced practice nursing (Lyon, 2003).

. CRNA
. CNM
- CNS
. NP

CODES: CONDUCT AND ETHICS

Nursing is a relational, moral activity (Volker, 2003). Nightingale used the term "high sympathies" to describe values and concern for the well-being of society (Nightingale, 1946). The Florence Nightingale Pledge, first recited by graduating nurses in 1893, guided nurses to "abstain from whatever is deleterious and mischievous . . . and devote [themselves] to the welfare of those committed to [their] care" (ANA, 2003). The Pledge is understood as the first nursing code of ethics (ANA, 2001). At the time of its composition, this promise might have seemed relatively straightforward. Early nursing's ethics literature was labeled "professional problems," "professional adjustments," "the art of conduct," and "friendly talks to nurses," touching on nurses' private and professional lives (Fowler, 1997, p. 18). Developments in medical science and technology that began in the 1960s make defining "deleterious" actions and the "welfare" of patients a very complex process. A poignant example of present-day nurses' ethical dilemmas is highlighted in *The Wall Street Journal* series revealing American nurses' unrecognized and undefined roles in health care rationing in an age of rising health care costs. According to that series, nurses make "daily battlefield decisions that influence whose lives should be prolonged and who should leave" in critical care units (Anand, 2003). Nurse managers use various means to decrease costly patient stays, influencing hospital pharmacy committees to relax guidelines restricting patients on certain drugs to stay in critical care settings, and prodding families to limit medical interventions and allowing patients to die (Anand, 2003).

Because of nurses' roles in health care delivery and their intimate relationships with the people in their care, nurses encounter ethical issues and dilemmas in daily practice. Professional codes, such as the ANA's (2001) *Code of Ethics for Nurses with Interpretive Statements* (Table 1.1), and position statements on ethical issues reflect a normative ethics approach, providing direction for straight thinking and right behavior for relationships of nurses to patients and clients, the community, and the profession. The *Code of Ethics for Nurses* evolved from efforts initiated in 1896 by the Nurses' Associated Alumnae of the United States and Canada (later the American Nurses Association) to establish and maintain a code of ethics (ANA, 2001). The first *Code for Professional Nurses* was accepted by the ANA House of Delegates in 1950. Subsequent revisions have occurred over the years, with the latest revision in this work in progress, the current *Code of Ethics for Nurses With Interpretive Statements*, released in 2001.

TABLE 1.1   American Nurses Association Code of Ethics for Nurses (2001)

1. The nurse, in all professional relationships, practices with compassion and respect for the inherent dignity, worth, and uniqueness of every individual, unrestricted by considerations of social or economic status, personal attitudes, or the nature of health problems.
2. The nurse's primary commitment is to the patient, whether an individual, family, group, or community.
3. The nurse promotes, advocates for, and strives to protect the health, safety, and rights of the patient.
4. The nurse is responsible and accountable for individual nursing practice and determines the appropriate delegation of tasks consistent with the nurse's obligation to provide optimum patient care.
5. The nurse owes the same duties to self as to others, including the responsibility to preserve integrity and safety, to maintain competence, and to continue personal and professional growth.
6. The nurse participates in establishing, maintaining, and improving health care environments and conditions of employment conducive to the provision of quality health care and consistent with the values of the profession through individual and collective action.
7. The nurse participates in the advancement of the profession through contributions to practice, education, administration, and knowledge development.
8. The nurse collaborates with other health professionals and the public in promoting community, national, and international efforts to meet health needs.
9. The profession of nursing, as represented by associations and their members, is responsible for articulating nursing values, for maintaining the integrity of their profession and its practice, and for shaping social policy.

Reprinted with permission from the American Nurses Association

The International Council of Nurses (ICN) adopted its initial *Code of Ethics for Nurses* in 1953. It has been revised and reaffirmed several times, with the most recent revision completed in 2000 (ICN, 2000). The preamble identifies a universal need for nursing and inherent values of respect for human rights, including the right to life, to dignity, and to be treated with respect. Basic elements of the Code cover nurses and people, nurses and practice, nurses and the profession, and nurses and coworkers (ICN). The ICN (2000) suggests that the Code is a guide for action based on social values and needs, and that its meaning derives from its application to the realities of nursing and health care in a changing society.

Despite recognition that nursing provides a unique service to society, there is no recognized definition of the term *nursing ethics*. The four traditional ethical principles of beneficence, nonmalfeasance, autonomy, and distributive justice, while central to nursing practice, are inadequate to address the countless moral phenomena that occur in contemporary nursing practice (Volker, 2003; Weis & Schank, 2002; Cameron, 2003; Milton, 1999). Current nurse scholars propose an ethical guideline for nursing service. Milton (1999), for example, suggests, "Nursing ethics is an examination of what it means to have straight thinking in carrying out the practice of the discipline of nursing." Whereas traditional ethical principles are aligned with the medical model of practice, a unique nursing ethos could be more consistent with philosophical beliefs and values of nursing.

CONCLUSION

The discipline of nursing has been, since its invention by Florence Nightingale, a work in progress. As global societal changes occur, nursing will necessarily change to meet the needs of patients and communities, reflecting the vision of nursing first articulated by Virginia Henderson (1960). Perhaps it is true of nursing in any era, but the profession holds unlimited potential now. Contemporary factors including the dynamic health care environment, changes in professional education and practice, new relationships among the health care professions and between nurses, individuals, and communities who use nursing services, and increased emphasis on efficacy and reducing costs of care make this time in our history as challenging as it is stimulating (O'Neil & Coffman, 1998). Opportunities for professional nursing and individual nurses abound. The shift from hospital-based nursing care to community-based services, and the ongoing globalization of health-related issues, set the stage for intelligent, imaginative nurses to explore the human need for nursing, and nurses' potential to meet those needs.

So, you want to be a nurse. You have chosen a noble profession, one with a long and honorable history based in science and the fundamental values of caring and compassion. Nursing is a profession in which diversity, creativity, and leadership skills are not just desirable traits; they are imperative to satisfying personal growth and to the future of the profession. Those individuals with intelligence, passion, commitment, courage, and imagination, who choose nursing can create a lifelong personal and professional journey filled with intellectual and spiritual challenges and rewards, and the exhilaration of serving humanity in profoundly meaningful ways.

REFLECTIVE QUESTIONS

- How would you describe the role(s) of nurses and nursing?
- How do you think the roles and responsibilities of nurses should be developed over the next ten years?
- Consider the issue of specialization. What are some of the positives and negatives associated with specialization?

RECOMMENDED READINGS

Halloran, E. J. (Ed.) (1995). *A Virginia Henderson reader: Excellence in nursing.* New York: Springer Publishing Company.

Henderson, V. (1960, 1997). *Basic principles of nursing care.* Washington, DC: American Nurses Publishing.

Nightingale, F. (1946). *Notes on nursing: What it is and what it is not.* Philadelphia: Edward Stern & Company, Inc. (Original work published 1859)

O'Neil, E., & Coffman, J. (Eds.) (1998). *Strategies for the future of nursing: Changing roles, responsibilities, and employment patterns of registered nurses.* San Francisco: Jossey-Bass Publishers.

Watson, J. (1999). *Postmodern nursing and beyond.* Edinburgh: Churchill Livingstone.

REFERENCES

Aiken, L. H., Havens, D. S., & Sloane, D. M. (2000). The Magnet Nursing Services Recognition Program: A comparison of two groups of magnet hospitals. *American Journal of Nursing, 100,* 26–35.

American Nurses Association (2001). *Code of ethics for nurses with interpretive statements.* Washington, DC: American Nurses Association.

American Nurses Association (2003). *The Florence Nightingale Pledge.* Press Release, retrieved September 14, 2003 from http://www.nursingworld.org/pressrel/nnw/nnwpled.htm

American Nurses Credentialing Center (2003). Frequently asked questions about ANCC certification. Retrieved September 11, 2003 from http://www.nursingworld.org/ANCC

Anand, G. (2003, September 12). The big secret in healthcare: Rationing is here. *The Wall Street Journal,* pp. A1, A6.

Ashley, J. (1976). *Hospitals, paternalism, and the role of the nurse.* New York: Teachers College Press.

Bureau of Labor Statistics, U.S. Department of Labor. (2003). Occupational Outlook Handbook, 2002–03 Edition, Registered Nurses. Retrieved September 12, 2003 from http://www.bls.gov/oco/ocos083.htm

Cameron, M. E. (2003). Our best ethical and spiritual values. *Journal of Professional Nursing, 19,* 117–118.

Cathcart, E. B. (2003). Using the NCLEX-RN to argue for BSN preparation: Barking up the wrong tree. *Journal of Professional Nursing, 19,* 121–122.

Christman, L. (1998). Who is a nurse? *Image: Journal of Nursing Scholarship, 30,* 211–214.

Clark, J. (1995). Expert nursing: A necessary extravagance. *European Journal of Cancer Care, 4,* 109–117.

Esper, P., Lockhart, J. S., & Murphy, C. M. (2002). Strengthening end-of-life care through specialty nursing certification. *Journal of Professional Nursing, 18,* 130–139.

Fowler, M. (1997). Nursing's ethics. In A. J. Davis, M. A. Aroskar, J. Liaschenko, & T. S. Drought (Eds.), *Ethical dilemmas and nursing practice* (4th ed.). Stamford, CT: Appleton and Lange.

Halloran, E. J. (Ed.) (1995). *A Virginia Henderson reader: Excellence in nursing.* New York: Springer Publishing.

Hamric, A. B. (1996). A definition of advanced nursing practice. In A. B. Hamric, J. A. Spross, & C. M. Hanson (Eds.), *Advanced nursing practice: An integrative approach.* Philadelphia: W. B. Saunders.

Henderson, V. (1960, 1997). *Basic principles of nursing care.* Washington, DC: American Nurses Publishing.

International Council of Nurses (2000). *The ICN Code of Ethics for Nurses.* Geneva, Switzerland. Retrieved July 28, 2003 from http://www.icn.org

Jacobs, L. A., DiMattio, M. J. K., Bishop, T. L., & Fields, S. D. (1998). The baccalaureate degree in nursing as an entry-level requirement for professional nursing practice. *Journal of Professional Nursing, 14,* 225–233.

Leighow, S. R. (1996). Backrubs vs. Bach: Nursing and the entry-into-practice debate, 1946–1986. *Nursing History Review, 4,* 3–17.

Long, K. A. (2003). Licensure matters: Better patient care requires change in regulation as well as education. *Journal of Professional Nursing, 19,* 123–125.

Lyon, B. L. (2003). Advanced Practice Registered Nurse Compact: A call to action with a primer on the regulation of CNS practice. *Clinical Nurse Specialist, 17,* 185–187.

Lynaugh, J. E., & Brush, B. L. (1996). *American nursing: From hospitals to health systems.* Cambridge, MA: Blackwell Publishers.

McClure, M. L. (2003). Another look at entry into practice. *Nursing Outlook, 151.*

Milton, C. L. (1999). Ethical issues from nursing theoretical perspectives. *Nursing Science Quarterly, 12,* 20–25.

National Council of State Boards of Nursing (NCSBN) (2003). *Nurse licensure statistics.* Retrieved September 1, 2003 from http://www.ncsbn.org

Nightingale, F. (1946). *Notes on Nursing: What it is and what it is not.* Philadelphia: Edward Stern & Company, Inc.

Nurse Licensure Compact Administrators (2003). *Nurse Licensure Compact: Just the facts.* Retrieved September 1, 2003 from http://www.ncsb.org

Oberle, K., & Allen, M. (2001). The nature of advanced practice nursing. *Nursing Outlook, 49,* 148–153.

O'Neil, E., & Coffman, J. (Eds.) (1998). *Strategies for the future of nursing: Changing roles, responsibilities, and employment patterns of registered nurses.* San Francisco: Jossey-Bass Publishers.

Peplau, H. (2003). Specialization in professional nursing (reprinted from *Nursing Science,* August 1965). *Clinical Nurse Specialist, 17,* 3–9.

Porter-O'Grady, T. (2000). Vision for the 21st century: New horizons, new healthcare. *Nursing Administration Quarterly, 25*(1), 30–38.

Reverby, S. M. (1987). *Ordered to care: The dilemma of American nursing, 1850–1945.* Cambridge, MA: Cambridge University Press.

Styles, M. (1997). Preface. In V. Henderson, *Basic Principles of Nursing Care.* Washington, DC: American Nurses Publishing.

Volker, D. L. (2003). Is there a unique nursing ethic? *Nursing Science Quarterly, 16,* 207–211.

Weis, D., & Schank, M. J. (2002). Professional values: Key to professional development. *Journal of Professional Nursing, 18,* 271–275.

Wesorick, B. (2002). 21st century leadership challenge: Creating and sustaining healthy, healing work cultures and integrated service at the point of care. *Nursing Administration Quarterly, 26*(5), 18–32.

2

The Evolution of Nursing Education and Practice in the U.S.

Vickie A. Lambert and Clinton E. Lambert

LEARNING OBJECTIVES

Upon completion of this chapter, readers should have gained insights into the:

- History of nursing in the United States of America (USA)
- Milestones that led to the development of nursing education and practice in the U.S.
- Social and political forces that shaped the evolution of nursing education and practice

KEY WORDS

Nursing education, nursing practice, milestones in nursing history

INTRODUCTION

When one explores the annals of history, it becomes apparent that some form of nursing practice has always existed with the intent of responding to the societal needs of the sick and infirm. During prehistoric times, nursing and medical practices were guided by magic, superstition, and religious beliefs. Primitive people believed that illnesses were the result of angry gods. Thus, the actions of individuals responsible for caring for the ill or infirm focused on appeasing the discontent of the gods. This attitude is still prevalent today among Native Americans and many immigrants who enter the United States. Traditional medicine has never ceased to exist and it continues to be based on the beliefs of many fundamental religions.

It was not until the ancient Greek, Hippocrates of Cos (460–370 BC), the "father of medicine," that the emphasis on care for the sick and infirm was seen as a natural phenomenon rather than a god-inflicted occurrence. Unfortunately, during the time of Hippocrates and continuing through the Middle Ages (476–1500 AD), the belief that the body was composed of four humors (blood, bile, phlegm, and black bile) prevailed and superseded the Hippocratic school of thought. These four humors were to remain in balance and were thought to correspond to the four elements of the world (fire, air, water, and earth). Depending upon the predominating humor, a person was either considered to be sanguine, choleric, phlegmatic, or melancholic. Using corresponding elements such as hot and cold, or wet and dry, health care practices focused on restoring the appropriate balance among the humors. None of these practices bore any relationship to actual physiology. Thus, the results were rarely, if ever, effective.

During the Renaissance (1438–1660) medical care was freed from ancient dogma and superstition, and began to be governed by a more rational and scientific manner of thought. By the early seventeenth century, the scientific method had evolved and many misconceptions of the ancients began to be refuted. Physicians began to observe things for themselves and to accept only evidence derived from personal experience. Medical practice began to be based upon accurate observations instead of the doctrines of the past. Nursing care, however, remained at a minimal, custodial level. With the exception of the members of certain religious orders, most individuals providing nursing care were poorly educated and ill trained.

One can discern that nursing and medical care, as we know them today, are the result of social, cultural, economic and political factors that have shaped our world. Since this chapter focuses on the evolution of nursing in the United States, the discussions of nursing education and practice will begin with colonial America and progress through historical timeframes that are reflective of American history.

COLONIAL AMERICA

Colonial America began with the exploration of the New World, in the fifteenth century, by the Spanish and the Portuguese. Health care at that time was extremely deficient. Physicians were poorly trained, life expectancy was low (35 years), smallpox and yellow fever were rampant, and health care practices (bleeding and purgatives) were often crude and tended to intensify any existing illnesses (Kalisch & Kalisch, 1995).

In an attempt to contend with the presence of poorly trained physicians, over 100 Americans were sent, during the end of the eighteenth century, to Great Britain to receive medical education. Thus, it was not until towards the end of the colonial period that two medical schools were established in America: The Medical College of Philadelphia (1765), which later affiliated with the University of Pennsylvania, and the Medical Department of King's College in New York City (1767). As a result, by the early 1770s, a handful of qualified and trained physicians were practicing medicine in colonial America. Nursing, however, remained predominantly in the hands of undereducated individuals.

The development of hospitals in colonial America was slow. The first hospital was started in Philadelphia in 1751 at the encouragement of Benjamin Franklin. A second hospital, New York Hospital, was founded in 1770 under a charter granted by King George III at the request of several New York physicians who were seeking to prevent the spread of infectious diseases. The colonial era hospitals, unfortunately, were seen as places for immoral and unfortunate people who required health care and as places where medical students could train. Hospital staff consisted of servants, attendants, coachmen, and others who may have had some nursing or housekeeping experience (Ellis & Hartley, 1988).

The development of health care facilities for the mentally ill was as slow or slower than the development of hospitals for the physically ill. The first hospital in the colonies for the mentally ill was established, in 1752 as a department of the Pennsylvania Hospital. A second hospital was founded in Williamsburg, Virginia in 1773, and a third, the Friends' Hospital near Philadelphia, was opened in 1817. By 1840, there were only eight hospitals for the mentally ill, which led to confinement of many mental patients in poorhouses and prisons. Like the hospitals for the physically ill, the hospitals for the mentally ill were deplorable. Dorthea Lynde Dix (1848), a schoolteacher from New England, worked to revolutionize the field of mental health care. Despite powerful public opinion against women in health care, she succeeded in bringing about improvements in mental hospitals and the training of attendants.

By today's standards, most American hospitals in the late eighteenth and early nineteenth centuries were disgraceful. They were dirty, poorly ventilated, and contaminated. These hospitals actually facilitated the spread of disease. Nursing care during this time was equally deplorable. The profession was considered an inferior and undesirable occupation. Individuals who provided nursing care often were drawn from the criminal classes or from among widows with large families who drowned their grievances in alcohol. It was not uncommon for these nurses to "assist" in the dying process of patients by removing pillows and bed-clothes or by performing other morbid activities designed to hasten death.

THE NINETEENTH CENTURY

Nursing in England

The arrival of the nineteenth century brought significant changes in nursing around the world. Florence Nightingale, a highly intelligent, talented, wealthy, well-travelled and well-educated young English woman, became interested in training as a nurse. Miss Nightingale attended a three-month training program for nurses at the Institution of Deaconesses in Kaiserwerth, Germany, where the modern movement for nursing education began. In 1854, she began training nurses at the Harley Street Nursing Home and served as superintendent of nurses at King's College Hospital in London (Nutting & Dock, 1912).

With the outbreak of the Crimean War, Nightingale's nursing career took a major turn. She was asked by the British Secretary of War to lead a group of nurses to Crimea and to work at one of the military hospitals. Nightingale assembled 38 individuals who were self-proclaimed nurses of varied experience and nuns from different Catholic and Anglican orders (Kelly & Joel, 1996). Upon her arrival in Crimea, Nightingale found deplorable conditions. There were no beds, food, blankets, or medications. Scurvy, starvation, and dysentery were rampant. Using her own money and the Times Relief Fund, Nightingale purchased medical supplies, food, and equipment. In addition, she assigned soldiers to repair and clean up the buildings housing the injured and infirm, and hired wives of the soldiers to manage and operate the laundry services.

Under the leadership and guidance of Nightingale, principles of asepsis and infection control, a system for transcribing physician's orders, and a procedure to maintain patient records were introduced (Pollard, 1902). Due to her outstanding record keeping, Nightingale was able to document that the British soldier death rate decreased from 42 percent to 2 percent. Most of this decrease was a result of her health care reforms emphasizing sanitary conditions. Nightingale's work in Crimea and her subsequent publication of *Notes on Nursing: What It Is and What It Is Not* (Nightingale, 1883), delineating the importance of appropriate training for nurses, were major factors influencing the advancement and evolution of professional nursing education and practice throughout the world.

The American Civil War (1860–1865)

Prior to the Civil War, health care and sanitary conditions in the U.S. were as deplorable as those described by Florence Nightingale during the Crimean War (Oermann, 1997). There were few physicians and trained nurses, and diseases such as smallpox, malaria, typhoid fever, syphilis, and gonorrhoea were at epidemic proportions.

At the start of the Civil War, there were no army nurses and no organized medical corps. Only a few hundred sisters from religious orders, who volunteered their services, were available to care for the sick and wounded. In April 1861, President Lincoln, in his call for militia volunteers, also heard from many wives, sisters, and mothers of the newly enlisted soldiers. These women volunteered to serve as nurses for the wounded Union soldiers. Out of the many hundreds of volunteers, 100 women were selected to take a special short nurse-training course under the direction of the physicians and surgeons in New York City (Kalisch & Kalisch, 1995). Two months later, in June 1861, Dorthea Lynde Dix, who was already well known for her humanitarian activities on behalf of the mentally ill, was appointed by the Secretary of War to supervise the newly trained Army nurses. Dix held rigid standards, accepting only young women (under the age of 30) and preferring women that were unattractive. Although these new army nurses were not required to wear a uniform, Dix insisted that they wear either a black or brown dress. Since the nurses had to work in settings where poor sanitation and primitive equipment existed, it was difficult to maintain asepsis. As a result, more lives were lost from diseases than from bullets. (Throughout the remainder of the chapter please refer to Table 2.1 for a list of individuals who were influential in the development of American nursing.)

TABLE 2.1   Leaders in the Evolution of Nursing Education and Practice in the U.S.

Dorthea Dix	• Was a pioneer in elevating the standards of care for the mentally ill • Served as Superintendent of Female Nurses in the Union Army
Mary Ann Bickerdyke	• Brought drastic improvements in sanitary conditions in the Union field hospitals
Clara Barton	• Developed the American Red Cross
Marie Zakrzewska	• Established the first formal training course for nurses
Linda Richards	• Was the first trained nurse in the U.S.
Mary Mahoney	• Was the first African-American professional nurse
Isabel Hampton Robb	• Established the Nurses' Associated Alumnae of the United States and Canada which later became the American Nurses Association • Served as a founder of the *American Journal of Nursing*
Lavinia Dock	• Created the organization "Society of Nursing School Superintendents" which later became the National League for Nursing • Served as a founder of the *American Journal of Nursing*
Sophia Palmer	• Served as the first editor of the *American Journal of Nursing*
Lillian Wald	• Founded the Henry Street Settlement in New York City • Served as first president of the National Organization for Public Health Nursing
Mary Nutting	• Served as a major leader in nursing education • Served as a founder of the *American Journal of Nursing*
Mary Breckenridge	• Was a pioneer in nurse-midwifery • Established the Frontier Nursing Service
Frances Payne Bolton	• Created the U.S. Cadet Nurse Corps
Lucile Petry	• Served as the first Director of the Division of Nurse Education
Esther Lucille Brown	• Called for major changes in nursing practice and nursing education

As the war progressed, several strong-willed women emerged as champions for change in the delivery of nursing care. Sojourner Truth, an African American abolitionist, and Harriet Tubman, a former slave who had escaped to the North in 1849, defied the boundaries of time, gender, and race. Both women cared for Union soldiers, in addition to smuggling slaves to freedom using the complex underground-railroad system.

Another famous untrained Civil War nurse was Mary Ann Bickerdyke, an uneducated, widowed housekeeper from Illinois, who was known locally for her nursing abilities. Over the strong objections of the physicians, Bickerdyke rallied the Union soldiers and brought drastic changes in the sanitary conditions of the Union field hospitals. Clothes were washed, soldiers were bathed, bedding was fumigated, and garbage was removed. Bickerdyke, a bold and outspoken woman outraged by the number of lazy and corrupt medical officers of the Union army, was often successful in securing their dismissals. Her success was primarily due to her firm friendship with two generals of the Union army, Ulysses S. Grant and William T. Sherman (Davis, 1886).

Soon after the Civil War broke out, Clare Barton, a Massachusetts woman working as a copyist in the U.S. Patient Office, began an independent campaign to provide relief for the soldiers. Not wanting to enlist in the military nurse corps headed by Dorthea L. Dix, Barton appealed to the nation for supplies of shirts, blankets, towels, lanterns, camp kettles, and other necessities (Barton, 1862). Since she was working outside the government, it was not until 1862 that Barton was permitted to take supplies to the battlegrounds of Virginia. Her efforts did not end at the close of the Civil War, but eventually led to the founding of the organization known as the American Red Cross.

Like the women of the North, the women of the South also responded to the news of war. However, unlike Northern women, Southern women did not have official governmental support for their activities. In addition, there was widespread public prejudice against women serving in hospitals. Nursing, an occupation involving intimate contact with strange men, was considered unfit for any self-respecting Southern woman to pursue. As a result, convalescing soldiers and untrained women volunteers cared for the sick and wounded during the first year and a half of the war. The lack of adequate nursing care for Confederate soldiers eventually lead to the granting, by the Confederate Congress, of official governmental status to the women working as nurses.

Despite the horrors of the Civil War, its impact helped to advance the cause of professional nursing. As a result of the successful reforms that took place in the military hospitals, doors were opened that would lead to reforms in civilian hospitals throughout the country (Rosenberg, 1977).

Establishment of Schools of Nursing

At the start of the Civil War, Florence Nightingale was establishing the first nursing school in England. When the nurse training school opened at St. Thomas' Hospital in London in June 1860, most London physicians opposed the project. They felt that nurses occupied much the same position as housemaids and, therefore, needed little instruction beyond poultice making, enforcing cleanliness, and attending to patients' personal needs. Although she was in ill health, Nightingale prevailed, and her school of nursing remains today as a major nursing educational force in England.

At the close of the Civil War, an increase in the number of informal nurse training courses occurred both in the North and in the South. As a result of segregation, African-Americans, however, had to establish their own hospitals and nursing courses to address the high rates of morbidity and mortality among the Black population. Unfortunately, all of the early nursing courses, developed for both Caucasian-Americans and African-Americans in the North and the South, offered little or no classroom education and relied heavily upon on-the-job-training. The students learned routine patient care responsibilities, worked long hours (six days a week), and served as supplemental hospital staff. After graduating, nurses tended to work as private duty nurses or hospital staff.

In 1868, at the meeting of the American Medical Association, the AMA president, Dr. Samuel D. Gross, advocated for the formal training of nurses. Throughout the nineteenth century, nursing services were haphazard and disorganized. Although some women developed an aptitude for nursing, most were uneducated and often morally unfit to care for patients. The better American hospitals used the services of Catholic nuns and Protestant deaconesses who, although superior in general skill to the women otherwise hired, were untrained and lacked adequate knowledge about nursing care.

It was not until 1862, when Dr. Marie Zakrzewska established and opened the New England Hospital for Women and Children, that the first formal training course for nurses developed. Students were required to attend the course for six months. After a probationary period of one month, students were granted a small wage, board, and laundry services (New England Hospital for Women and Children, 1863). However, despite these incentives, few women were willing to invest the required six-months for training. No doubt this was a result of the extreme patriarchal attitude that prevailed during the nineteenth century. Women were educated for marriage and were expected to have little formal education. Any young woman of "genteel background" who desired to seek an opportunity for self-development faced a real problem. Aside from teaching as a private governess or engaging in handiwork such as dressmaking or embroidery, few occupations, nursing included, were considered proper for a woman to undertake. However, the nursing course prevailed and ten years later it was expanded into the first general training school for nurses in America. On October 1, 1873, 32-year-old Linda Richards, America's first professionally trained nurse, graduated. In 1879, America's first professionally trained African-American nurse, Mary Elizabeth Mahoney, graduated. Mahoney has been credited with providing the necessary leadership that led to the acceptance of African-Americans as professional nurses. In a philanthropic move to further prepare African-American nurses to meet the needs of the black population, John D. Rockefeller funded the creation of a school of nursing specifically for African-American women at the Atlanta Baptist Seminary, now known as Spelman College (Salzman, Smith, & West, 1996).

Even as Linda Richards was graduating, three more nurse training schools were opening in New York, New Haven, and Boston. These schools included The New York Training School, attached to Bellevue Hospital, The Boston Training School for Nurses, and The Connecticut Training School for Nurses at New Haven State Hospital (Bacon, 1895; New York State Charities Aid Association, 1872). The New York Training School was recognized as the first nursing program in the U.S. to be modelled after the Nightingale school in London and to have a published nursing textbook, *A Manual of Nursing*. The curricula for these programs were from 18 months to two years. By 1873, graduates of the Nightingale school of nursing migrated to the U.S. where they became supervisors in these three nursing programs.

The New York Training School for Nurses at Bellevue Hospital also was the first school to adopt a standard uniform for student nurses. Not until the 1890s was a regulation uniform generally established as a distinguishing mark of each nurse training school. The practice of wearing a uniform and a cap (for the purpose of covering the long hair styles of the nineteenth century) had its origins from the military and religious orders where high value was placed on standardized dress. As reflected in the 1905 commentary published by Oldfield, "The adoption of a pretty and distinctive uniform, worn in public, was the real starting point of the modern professional nurse. . . . The uniform gave a status, an attractive status, to those thousands of young women who wanted occupation and status" (pp. 655–656).

The Movement Toward Professionalism

An important movement toward professionalism in nursing occurred in 1893 at the Chicago World's Fair. Some of the most influential nursing leaders of the century gathered to share ideas and discuss issues pertaining to nursing education. As a result of their discussions, groundwork was laid for the future establishment, by Lavinia Dock, of the American Society of Superintendents of Training Schools (later to become known as the National League for Nursing Education and then the National League for Nursing) and the establishment, by Isabel Hampton Robb, of the Nurses' Associated Alumnae of the United States and Canada (later to become known as the American Nurses Association) (Nutting & Dock, 1912).

Despite strong opposition from the medical profession toward the training of nurses, professional nursing thrived and flourished. The origins of professional nursing in the U.S. can be attributed to the desire of respectable women for a broader occupational role, pioneering efforts of female physicians, humanitarian sentiments expressed by journalists, and the financial support of various philanthropic groups in New York, New Haven, and Boston.

End of the Nineteenth Century

At the end of the nineteenth century, the movement for increasing the rights of women began. As a result, there was a rapid increase in the number of jobs for women. This amounted to a form of female emancipation that allowed women more independence and the ability to be self-sufficient. However, nursing did not fare well compared with many other forms of work that were opening to women. After graduation from a school of nursing, a nurse could work either in a home, as a private-duty nurse, or in a hospital as a head nurse or superintendent.

The practice of nursing included many housekeeping tasks. The nurse was expected to maintain the room temperature, humidity, and ventilation, as well as cook and serve food to patients. Scrubbing, cleaning, polishing furniture, controlling insects, washing clothes, folding linen, and making bandages were all considered to be within the domain of nursing practice. In addition to all of these housekeeping tasks, nurses were expected to make beds, give baths, prevent and care for bedsores, give enemas, insert catheters, bandage wounds, dress blisters/burns/sores, observe secretions, monitor vital signs, observe effects of diet and medications, and administer medications and treatments ordered by the physicians. Treatments often carried out by nurses included the application of leeches, cups, poultices, counter-irritants, and blisters. The dominance of the physicians, however, prevailed. Wherever the nurse worked, it was always emphasized that the physician was in charge and that there was no greater function than to perform the orders dictated by the physician.

The nineteenth century ended with the United States Congress declaring war on Spain. Once again, as demonstrated in the Civil War, nurses would have a major role in caring for the sick and wounded. This was the first use of trained nurses in a war. As a result, the stage was set for the development, in the future, of both a permanent Army Nurse Corps (1901) and a Navy Nurse Corps (1908).

THE TWENTIETH CENTURY

The First Decade

In the early twentieth century, nurses in the U.S. began to gain control of their profession. After years of dedicated work by Robb, Nutting, Dock, Palmer, and Davis, the *American Journal of Nursing* was finally published. Sophia Palmer, the director of nursing at Rochester City Hospital in New York, was appointed as editor of the journal. Nurses now had both a professional organization and an official journal through which they could communicate. The editorial in the first issue stated:

> It will be the aim of the editors to present month by month the most useful facts, the most progressive thoughts and the latest news that the profession has to offer in the most attractive form that can be secured. (Palmer, 1900, p. 64)

In 1903, state legislatures in North Carolina, New Jersey, New York, and Virginia passed licensure laws for nursing, all within a period of two months. By 1910, most states had passed similar legislation requiring nurse registration before entering into practice. The roots of professionalism had begun to take hold! The reader is advised to refer to chapter 13 which discusses, in further depth, aspects of professionalism.

While nursing was addressing important professional issues, communicable diseases became a major health problem in the overcrowded slums of the major cities. Between 1820 and 1910, nearly 30 million immigrants entered the United States. Ninety-one percent of these immigrants came from Europe. With the rapid growth in population came the necessity for adequate housing and numerous tenement houses were built. However, it was not uncommon to find in New York City, as many as 550 people living in no more than 95 rooms. To make sanitary conditions even worse, immigrant families often would convert their apartments into "sweatshops," where garments or cigars were manufactured. As a result, slum dwellers were ravaged by typhoid fever, scarlet fever, and smallpox. Many of them died or developed tuberculosis or other communicable diseases.

To address the public health problems that were occurring in the slums of the cities, the Women's Branch of the New York City Mission, as early as 1877, began sending trained nurses into the homes of the indigent. By 1890, there were 21 organizations in the U.S. engaged in working as visiting nurses, most employing no more than one nurse each. However, it was not until Lillian Wald and Mary Brewster created the Nurses' Settlement House in one of the slum sections of the Lower East Side of Manhattan (later known as the Henry Street Settlement House) that public health nursing for the entire county was born. The primary aim of the Settlement House was providing nursing care to the sick in their homes, with health instruction being a secondary aim. By 1909, the Henry Street Settlement House staff consisted of 37 nurses, with ten of them actually living in the Henry Street headquarters. The Settlement House grew from only two nurses into a highly organized social enterprise consisting of many departments. In 1912, a handful of visiting nurses formed the National Organization for Public Health Nursing (NOPHN) with Lillian Wald as its president. The nurses forming the NOPHN favored the title "public health nurse" over the title "visiting nurse." They felt that the term was more inclusive and allowed for future extension of nursing services to a much larger proportion of wage-earners and people of moderate means (Gardner, 1912).

Nursing Education Reform

In the early twentieth century, the nebulous concept of postgraduate training for nurses came to light. This training basically consisted of learning new skills through on-the-job training or attending lectures for nursing students, but there was no consistency among the various programs as to what was offered or how the content was presented. Of the 26 hospitals that offered postgraduate training courses, only three had any provision for a regular course of lectures and class work (Allenson, 1904).

To address the need for some type of uniformity in providing postgraduate nursing education and to prepare graduate nurses for the role of superintendent for either a training school for nurses or a hospital, Teachers College, Columbia University developed a one-year postgraduate program that consisted of eight months of classes and three to four months of private-duty nursing experience. In 1910, a sizable endowment was provided to Teachers College that allowed for expansion of the length and quality of the program. A new department of nursing and health was created within the College which focused on the preparation of nurses for teaching and supervision in nursing training schools, for administration in hospitals and training schools, and for work in the social and preventive branches of nursing. Under the leadership of Adelaide Nutting, who had come to Teachers College from the Johns Hopkins Hospital three years earlier, the new postgraduate nursing program soon became the world leader in preparing nurse educators.

World War I

When the United States entered World War I in 1917, three years after its start in Sarajevo, Serbia, nurses were needed desperately to care for the sick and wounded suffering from the results of trench warfare (Stanhope & Lancaster, 1996). Once the American government declared that the country would enter the war, the interest in nursing, among American women, began to rise. The Army Nurse Corps rapidly expanded. The Navy Nurse Corps also expanded, but at a much slower rate because the fighting was taking place primarily on land. Six months after the U.S. entered the war, approximately 1,100 nurses were overseas, with nearly half of them stationed in British general hospitals.

As the need for nurses grew, action was taken to increase the supply of student nurses. Major marketing efforts were mounted, including posters, motion pictures, photographs, pamphlets, newspaper publicity, and magazine articles. The intent was to make the American population aware of the need for nurses and to create a positive attitude toward the nursing profession. Seven hundred of the leading schools of nursing were asked to enlarge to the maximum capacity their resources and clinical facilities. This was the first time that a publicity campaign for student nurses was implemented on such a large scale. No doubt, its effectiveness was a result of its patriotic wartime appeal. As a result, the number of students entering nursing schools, in 1917–1918, increased by 25%.

As a result of unfavorable reports on nursing conditions in the Army, a proposal to establish an Army School of Nursing was drafted. It was the intent of the proposal to provide students who could care for patients in Army hospitals in the same manner that students were providing care to patients in civilian hospitals. The school was to be centralized in the Surgeon General's Office, under the supervision of a dean, with training units and teaching staff in many of the camp hospitals. On May 25, 1918, creation of the proposed school was approved.

Another attempt to increase the number of available trained nurses was implemented through an experimental program at Vassar College. The program, known as the Vassar College Training Program for Nurses, was designed to attract college graduates and to train them as nurses within two and a half years. Preparatory courses in such areas as anatomy/physiology, nutrition, psychology, chemistry, hygiene/sanitation, bacteriology, and nutrition, along with nursing courses and clinical practice, made up the curriculum. The standard of teaching was much higher than that available in most other nursing programs. The program was shortlived and the school was closed when peace was declared in 1919. However, the most important long-term effect of this experimental program was the change in philosophy by many nurse educators. Having prenursing or preparatory course work in the sciences, conducted under the auspices of a recognized college or university, was seen as an important move toward elevating the standards of nursing education (Kalisch & Kalisch, 1995).

While World War I was raging, another insidious force was gathering momentum. Between 1918 and 1919, a massive influenza epidemic spread across the U.S. and around the world. The U.S. experienced the highest death rate in its history. Ninety-two percent of deaths were directly attributed to influenza (Kalisch & Kalisch, 1995). Often physicians were not available, leaving nurses to deal with the sick and dying. When the epidemic ended, data revealed that the death toll in the U.S. alone was five times greater from influenza than from war-related causes.

The 1920s

World War I provided nurses with an opportunity to enter new areas of activity. In addition, the war demonstrated that nurses were able to manage and care for patients in an effective manner. As a result, in 1920, Congress passed a bill allowing nurses to hold military rank (Dock & Stewart, 1920). The passage just one year earlier of the Woman Suffrage Amendment of the United States, allowing women the right to vote, also allowed for new and unheard of freedoms for women. Short hairstyles, rising hemlines, and the use of cosmetics were all reflections of this "newfound" freedom.

Amidst all of these social changes, nursing was progressing in two directions: advocating for the establishment of collegiate schools of nursing, rather than hospital-based diploma programs, and developing rural midwifery programs. The first attempt to establish a nursing program that was an integral part of a university occurred at the University of Minnesota. Although the program offered only a three-year diploma, it was still a significant step forward. Previously, schools of nursing based on college campuses functioned as "offshoots" of the university hospitals and not part of the academic organization.

By 1916, several colleges and universities maintained schools, departments, or courses in nursing education. Upon completion of high school, a student took two years of preliminary work in a university or college and then completed two years of nurse training in the hospital. This was followed by a year of clinical work and study to become specialized in some aspect of nursing. Successful students graduated with a diploma in nursing and a bachelor of science degree. By 1925, twenty-five colleges and universities were granting an BA or BS degree in nursing. The total enrollment in these programs was just under 400 students.

It was not until 1924 that the Yale School of Nursing was opened as the first autonomous collegiate program in nursing. Founded as a pioneering and experimental venture funded by the Rockefeller Foundation, the five-year program correlated nursing theory with practical experience and emphasized preventive aspects of health care. The Yale School of Nursing was so successful that it went on to offer a 30-month course leading to a master of nursing degree.

In the early 1920s the number of college-based nursing programs slowly began to grow in such prestigious universities as Case Western Reserve University, The University of Chicago, and Vanderbilt University. Not surprising, however, was the strong opposition by physicians to higher education for nurses! The physicians argued that nurses in collegiate programs were being overtrained, that the service they provided was too costly, and that women with brief training in bedside routines were just as satisfactory (Davis, 1921). They felt that intelligence and sound knowledge of theory were unnecessary for the student nurse and might handicap her as a prospective practicing nurse. Unfortunately, veteran nurses supported some of these beliefs by indicating that the old-fashioned training of nurses had been simple, rigorous, and sufficient. As a result of the weight of such attacks by physicians and many veteran nurses, efforts to improve nursing education standards lagged in many states.

The early part of the decade brought the passing of the Shepard-Towner Act, one of the first pieces of legislation to allow for federal funds to assist in the care of special populations. The funding provided public health nurses with the resources necessary to promote the health and well-being of women, infants, and children (U.S. Department of Labor, Children's Bureau, 1923). Following this major improvement, Mary Breckenridge, a nurse and midwife, established the Kentucky Committee for Mothers and Babies, later known as the Frontier Nursing Service (FNS). This service was the first organized midwifery program in the U.S. The FNS eventually attracted physicians and nurses who provided medical, dental, surgical, nursing, and midwifery care to the rural poor. The FNS remains in operation today and continues to provide vital services to the rural residents of Kentucky.

The 1930s

The U.S. experienced economic prosperity during World War I and into the 1920s. However, in October 1929, the American economy disintegrated with the crash of the stock market. One year after the crash, over six million men and women were unemployed (Karger & Stoesz, 1994). The Great Depression had a profound impact on the profession of nursing. Up until this time, hospitals tended to be staffed by student nurses with most graduate nurses working "private duty" in the homes of their patients. Families without an income could no longer afford to hire private duty nurses. Thus, many nurses joined the ranks of the unemployed.

The depression also affected many hospitals, which were forced to close their schools of nursing as a result of the economic times. The poor economy led to an increased number of charity cases requiring hospital-based nursing care. As a result, the unemployed nurses, who were willing to work for minimum wage, were recruited to work in the hospitals rather as private duty nurses. In the staffing of hospitals, this led to a change from student nurse to graduate nurse. The work hours were long and the working conditions often were not desirable or pleasant. This staffing change, however, had a lasting effect on the profession by moving the hospital workforce out of the realm of the student nurse into the realm of the graduate nurse.

As the depression worsened, a new field opened for a limited number of nurses. Air travel was becoming more common. However, its growth was not increasing markedly because of the publicity around the number of airplane crashes that were occurring. In an attempt to make air travel appear safe, airlines such as United, American, Eastern, and Delta, hired nurses to be available for all emergencies. The nurse-stewardess role, at the time, was one of the most appealing jobs that nurses could find.

The middle to late 1930s brought massive unemployment, uneven distribution of nursing services, and depression-stricken hospitals. These changes called for major revisions in the curricula of schools of nursing. Subsequently, the third edition of the National League for Nursing Education's *Curriculum Guide for Schools of Nursing* (1937) was published. The guide stated two major assumptions, the first assumption being that the primary function of a nursing school should be to educate the nurse. This was different from the earlier assumption that schools of nursing existed to provide nursing services for hospital patients. The purpose of the newly drafted assumption was to point out to the public that the educational preparation of the future nurse should not be sacrificed to meet the immediate needs of patient care. The second assumption was that the nurse should be serving the total community rather than just the hospital. Public health nursing, mental health nursing, and occupational health nursing all were considered to be aspects of this concept.

On the Hollywood scene, the role of the nurse in major motion pictures was changing. No longer was nursing being portrayed as a temporary job for women interested in a little humanitarian activity prior to marriage, but as a profession that espoused high ideals and rigorous self-discipline. Although the characters in these movies engaged in minimal realistic nursing activities, what was important was that the image of nursing, being portrayed to the public, was relatively positive.

World War II

After the bombing of Pearl Harbor by the Japanese, the U.S. officially entered World War II. Unfortunately, all military branches had inadequate numbers of nurses. In an attempt to address this nursing shortage, Congress passed the Labor-Federal Security Appropriation Act in 1941. This act provided funds to schools of nursing for: a) provision of refresher courses in modern practices for retired nurses; b) creation of courses in special fields of nursing; and c) facilitation of an increase in the enrollment of basic nursing students.

Because of the growing concern that there would continue to be an insufficient number of nurses to care for the sick and wounded, programs also were developed to prepare additional nurses' aides. The aides were to be intensively trained, to serve an adequate number of hours in a hospital or clinic or in field service, to conform to the discipline of the organization in which they worked, to render service without pay, and not to replace paid hospital personnel while serving specifically as nurses' assistants (Commentary, 1941).

To further bolster the number of available military nurses to serve the country's war efforts, the Bolton Act of 1943 was passed to create the U.S. Cadet Nurse Corps. The act stipulated that the total cost of the education of nursing students (tuition, fees, books, uniforms, and monthly stipends) be provided. The student did not have to demonstrate a need for these funds, but only promise to engage in military or civilian nursing for the duration of the war. Immediately following the passage of the Bolton Act, the Division of Nurse Education was established within the U.S. Public Health Service. The division was made directly responsible to the Office of the Surgeon General. Quotas for the number of military nurses required to meet the needs of the war effort were established. Under the direction of Lucile Petry, the first director of the Division of Nurse Education, along with the War Advertising Council, the quotas were exceeded. Nursing had become an essential part of the military advance. Working under combat conditions and adapting patient care to the challenges of climate, facilities, and supplies, nurses finally had been recognized as an integral part of the military force. In 1944, Congress passed a law providing members of the Army Nurse Corps and Navy Nurse Corps with officer rank.

World War II created a new career option for nurses, that of flight nurse. When the war began, it was thought that only cargo or bomber-type aircraft would be used to transport sick and wounded soldiers.

Thus, since enlisted men in the Medical Corps were taught first aid, it was not considered necessary to assign nurses to accompany the wounded while being transported in an aircraft. However, this policy quickly changed with the establishment of a Nursing Division in the Air Surgeon's Office for the development and special training of flight nurses.

In the civilian sector, nurses were becoming aware of the massive defense spending that was occurring to support the war effort. One of the more striking effects of the war on the nursing profession was the massive increase in the number of nurses employed in industry as public health nurses. These nurses generally were employed by a company to engage in preventive health care and provide health education to the company's employees. Nurses in particular were sensitive to the special health care needs of the large number of women who had entered the industrial work force as a result of the war. For example, safe attire for women presented a problem. Since it was fashionable at the time to have long hair, nurses encouraged female workers, even against their expressed reluctance, to adequately cover their hair.

As a result of so many nurses leaving the civilian sector to serve their country as military nurses, an acute shortage occurred in nursing personnel during the winter of 1944–1945. More than 65,000 nurses, most of whom came from civilian hospitals, were in the Army or Navy Nurse Corps, with another 13,800 nurses working in industry in the civilian sector (Kalisch & Kalisch, 1995). Thus, to fill the void of registered nurses in civilian hospitals, the majority of the workload was carried out by student nurses.

World War II finally ended in 1945. The Third Reich had fallen in Europe and the conflict with the Japanese was brought to closure. Despite all the bloodshed and horrors of war, the profession of nursing had prevailed and had made advancements in demonstrating its importance to the health and welfare of Americans. In 1948, since massive numbers of military nurses were no longer needed, the U.S. Cadet Nurse Corps was terminated.

Postwar Era

The postwar era was a time of prosperity for the average American. However, the end of the war did not ease the demand for nurses. Civilian hospitals were eagerly awaiting the return of all of the nurses who had left their ranks to serve in the Nurse Corps. However, many military nurses indicated that they did not want to return to general duty in civilian hospitals. They had become accustomed to having considerable responsibility in the Army or Navy, and had found real satisfaction in the more flexible, autonomous roles that they had held. In addition, many of the women returning from the battle front wanted to start a family. Thus, over 65% of the hospitals reported acute nursing shortages.

In 1946, the average starting salary of the staff nurse was $35.75 a week, with the workweek being 48 hours. Most nurses wanted the workweek cut to 40 hours and an increase in pay to at least $40. Typists, bookkeepers, and seamstresses were making a higher salary than were nurses. Although nurses had achieved the status of "professionals" as a result of the war, physicians, administrators, and the public did not treat them accordingly. Thus, few nurses saw hospital nursing in terms of a professional career.

Many saw such work as a means to earn "pin money" or simply as a means to supplement their husband's income. The majority of hospital nurses surveyed were dissatisfied with the quality and quantity of nonprofessional help, the unevenness of the workload, the time spent on nonprofessional work, the number of duties required, the quality of supervision, the lack of educational opportunities, the long hours, the lack of a retirement plan, and poor employment security (U.S. Department of Labor, Bureau of Labor Statistics, 1948).

A decline in enrollment in schools of nursing was occurring. Young women were not choosing an education in nursing. Schools of nursing were encountering great difficulties in filling their classes. Controversy was occurring as to whether nursing education belonged in colleges and universities. Physicians, once again, were advocating that student nurses spend less time in classroom learning and more time in direct patient care. According to the 1947 postwar survey made by the American College of Surgeons, less expensive nursing care was needed, and could be carried out by auxiliary help. This attitude on the part of physicians and hospital administrators subsequently led to the widespread introduction of more nurses aides and licensed practical nurses in the hospital workforce (Commentary, 1947).

Occurring almost simultaneously were the recommendations proposed by Esther Lucille Brown (1948), which called for far-reaching changes in nursing practice and nursing education. Brown, a member of the research staff of the Russell Sage Foundation, recommended that the nursing profession: a) implement an official examination of every school of nursing leading to accreditation; b) publish and distribute the names of all accredited schools; c) mount a nationwide campaign for the purpose of rallying public support for having accredited schools of nursing; d) provide for a periodic re-examination of all accredited schools, as well as an accreditation process for all new schools of nursing; and e) obtain public support for a substantial part of the financial burden of implementing the accreditation process. Not surprisingly, most physicians and hospital administrators were hostile to these aspirations. Through the Committee to Implement the Brown Report, soon renamed the National Committee for the Improvement of Nursing Services, Brown's recommendations were implemented. At the completion of the analysis, schools that were rated in the upper 25% were classified as Group I, those in the middle 50% were placed in Group II, and those in the lowest 25% were placed in Group III. All of the college-controlled nursing programs participated and were classified in either Group I or Group II. The findings were published in a report entitled *Nursing Schools at the Mid-Century* (West & Hawkins, 1950). In response to the report's development of the classification system and the statements advocating movement toward nursing in institutions of higher education, the National Organization of Hospital Schools of Nursing (NOHSN) was formed. NOHSN assumed responsibility for assisting hospital schools of nursing to deal with what was termed their "struggle for existence."

The Mid-Twentieth Century

The mid-twentieth century brought the persistent problem of an acute shortage of professional nurses. Some of the factors contributing to the dilemma were that there were fewer women between the ages of 18 and 19 years of age in the 1950s than in the 1940s, that unlike most other professions, nurses did not stay in their chosen profession until retirement, that schools of nursing would not accept married women as students, that most hospitals and health care institutions preferred single nurses, and that married nurses with children tended to be strongly committed to their families. Because of the nursing shortage, there was a very high degree of job mobility. In some hospitals, annual turnover exceeded 66% (Kalisch & Kalisch, 1995).

In an attempt to address the nursing shortage, in 1956 associate degree programs in nursing were developed. It was the purpose of these two-year programs to prepare bedside nurses for beginning, general-duty positions at a faster rate than was being done by the diploma schools of nursing, which remained the backbone of nursing education. In addition, it would help move nursing education into the overall system of higher education. Diploma schools of nursing perceived this new type of nursing program as a threat. Some diploma nurse educators indicated that unless changes were made in diploma programs, they would not continue to attract desirable candidates in sufficient numbers. The movement to create associate degree programs in nursing proved to be very successful and these programs grew markedly in number, while hospital-based diploma programs began to close.

The postwar movement that greatly enhanced the standards in nursing schools was the development of the State Board Test Pool. During the 1930s, state board examinations were poorly constructed and unreliable (Florida State Board of Nursing, 1939). With the outbreak of World War II, increased pressure was placed on the individual state licensing authorities. Schools found that preparing students to meet the minimum standards for their own state licensing examination was no longer adequate. A national norm for competency in nursing had to be considered. The National League for Nursing recommended that assistance be offered to states in the development of a standardized examination (Department of Measurement and Guidance, National League of Nursing Education, 1952). As a result, the State Board Test Pool was created. By 1950 all state boards were participating, and continue to do so today.

The peacetime calm of nurses was suddenly halted in June 1950 when the Korean War broke out. One year prior to the war, army nurses had been transferred from the Department of the Army to the new Department of the Air Force. Thus, just as the Air Force nurses were preparing to celebrate their first anniversary, they were deeply involved in carrying out air evacuations of patients. The air evacuations basically eliminated hospital ships as a means of transporting the wounded.

The Korean War provided the first test for the use of the Mobile Army Surgical Hospital (MASH) units. Designed to be movable, these hospitals were located as close to the front line as was safely possible. The MASH unit was the first hospital to which wounded soldiers were sent for evacuation. As a result of the MASH units, the mortality rate among the wounded soldiers who reached the hospitals in Korea was half that of the mortality rate of soldiers during World War II.

Need for Equality

One of the most important and emotionally charged domestic issues in the U.S. during the mid 1950s was the Supreme Court's ruling in

Brown vs. Board of Education of Topeka. This 1954 ruling outlawed racial segregation in public schools. The doctrine overturned the old "separate but equal" mandate by asserting that separate educational facilities were unequal. At this time, about 6% of all graduate and student nurses in American were African-American.

In 1950 approximately 200 nursing schools had at least one African-American student enrolled. Schools with African-American students described such difficulties as having to hold picnics in private homes since public parks prohibited entry by black students, finding clinical placements since some clinical facilities refused to accept African-American students, and locating housing in locales where segregation continued to be enforced since black students could not be placed in the nurses' residence and could not eat in the school cafeteria.

A ground breaking event took place in 1951, when the 42-year old National Association of Colored Graduate Nurses was dissolved and merged with the American Nurses Association (ANA). This was truly an act of faith, but it created for the ANA the new responsibility of removing membership barriers in districts and state associations.

The male nurse and nursing student also suffered from minority status. Some schools of nursing would not admit men. Schools that did admit men would not allow them to care for female patients or utilize the same resources as those provided for the female students, such as the dormitories. What the public and the health care industry failed to recognize was that, during medieval times, men carried out the majority of nursing care (Kalisch & Kalisch, 1995).

During World War I, a large percentage of nurses who volunteered for military service were men. However, they were absorbed into army divisions where there was no opportunity for them to make a contribution to nursing care. This was due, in part, to the existing law that barred men from the Army Nurse Corps. Thus, male nurses who were employed in military service had no official status. They were not recognized as nurses and had no distinction that identified them as being qualified to care for the sick and wounded.

The ANA made attempts to change the biases against men in nursing. However, despite the appeals that were brought forward, registered male nurses were inducted into the military as either a private in the army or as a pharmacist's mate, third class, in the navy. After the war, male nurses strongly recommended that the ANA continue its efforts to obtain commissions for male nurses. It was not until 1954 that male nurses finally achieved official status as commissioned officers in the Army and Navy Nurse Corps (Bullough, 1976).

A Movement in Professionalism

In a move to advance the ability of nursing to improve its educational level, Congress passed the Health Amendments Act of 1956. For the first time since World War II, federal aid to nurses was provided. As a result of this federal funding, many nurses studied at the graduate level, some even earning a doctoral degree. The available funding was so well received that some schools used traineeship funds to support students at two or more academic levels.

Research into the practice of nursing began to become a recognized necessity and one that was essential if the health care needs of modern society were to be met. To facilitate the dissemination of research findings generated by nurses, the scholarly journal, *Nursing Research,* was launched in the early 1950s. To further facilitate nursing research, the U.S. Public Health Service, Division of Nursing Resources was created in 1956 for the purpose of providing competitive funds with an emphasis on applied research.

Scholarly nursing endeavors were further facilitated by expansion in the development of doctoral programs in nursing. The first nursing doctoral programs were developed within the schools of education at Teachers College, Columbia University and at New York University in 1920 and 1934, respectively. However, the growth of doctoral programs was extremely slow. The first comprehensive movement in the development of doctoral education did not occur until the mid 1970s. Since the 1960s, doctoral education in nursing has grown extensively. By the end of the twentieth century, 73 recognized programs were in existence (American Association of Colleges of Nursing, 2003). There are now more than 90 such programs.

The 1960s and 1970s

The 1960s brought many changes in social and political policies. The federal legislation that was enacted during this period had a major and lasting impact on the nursing profession. The Community Mental Health Centers Act of 1963 provided funds for the construction of community outpatient mental health centers. As a result, opportunities for mental health nurses were enhanced.

Another piece of important legislation was The Nurse Training Act of 1964, which expanded federal aid for professional nursing education. The act provided funds for construction of schools of nursing, student loans, and student scholarships. By providing support for students to finance their education by way of long-term, low-interest loans, Congress felt that the number of nursing students would increase.

In 1965, the Medicare and Medicaid Acts were passed. Medicaid provided medical coverage for families, primarily women and children, with an income at or below the poverty level. It soon became the largest public assistance program in the nation (Karger & Stoesz, 1994). Medicare provided hospital insurance, Part A, and medical insurance, Part B, for all people 65 years of age or older who were eligible to receive Social Security benefits, people with total permanent disabilities, and people with end-stage renal disease. Since all hospital charges, regardless of amount or appropriateness, were reimbursed through the Medicare Program, treating Medicare patients became very attractive to hospitals. Thus, hospital occupancy increased. With increased hospital occupancy came an increased need for hospital nurses.

At the same time that Medicaid and Medicare were enacted, the ANA was taking a position regarding nursing education. The ANA, in their first position paper on education for nursing, stated that education for those employed in nursing should take place in institutions of higher learning (American Nurses Association, 1965). The impact of the associate degree in nursing programs was beginning to be felt by the diploma programs. The trend away from hospital-based diploma nursing education was becoming evident. Hospitals were realizing the high cost of operating a school of nursing (National League for Nursing, 1966). The changing patterns in nursing education were being reflected by student admissions. There was a decline in admissions to the diploma programs, a marked increase in admissions to the associate degree programs, and a small increase in admissions to the baccalaureate programs.

Two of the most progressive events of the 1960s, which expanded the role of the professional nurse, were the development of coronary care nursing and the creation of the first educational program for nurse practitioners. Newly created coronary care units (CCUs) provided an environment in which nurses could begin to work collaboratively with physicians and share their knowledge about the diagnosis and treatment of cardiac arrhythmias. It was not long before nurses were recognized for their expertise in the care of critically ill patients. They began to administer intravenous drugs and to defibrillate patients according to written protocols. The nurses in the CCU set the stage for more independent practice among nurses working in such subspecialties as dialysis, oncology, and intensive care.

In 1965, the first nurse practitioner program was started as a pilot project at the University of Colorado. The program was to prepare professional nurses to manage common childhood illnesses and provide well-child care. The outcome of the program demonstrated that nurse practitioners were able to manage 75% of pediatric patients' problems in community clinics (Ford & Silver, 1967). These findings attracted considerable attention that eventually led to the provision of federal funds to support the nurse practitioner role.

The 1960s brought yet another war, Vietnam. It was one of America's longest (1962–1974) and most controversial wars. Nurses once again rose to the occasion by serving their country in the treatment of the sick and wounded. They worked in inflatable medical units in the jungles of Vietnam, performed emergency tracheotomies, inserted chest tubes, administered blood, and gave morphine without orders when physicians were unavailable. Like their military comrades on the battlefield, nurses faced the intense struggle of dealing with the lack of support they were receiving from large segments of society. After returning home, the traumas of the battlefield were only intensified by the chastisement they encountered from many Americans for taking part in the war. As a result, many of them experienced post-traumatic stress disorder.

The 1960s and 1970s brought a marked increase in the number of elderly Americans. Advances in medical technology and the provision of good health care contributed to the longevity of U.S. citizens. However, with this increase in longevity came the problem of caring for the elderly. Although nursing homes, which were developed for the purpose of providing care for the elderly, had existed for some time, they markedly increased in number between 1960 and 1970. By the end of the 1970s over eighteen thousand nursing homes were in operation. Medicaid became the nation's primary payer of nursing-home care. Although the primary care providers in nursing homes were nurses' aides and licensed practical nurses, an interest in graduate preparation in gerontology nursing began to grow.

The 1970s brought continued change in the role of nurses. Nurses demanded fairer wages from hospitals, played a major role in providing care to communities, and were instrumental in the development of hospice programs, birthing centers, and day care centers for the elderly. As disease prevention gained prominence among the health care community and the public, nurse practitioners were seen as viable, cost-effective providers (U.S. Department of Health, Education, and Welfare, Secretary's Committee to Study Extended Roles for Nurses, 1972).

The movement to expand the traditional role of nurses gained momentum in the 1970s. As a result of the success of the initial nurse practitioner programs, federal and private funding stimulated the further development of programs. The Nurse Training Act of 1971 provided funds that were used to develop training programs for nurse practitioners. During the 1970s, nurse practitioners worked cooperatively with physicians in increasing their contributions to overall patient care. Thus, nurse practitioners gained and received acceptance by physicians and patients. State Nurse Practice Acts, as a result, were amended to provide for the monitoring and authorization of this newly created advanced practice role.

The 1980s

The types of patients requiring health care in the 1980s changed. The number of individuals and families who were homeless became a common problem across the country. Unstable economic times contributed to an increase in the indigent population and acquired immune deficiency syndrome (AIDS) emerged as a frightening and fatal disease.

Nurse practitioners had expanded their areas of practice, which included hospitals, outpatient clinics, health maintenance organizations, health departments, occupational health centers, schools, homes, and physicians' offices. In the area of prescriptive drugs, the nurse practitioners were finding it difficult and cumbersome to function under the state laws that required prescriptive authority using standing orders or protocols set down by physicians. Independent prescriptive authority would allow nurse practitioners the ability to prescribe medications on their own. In the early 1980s, Oregon and Washington provided nurse practitioners with "independent" prescriptive authority. A number of states followed suit and put into place similar provisions for their nurse practitioners. By the end of the twentieth century, all states had some form of prescriptive authority in place, even if somewhat dependent in nature. Most states still do not have independent prescriptive authority for nurse practitioners.

In the 1980s, escalating health care costs became a national issue. Medicare was still reimbursing hospitals for any and all types of services that they provided. Between 1966 and 1981, the federal contribution to hospital care had risen from 13% to 41% (Karger & Stoesz, 1994). In an attempt to control escalating hospital expenditures, Congress passed the Diagnosis-Related Group System (DRGs) for reimbursement.

The purpose of DRGs was to provide prospective payment for hospital services based upon the patient's admitting diagnosis. Since reimbursements would be based upon diagnosis and not on actual hospital charges, overall hospital costs would be reduced. Reimbursement was to be based upon diagnostic classifications related to expected length of stay and costs of procedures associated with the diagnosis (Williams & Torrens, 1993). To deal with DRGs, hospitals were forced to increase efficiency and more closely manage the services they provided. Case management was developed to address the efficiency of patient care, which opened a new area of specialization for nurses.

Outpatient services such as outpatient surgical units were created to reduce hospital expenditures. Such services required fewer staff and supplies, and lower facility costs. Working in outpatient facilities was seen as desirable by nurses, since it provided an opportunity to work Monday through Friday with no weekend commitments.

Another action to reduce health care expenditures occurred on the patient side of the equation. As a result of the programs developed by nurses, physicians, and health care agencies, patients began to address their unhealthy daily practices, such as smoking, drinking, sedentary lifestyle, and unhealthy diet. The word "consumer" soon took the place of the term "patient" regarding individuals interested in and concerned about good health practices.

The End of the Twentieth Century

The 1990s began with grave concerns about the economy of the United States. The national debt was increasing and the growth of the economy was slowing. Many women with families, who were not employed, were forced to find a job to help "make ends meet." Increasing numbers of nurses looked for jobs that provided more work hours in fewer days for higher pay. Often this was at the cost of losing fringe benefits. However, being able to work more hours in a compressed timeframe allowed nurses to work a second job. Some nurses requested hospital shift work, in order to receive the available pay differential that was given if one worked evenings or nights. Creative work shifts, such as ten-hour days or four-day workweeks consisting of twelve-hour shifts, became common.

AIDS was continuing to be a major health care concern. As a result, radical changes occurred in the way that infection control among health care workers was carried out. Health care providers were required to institute universal precautions and considered contact with blood and body fluids from all patients potentially infectious. Members of law enforcement even exercised the use of precautionary measures.

In addition, health care providers had to change the focus of their care from one of "cure" to one of "caring." Death as a result of AIDS was inevitable for most patients. Some physicians, in particular, had developed a more impersonal attitude toward patients, largely due to their reliance on medical technology to cure illnesses and diseases.

Exposure to hazardous materials also was a major concern at the close of the twentieth century. More individuals were being exposed to chemical and radioactive substances in the workplace. Thus, employers were becoming legally accountable for informing employees of the actual or potential risks, providing adequate training of employees to reduce potential risks, and ensuring the appropriate use of protective equipment.

A glaring void in the efforts to improve efficiency and productivity in health care delivery was the limited use of new information technologies. By 1993, only an estimated 15% of hospitals had a clinical information system in place (Kalisch & Kalisch, 1995). It was estimated that nearly one-half of nurses time and about one-third of physicians time was spent doing paperwork. Computers could reduce that time considerably. Despite the clear benefits of computerization, many medical personnel resisted. However, by the mid 1990s the use of computers had gained momentum. At the close of the twentieth century, hospitals, insurance companies, payers, and regulators all realized that computerization facilitated the process of managing care, controlling costs, and measuring outcomes.

Although DRGs had been instituted in the 1980s in an attempt to control health care costs, health care expenditures continued to rise in the 1990s. Fifteen percent of the gross national product was related to health care expenditures, and more than twice as much was being spent on health care services in the U.S. than in any other industrialized nation. Furthermore, there was growing demand for Medicare as a result of Americans living longer. To control spiraling health care costs, managed care, a prepaid plan providing comprehensive coverage to voluntarily enrolled members, was instituted.

Managed care consisted of various forms of health maintenance organizations (HMOs) and preferred provider organizations (PPOs). These systems included a) HMOs, allied clinics, hospitals, and health care providers that charged a fixed fee per year and provided all health care services deemed necessary; b) PPOs, a collective of private physicians and hospitals that contracted with private insurance companies to provide health care at a discounted rate; c) individual practice associations (decentralized HMOs), where physicians, not salaried employees of the plan, shared in the risks and profits of providing health care services at a discounted rate; and d) point-of-service systems (open-ended HMOs), where enrollees go to physicians outside of the plan's network, but have to pay 30% of the medical bills, with a deductible often running as high as $1000.

With the floundering economy and the rise in the homeless and indigent population, an increase in the number of uninsured resulted. The absence of adequate health care insurance coverage created one of the largest barriers between the poor and the health care services they needed. Thus, a sizable number of Americans was unable to obtain adequate health care as a result of limited resources. Having limited access to appropriate health care in hospitals and clinics led patients to ultimately seek care through hospital emergency rooms, one of the most expensive health care environments in the American health care industry. Such actions drove the costs of health care even higher, but the patients' health care outcomes would continue to deteriorate. Health care disparities were a major problem at the close of the twentieth century.

THE TWENTY-FIRST CENTURY

A New Beginning

The start of the twenty-first century marked a new beginning for Americans. However, many of the problems present at the close of the twentieth century continued into the new century. Health care disparities continued among the poor and marginalized members of the population. Approximately 41 million Americans (over 15% of the population) remained uninsured (Lieberman, 2003). AIDS remained a serious health care concern. Increasing health care costs remained. Problems related to an increasing elderly population continued (Eastman, 2003). All of these problems remained to be addressed.

On September 11, 2001, however, Americans were faced with a totally new problem, international terrorism. With the destruction, by terrorists using commercial airplanes as weapons, of the World Trade Center in

New York City and one section of the Pentagon in Washington, D.C., along with the downing of a plane in Pennsylvania that was intended to crash somewhere in the nation's capital, new issues of health and welfare faced the nation. Health care providers were confronted with exploring and understanding means of dealing with the impact of terrorism on mental health, not to mention the physical health care problems related to such actions. Examining how massive numbers of citizens could be cared for in the event of terrorist acts involving nuclear weapons, the dispersion of bacteria and viruses that cause contagious diseases, and the dispersion of poisonous gases, has become a priority for all health care providers as the twenty-first century unfolds.

Although the aforementioned social and health care issues remain, as history has already shown, the profession of nursing will rise to the occasion. Nurses will continue to contribute significantly to the health and welfare of the citizens of America through education, practice, and research.

REFLECTIVE QUESTIONS

1. How have the various wars influenced the evolution of nursing education and practice in the U.S.?
2. How has nursing education changed throughout the history of the U.S., and what have been some of the major factors that have influenced this change?
3. Who were some of the leaders in U.S. nursing and what were their contributions?

RECOMMENDED READINGS

Kalisch, P., & Kalisch, B. (1995). *The advance of American nursing.* Philadelphia: Lippincott.

McGann, S. (1990). *Battle of nurses: A study of eight women who influenced the development of professional nursing, 1880–1930.* London: Scuturi Press.

Schorr, T., & Kennedy, M. (1999). *100 years of American nursing: Celebrating a century of caring.* Philadelphia: Lippincott.

REFERENCES

Allenson, M. (1904). My impressions as a post-graduate. *American Journal of Nursing, 5,* 100–103.

American Association of Colleges of Nursing (2003). *Doctoral programs in nursing.* Washington, DC: The Association.

American Nurses Association (1965). *American Nurses Association's first position on education for nursing.* New York: The Association.

Bacon, F. (1895). Founding of the Connecticut Training School for Nurses. *Trained Nurse, 15*, 187–189.

Barton, C. (1862). *Diary: The papers of Clara Barton (1812–1912).* Washington, DC: Library of Congress.

Brown, E. L. (1948). *Nursing for the future.* New York: Russell Sage Foundation.

Bullough, B. (1976). The lasting impact of WWII in nursing. *American Journal of Nursing, 76*(1), 118–120.

Commentary (1947). College of Surgeons survey the nursing situation. *Modern Hospital, 69*(2), 59.

Commentary (1941). Training program announced for 100,000 nurses' aides. *Hospital Management, 52*(3), 44–51.

Davis, L. (1921). *Immigrant health and the community.* New York: Harper & Brothers.

Davis, M. (1886). *The women who battled for the boys in blue—Mother Bickendyke.* San Francisco: Pacific Publishing House.

Department of Measurement and Guidance, National League of Nursing Education (1952). State Board Test Pool Examination. *American Journal of Nursing, 52* (May), 613–615.

Dix, D. (1848). *Memorial of D. L. Dix: Praying for a grant of land for the relief and support of the indigent curable and incurable insane in the United States.* Washington, DC: Tippin & Strapper.

Dock, L., & Stewart, I. (1920). *A short history of nursing.* New York: Putnam.

Eastman, P. (2003). Restoring the inner self. *AARP Bulletin, 44*(3), 16–18.

Ellis, J., & Hartley, C. (1988). *Nursing in today's world: Challenges, issues and trends.* Philadelphia: Lippincott.

Ford, L., & Silver, H. (1967). The expanded role of the nurse in childcare. *Nursing Outlook, 15*(98), 43–45.

Florida State Board of Nursing (1939). *Registered Nurse Examination of 1939.* Miami: Archives of the Jackson Memorial Hospital School of Nursing.

Gardner, M. (1912). The National Organization for Public Health Nursing. *Visiting Nurse Association of Cleveland, 4* (July), 13–18.

Kalisch, P., & Kalisch, B. (1995). *The advance of American nursing.* Philadelphia: Lippincott.

Karger, H., & Stoesz, D. (1994). *American social welfare policy: A pluralist approach.* New York: Longman.

Kelly, L., & Joel, L. (1996). *The nursing experience: Trends, challenges and transition, 3rd Edition.* New York: McGraw-Hill.

Lieberman, R. (2003). Bruised and broken U.S. health system. *AARP Bulletin, 44*(3), 3–5.

National League for Nursing Education (1937). *Curriculum guide for schools of nursing, 3rd edition.* New York: The League.

National League for Nursing (1966). *Study on cost of nursing education, Part I: Cost of basic Diploma programs.* New York: The League.

New England Hospital for Women and Children (1863). *Annual report of the officers to the society and friends, 1862–1863.* Boston: The Hospital.

New York State Charities Aid Association (1872). *Report of the committee on hospitals on the Training School for Nurses to be attached to Bellevue Hospital.* New York: The Association.

Nightingale, F. (1883). *Notes on nursing: What It Is and What It Is Not.* New York: Appleton.

Nutting, M., & Dock, L. (1912). *A history of nursing: The evolution of nursing systems from earliest times to the foundations of the first English and American training school for nurses (4 volumes).* New York: Putnam.

Oermann, M. (1997). *Professional nursing practice.* Stamford, CT: Appleton & Lange.

Oldfield, J. (1905). The nurse of the future. *The Westminster Review, 64,* 655–656.

Palmer, S. (1900). The editor. *American Journal of Nursing, 1*(1), 64.

Pollard, E. (1902). *Florence Nightingale.* London: S. W. Patridge Co.

Rosenberg, C. (1977). And heal the sick: The hospital and the patient in nineteenth century America. *Journal of Social History, 10,* 428.

Salzman, J., Smith, D., & West, C. (1996). *Encyclopedia of African-American culture and history, Volume 3.* New York: Simon & Schuster Macmillan.

Stanhope, M., & Lancaster, J. (1996). *Community health nursing: Promoting health of aggregates, families and individuals.* St. Louis: Mosby.

U.S. Department of Health, Education, and Welfare, Secretary's Committee to Study Extended Roles for Nurses (1972). *Extending the scope of nursing practice: A report of the Secretary's Committee.* Washington, DC: Government Printing Office.

U.S. Department of Labor, Bureau of Labor Statistics (1948). *The Economic Status of Registered Professional Nurses, 1946–1948.* Washington, DC: Government Printing Office.

U.S. Department of Labor, Children's Bureau (1923). *Annual report of administration of the Maternity and Infancy Act.* Washington, DC: Government Printing Office.

West, M., & Hawkins, C. (1950). *Nursing schools at the mid-century.* New York: National Committee for the Improvement of Nursing Services.

Williams, S., & Torrens, P. (1993). *Introduction to health services, 4th edition.* Albany, NY: Delmar Publishing.

3

The Art and Science of Nursing

Judith M. Parker

LEARNING OBJECTIVES

Upon completion of this chapter, students should have gained:

- An understanding of the development of ideas about nursing as an art and a science within the historical context
- An appreciation of the meaning of the art of nursing within the Florence Nightingale school of thought
- An appreciation of debates about the art and science of nursing in the U.S. context
- An appreciation of emerging ideas about art and science and the relationships between them in the current context of health care
- Insight into the implications of these ideas for current nursing education, practice, and research

KEY WORDS

Art, science, nursing, gender, aesthetics, enlightenment, contemporary

INTRODUCTION

What is nursing? Is nursing an art? Is nursing a science? Is nursing both an art and a science? Is nursing neither an art nor a science? Over the years there has been extensive debate in the nursing literature about the art and science of nursing. Why are questions about the nature of nursing posed in these terms? What is it about how knowledge and practices are understood in our society that invites us to ask these questions about nursing? What are the implications of these perceptions for education, practice, and research in nursing?

This chapter seeks to explore some of these questions. It considers some of the history of the development of ideas about modern nursing as an art and as a science. More specifically, it examines the division between art and science and explores the impact that this separation has had upon ideas about nursing.

Two particular developments in the history of nursing ideas are discussed, one stemming from the United Kingdom, and the other from the United States. The first, often described as the Florence Nightingale school of thought, represents the first expression of nursing as an art in modern times. In this development, nursing as an art is conceived of in relation to the character of the nurse and the importance of character training in nursing education programs.

The second is the impact of the development of nursing ideas within the university context in the United States. Of particular note in this discussion are the attempts to construct systems of thought through nursing theory development and the production of nursing science. It was in this context that tensions between nursing as an art and as a science began to be recognized and attempts made to reconcile the two.

The chapter then examines some of the implications of these ideas for nursing in the contemporary context where many of the binary divisions that occurred historically, including those between art and science, are collapsing. It concludes with a discussion of the art and science of nursing within the changing environments of health care delivery.

WHAT IS AN ART? WHAT IS A SCIENCE?

Many modern ideas about art and science have their origins in the scientific revolution of the seventeenth century, and the eighteenth century "Age of Reason" that was generated by the philosophical movement known as the French Enlightenment.

The scientific revolution was a quest to understand, control, and manipulate nature through rational, empirical means. As Capra pointed out in 1982:

This development was brought about by revolutionary changes in physics and astronomy, culminating in the achievements of Copernicus, Galileo and Newton. The science of the seventeenth century was based on a new method of inquiry, advocated forcefully by Francis Bacon, which involved the mathematical description of nature and the analytical method of reasoning conceived by the genius of Descartes. (p. 54)

The Enlightenment project had the aim of civilizing all, of implementing its ideal of social betterment through the power of reason. It was based on beliefs in the universal superiority of the knowledge and values produced by Western science and culture. Those who believed in the democratic ideals of the Enlightenment sought to perfect humankind through reason and create a better world, a civilized and cultured one aided by the new knowledge produced by science (Parker & Gibbs, 1998). Two ways of thinking about art can be linked to the Enlightenment, one concerning the cultural production of knowledge, and the other, the art of living.

A separation of the arts and the sciences occurred in the educational structures and processes that emerged in the wake of the Enlightenment and with the rise of modern professions. Knowledge came to be packaged into the two domains of the sciences and the arts within university faculties, and a division emerged between those who were educated in the sciences and those who were educated in the arts (humanities). Each of these produced different ways of thinking and acting, and different types of knowledge. According to C.P. Snow (1964), writing of the United Kingdom, scientific training produces "doers" and training in the arts produces "thinkers" (intellectuals). He argued that by the 1950s, the science/art professional rift was so deep that the two groups worked completely independently of each other, a trend he saw as potentially dangerous for society.

Another way of thinking about art that emerged out of the Enlightenment concerns the art of living. The search for human perfectibility, which was a major plank of the Enlightenment, became linked to a philosophy of humanism, which, as Nelson (1995) points out, "stresses the centrality of the human subject and sets freedom as the subject's destiny" (p. 53). The human subject, however, was deemed to be male, and rationality was understood to be a masculine attribute. The art of living for men was linked to the pursuit of freedom through rationality, as "doers" and "thinkers."

Women were seen as neither free, nor rational. They were understood "as an essential nature defined by purposeful organic functions" (Berriot-Salvadore, 1993, p. 387). Medical discourse defined the feminine ideal in terms of natural determinism as "the mother, the guardian of virtues and eternal values" (p. 388). Thus while men, defined as human subjects, were separated and freed from the constraints of nature via reason and culture, women, defined in relation to nature and the feminine, were not. Nature and culture merged in this understanding of the feminine, and women were defined in natural and moral terms. Good women exercised their womanly arts and civilized others through the exercise of these arts. By and large, women were excluded from education into the professions.

ART, SCIENCE AND MODERN NURSING

The nature of modern secular professional nursing as it has evolved since the days of Florence Nightingale has been influenced by some of these ideas. Of particular importance to this discussion is how the divisions that occurred between art and science were managed in nursing. These will be considered first in relation to the Florence Nightingale school of thought stemming from Britain, and then in relation to university-based nursing in the United States.

THE FLORENCE NIGHTINGALE SCHOOL OF THOUGHT

The Florence Nightingale school of thought developed and was sustained within the nurse training schools that sprang up in hospitals, not only in Britain but also in Australia, New Zealand, the U.S., and other countries. I argue that within nursing education and practice, nursing as an art was seen to involve the character of the nurse in the exercise of feminine virtues, and the importance of character training in the development of nursing as a female profession/occupation. In this context, science was out of place; the scientific enterprise was a male one and, in the hospital and medical context, belonged to the doctor.

Nursing in nineteenth century industrial England was regarded as an inferior, undesirable occupation practiced by morally suspect women. In

Martin Chuzzlewit, Dickens epitomized the 19th century English nurse in the character of Sairey Gamp, writing that "it was difficult to enjoy her company without being conscious of a smell of spirits" (1910, pp. 312–313). The contrast of Florence Nightingale's work in Crimea, and the subsequent publicity, brought about her identification in the public mind as a "ministering angel" (*The Times,* 1854). This image was instrumental in elevating secular nursing to the status of a female vocation based on Enlightenment ideals of the womanly virtues and the exercise of the womanly arts through the care of the sick. Indeed, Florence Nightingale described nursing as "the finest of the fine arts" (Donahue, 1996).

Enormous effort went into the attempts to position nursing as epitomizing feminine ideals of the good woman. Nursing transgressed many prevailing ideas about the role of women in society, and it was extremely difficult for nursing to gain acceptance as a legitimate and respectable occupation. Sairey Gamp and the "bad woman" were never far beneath the surface; it is therefore not surprising that Florence Nightingale and her followers placed so much emphasis upon ensuring appropriate character formation among nurses in training (Parker 1990).

The first Florence Nightingale training school began at St. Thomas Hospital in London in 1860 and became the model for many training schools in Britain and its overseas territories in the latter half of the nineteenth century (Trembath & Hellier, 1987). Student nurses were judged on their qualities of trustworthiness, neatness, quietness, sobriety, honesty, and truthfulness (Smith 1982). Additionally, nurses were trained to ensure that they did not wish to usurp any of the doctor's functions. Isabella Rathie, the first trained Matron of the Melbourne Hospital, noted, "we are in a great measure the handmaid of the medical man and our function in this particular is to be obedient in every detail" (quoted in Trembath & Hellier, 1987, p. 19).

Thus, the division between art and science manifested within modern secular professional nursing of the Nightingale school of thought can be described as a gendered division. Nursing as a feminine art was developed through character training that resulted in nonassertiveness, obedience, and compliance with medical directives. Specific nursing arts comprised procedures such as bathing, bed-making, positioning patients, and comforting techniques. While some science content was included in nursing courses, "(t)here was minimal, if any, application of science content in nursing practice" (Peplau, 1988, p. 8). Nor were nurses educated in the arts subjects of the university, which produced the thinkers of society, for that belonged to the sphere of men. Rather, they were instilled with womanly virtues.

Nursing education was a process of systematically inculcating a task orientation and the moulding of a set of appropriate attitudes within hospital training schools to produce nurses who exemplified the feminine ideal. Science belonged to the rational and objective world of men, of which medicine was one domain. Men were subjects (minds), women objects (bodies); nurses were therefore not positioned as rational subjects shaping the Enlightenment project and their own destinies, but rather as passive and compliant objects, subservient to medicine.

Hospital-based nurse training lasted for more than one hundred years in Australia and the U.S., and much longer in Britain. Many changes occurred over that time, including considerable strengthening of the science content, particularly from the 1950s onward. However, the gendering of nursing as a feminine art, developed in the restrictive environment of the hospital, placed limitations upon the possibilities for nursing to develop as a modern profession. It also limited the possibilities for nurses to develop knowledge, skills, and attitudes in ways that would enable them to act as independent subjects. Nevertheless, it equipped them powerfully to work as moral agents engaged in socially significant work and to develop in-depth knowledge of the human condition in sickness and in suffering, although in an unarticulated, scientifically untested form.

NURSING IN THE UNIVERSITY

In the United States, a four-year entry-to-practice program had been established within a university by 1919. Within this system, it was possible to ensure the development of knowledge in a systematic and orderly way. By the late 1950s, programs for training nurse scientists had developed in a number of major universities, which stimulated interest in theoretical and scientific bases of practice. These developments were supported by a huge federal investment in nursing education during the 1960s and early 1970s (Gortner, 1983). In the period from the late 1950s to the early 1980s, theories of nursing proliferated as nurse scholars sought to include in the concept of nursing an understanding of biological, behavioural, social, and cultural factors in health and illness. Of particular note in this discussion were the attempts made to produce systems of thought through the development of nursing theory and the creation of nursing science.

This scientific orientation in nursing, however, came into conflict with ideas about the art of nursing. These stemmed not only from the Nightingale school of thought, but also from consideration of the art of nursing in relation to humanism and the nature of the human subject, by this time conceived of as including women. It is in this context that most of the debates about the art and science of nursing have occurred.

NURSING AS A SCIENCE

As has already been noted, a significant feature of the modern era has been the rise of professions, each clearly delineated by a separate body of knowledge. In the early modern era, nursing could not be regarded as a profession because it was seen to be subservient to, and part of, the medical tasks of diagnosis and treatment. With the location of nursing education within universities, and with the goal of securing professional status for nurses, a major task was to establish its own scientific base, separate from that of medicine.

One early nursing theorist, Johnson (1980), distinguished medicine from nursing by arguing that, while the scientific basis of medical knowledge was biological systems, the scientific base of nursing was behavioral systems. She proposed a behavioral subsystem model of the person "with behaviour understood as the sum total of physical, biological and social factors/behaviours" (Parker, cited in Gray & Pratt, 1995, p. 334). These ideas were further developed by Roy (1980), who conceived of the person as an open adaptive system and nursing as the science and practice of promoting adaptation.

Other theorists, however, argued that these approaches did not sufficiently distinguish nursing from medicine. Like medical knowledge, the knowledge produced through study of systems was overly simplistic and mechanistic. Nursing, by contrast, needed to be conceptualized in much broader, more encompassing terms (e.g. Levine, 1971). Ideas about nursing as a holistic science were developed by writers such as Rogers (1970) who conceived of the whole person as an energy field, coextensive with the environment, identified in terms of unified wholeness, openness, pattern, organization, and sentience.

Other writers further differentiated nursing science from medical science by emphasizing nursing's caring function in opposition to medicine's curative function. Watson, for example, pulled together two of the central ideas of the modern era by describing nursing as a humanistic science, with caring the central unifying dimension of nursing (Cohen, 1991).

Thus, with the shift of nursing education to universities in the United States, strong schools of nursing thought emerged. Each was developed in opposition to medicine, and understood nursing as a behavioural science, a holistic science, or a caring science. These conceptual models for nursing practice were the work of a number of nursing intellectuals who had undertaken higher degree work in a range of disciplines, particularly in social sciences and education. Each model was designed to capture the complex dimensions of nursing, although naturally enough, each one tended to reflect the disciplinary base of its author.

Following the establishment of the basis for nursing science through these models, there were calls to test the models against practical experience and refine them. However, progress was slow, as Flaskerud and Halloran (1980) and Fawcett (1984) pointed out. There was also concern that the proliferation of models would weaken nursing's claims to be seen as a profession based in a single unique body of knowledge. Fawcett noted that "(t)he discipline of nursing will advance only through continuous and systematic development and testing of nursing knowledge" (p. 84). Nursing authors sought to concentrate on the common ground in nursing conceptual models. Fawcett, for example, proposed a "metaparadigm" (an explanatory framework) for nursing, built on the central concepts of the discipline—person, environment, health, and nursing—and attempts were made to further unify nursing knowledge around these concepts.

Many nurses, however, rejected nursing theories altogether as a means of establishing a science base for nursing. Nursing administrators and clinicians were particularly vocal in their rejection of the theories following frustrating experiences of trying to implement them in practice. Nursing theories were seen to reinforce the splits between the theory and practice of nursing, between the education students received and the realities of providing health care service, and between nursing thinkers (academics in universities) and nursing doers (nursing administrators and clinicians). While nursing theory was being elaborated, attempts were also being made to develop nursing science knowledge in ways that were linked more closely to practice. The nursing diagnosis movement attracted strong support following the First National Conference on the Classification of Nursing Diagnosis held in Missouri in 1973. Nursing diagnosis sought to identify and classify the phenomena of nursing, to develop a common language for nursing, and to facilitate the development and testing of nursing concepts and techniques. However, by 1983, the first broad-scoped critical rejection of nursing diagnosis emerged (Kritek, 1985).

This more practice-focused approach to developing nursing science suffered from the same fundamental problem as the theory-based approach. Once again, nursing was attempting to develop its science in opposition to medicine by identifying a discipline-specific scientific knowledge base that would legitimize nursing's claims as a separate profession. In doing this, nursing opened itself to some of the same critiques that were made of medicine. The development of a dedicated nursing language separated nursing not only from medicine but, more important, from patients. When viewed through the nursing diagnosis lens, the patients were reduced to objects of nursing diagnoses and treatments, a positioning that was contrary to nursing's understanding of the patient as a holistic subject.

Two broad approaches to the development of nursing science have been identified: one that focused on defining the domain of nursing theoretically and then testing propositions empirically; another that focused on the phenomena of nursing practice and on developing ways of defining and classifying them. Both approaches were consistent with prevailing philosophies of science. Neither appears to have been successful in providing a discipline-specific body of knowledge that would justify nursing's claims to professional autonomy and power.

NURSING AS AN ART

Ideas that stem from the Nightingale school about the nature of nursing art as an expression of the essential goodness of feminine virtues persist in contemporary nursing practice. Peplau (1988), writing about the United States but presenting a view widely held internationally, points out that nursing has been called the conscience of the health care system, which "suggests that nurses are major keepers of the morality, goodness, honesty, and ethics of client care" (p. 9). This positioning of nurses on the moral high ground in the battlefield of health care provision has been sustained by beliefs that nurses exemplify feminine ideals, and appears to have wide community support. It points to a persistent belief in the Nightingale legacy that presents nurses as good women. It also suggests that nurses and nursing organizations recognize and exploit the ways in which this characterization of nursing serves wider political agendas and social functions. Additionally, it supports the idea of nursing as a caring and holistic art that sets itself in opposition to the rationality and reductive practices of scientific medicine and health care organization. As Tanya Buchanan (1999) has noted, the "Nightingale discourse generates myths about nursing that . . . appear to be eternal truths. We need to see past it" (p. 30).

And indeed, ideas that the art of nursing stems from essential female virtues have been challenged within the university setting. The essence of nursing has been claimed to lie in its humanistic philosophy and the artistic practice that flows from this philosophy. In a much-quoted paper, Munhall (1982) argued that nursing has identified itself as a humanistic discipline, adhering to a basic philosophy "that focuses on individuality and the belief that the actions of men (sic) are in some sense free" (p. 176).

Munhall focuses attention on the extent to which university-based nursing education in the United States moved away from the Nightingale school of nursing thought based on female character training, and drew more upon a precisely set out philosophy of the discipline to provide the basis for artistic practice. However, this placed nursing philosophy in opposition to prevailing notions of nursing science. As Munhall pointed out, because nursing subscribed to a humanistic philosophy as well as a scientific research orientation "incongruities, paradoxes, and conflicting ideologies resulted between philosophy and research."

She also draws attention to the attempts made within nursing education to accommodate both a scientific and humanistic (arts) orientation. This suggests that professional, university-based nursing education in the United States attempted to bridge the divide between the sciences and the arts that had been identified by C. P. Snow in the British higher education context. Nursing in the university aimed to produce practitioners who were both scientists in orientation and humanists in practice. However, in educational preparation, the aims and scope of science and the arts differ significantly, and the transfer of both scientific and humanistic orientations to the realities of practice is a complex process.

Many writers have noted that the differing orientations of art and science have resulted in problems for nursing practice. Peplau (1988), for example, notes that science and art are both essential for excellence in the performance of nursing's mission, but points out the difficulty for a discipline to accommodate these two forms of professional behavior.

"Combining both the art and science of nursing, seeing and bringing to bear the distinctive characteristics of each form and of the relation between them, imposes a complexity in professional nursing that virtually defies description" (p. 9).

Holden (1991), an Australian nurse, argues that the split between the arts and the sciences seriously complicates the notion of nursing. She points out that the caring role in nursing pushes nursing into the domain of the arts, while nursing that embraces high technology is pushed into the domain of science. Jennings (1986) suggests that it is not a matter of choosing *either* art *or* science, but rather of skillfully blending both for the betterment of nursing.

Peplau (1988) supports Jennings' view, pointing out that both science and art come together in practice, so that "(t)here is surely a seamless quality, a graceful and delicately balanced movement between art and science portrayed by experienced expert nurses that transcends as it uses the differences between these forms" (p. 14). She suggests further that this transcending of the differing forms of art and science enables nursing to be practiced not only as a helping art, but also as "an enabling, empowering or transforming art." People, she notes "are touched (literally and figuratively) and sometimes changed at a very personal level by the art nurses practice" (p. 9).

The aesthetic dimension—the creative expression—of nursing has received increasing attention over the last two decades. It has built particularly upon the work of Carper, who noted in 1978 that the primary emphasis in the professional literature of the time was being placed on the development of the science of nursing. She pointed out:

> There is, nonetheless, what might be described as a tacit admission that nursing is, at least in part, an art. Not much effort is made to elaborate or to make explicit this aesthetic pattern of knowing in nursing—other than to vaguely associate the 'art' with the general category of manual and/or technical skills involved in nursing practice. (p. 16)

Peggy Chinn and Jean Watson (1994) have been very influential in further developing ideas about aesthetics and nursing, drawing upon notions of nursing as a caring science. Later, Chinn, Maeve, and Bostick (1997) described the development of aesthetic inquiry in nursing and the conceptualization that has emerged of nursing as an art form. (1993, 1994, 1996a, 1996b) undertook a philosophical analysis of conceptualizations of nursing art as a means of contributing to debate on the specific abilities required for artistic creation in nursing.

Despite these developments, other writers (e.g., Darbyshire, 1994a, b; Lafferty, 1997) suggest that science content is still emphasized in nursing curricula at the expense of humanities content, and that, as a result, humanistic aspects of care believed to be essential to the artistic component of nursing are not being addressed sufficiently. Lafferty argues that nursing's dual identity as an art and a science requires a balance, and calls for the promotion of aesthetic knowledge and its acquisition by nursing students. She suggests that studying literature is a way of fostering this. Darbyshire makes a similar point, arguing that nursing as an art and a science is in danger of becoming a cliché unless attempts are made to reverse the marginalization of arts and humanities within nursing curricula.

It can be seen that nursing as a contemporary secular profession has developed out of ideas about the essential nature of women, wherein nursing has been regarded as an art practiced by virtuous women. This essentialist notion of nursing as a gender-based art may help account for the continuing failure to attract equal numbers of men into nursing. This view has also resulted in nurses sometimes regarding themselves, and being regarded by others, as the conscience of the health care system. The concept of nursing as a gendered art is a continuing thread in professional nursing and appears to be a primary source of its moral claims.

However, this notion was challenged by the shift of nursing education into universities in the United States and by the attempts that have been made to discuss nursing as a science and a humanistic art. The literature explored indicates that nursing lies somewhat uneasily in the domains of science and art, a division which stemmed from dividing practices in the cultural production of knowledge. Nursing developments, too, have replicated many of these dividing practices.

NURSING AND CONTEMPORARY HEALTH CARE

Many of the old divisions of the modern era are collapsing in both contemporary higher education and the health sector. The clear division between arts and sciences in higher education that reinforced the arts/sciences divide in knowledge development and the professions is clearly breaking down. It is becoming less possible for professions to define themselves in relation to discrete bodies of discipline-specific knowledge. The continuing knowledge explosion resulting in new fields of scientific enquiry and the development of information technologies have resulted in the proliferation of new professions that draw upon knowledge from a range of sources.

The nexus between professional knowledge and power is being subverted in a number of ways, not least through mass higher education and the access consumers now have to information enabling them to make their own decisions independent of professional advice. These changes are taking place in a wider context in which global market influences are strengthening and humanist principles are weakening. This is an era of market contestability, privatization, accountability, and competition. It is an era in which performance is measured and evaluated on the basis of outcomes.

THE "REINVENTION" OF NURSING

The health care sector is rapidly transforming in response to demands for identifiable, quantifiable indicators of cost-effective quality outcomes. Clinical areas are responding to the changes in diagnosis and treatment as a result of new investigative and surgical technologies. Nursing, like many other professions, is seeking to "reinvent" itself to meet emerging challenges (Parker & Rickard, 1999).

The reinvention of nursing, I would suggest, is occurring on several fronts, all of which have implications for the art and science of nursing. Measures are being undertaken in nursing education, research, and practice to ensure that nurses have the necessary repertoire of knowledge and skills to play a part in the transformations currently underway that are aimed at cost-effective quality outcomes. Efforts are being made to identify the nursing practices that positively influence health outcomes. Nurses are investigating traditional nursing practices to determine both their continuing appropriateness and the skill level necessary for their implementation.

Competencies for general, specialist, and advanced practice are being refined to ensure greater accountability in relation to consumers, within the profession, in relation to other health professionals, and with regard to various contexts of practice (ANCI, 1998). Nurses, in collaboration with other health professionals, are also contributing to the development, testing, implementation and evaluation of standardized clinical pathways. They are developing evidence-based nursing practices and contributing to developments in evidence-based health care. They are working with consumers of health services to satisfy their learning needs.

As it moves into an interdisciplinary, team-based, and consumer-oriented approach to practice and research, nursing is drawing upon current science/technology and information systems and focusing upon nursing contributions to health outcomes and accountability for practices.

Nurses today need to draw substantially upon scientific knowledge to inform their practice, and scientific training needs to be a significant component of nursing education programs. At the same time, nurses can contribute to the development of scientific knowledge in interdisciplinary and nursing-specific research projects. Questions for—and about—nursing emerge from what nurses themselves ask about their practices and the people and communities that they serve.

But how is the art of nursing manifest in this reinvention of the discipline? In a multitude of ways, I would suggest. We live today in an era of diversity, multiplicity, and hybrid practices. Nursing can be practiced as a gendered art, as a humanistic, aesthetic endeavour, and it can take fragments from both of these traditions and draw upon others as well. It can take up aspects of traditional art forms such as music, movement, and touch, and incorporate them in diverse ways into repertoires of skillful practice.

In all of the multiplicity that is the art of nursing there is, however, a continuous thread, expressed as support of the sense of wholeness and integrity of individuals and communities rendered vulnerable through sickness and suffering.

CONCLUSION

In the current climate many nurses are expressing reservations about the market-driven approach and the economic motives that underlie health reforms. They are concerned that standardized approaches to care will compromise their ability to meet the demands of particular and unique situations. They also are concerned that the increasing rationalization of health services is causing fragmentation of those services, despite the rhetoric of continuity of care. Finally, they are concerned that greater reliance upon advanced technologies is resulting in delivery of dehumanized services.

It is important that compliance with current health care reforms and resistance to them not be seen as mutually exclusive endeavours. We can no longer claim that nursing is a holistic and artistic enterprise with humanistic and expressive concerns developed in opposition to the scientific, technical, and instrumental dimensions of care (Parker, 1995). The therapeutic tools and technologies of care we use are not separate from us; they are part of us and we are part of them. As they change, so we change. As we change, they change, too. They are integral to our self-expression as nurses. The art of nursing, then, involves the perception and understanding of the inseparability of expression and technology.

Working within the framework of a standardized pathway does not prevent a nurse from recognizing the individual and the unique needs of particular patients. An aesthetic sensibility recognizes the extent to which there is congruence between the standard (form) and the individual (content). Aesthetic integrity is responsive nursing in which standard and individual, form and content, become shaped into wholeness. An aesthetic sensibility facilitates expression of the art of nursing as part of the complex, ambiguous, and technologically expressive milieus in which nurses work. An aesthetic sensibility responds to unified experiences both for recipients and providers of health care. It resists fragmented experience and can also "empower people who are . . . sick, weak, vulnerable, or disturbed to demand that attention is given to the particularities, complexities, and ambiguities of their individual situation" (Parker, 1995, p. 2).

Nursing as art and/or science has been addressed somewhat differently at different times and in different contexts. A continuous thread nonetheless exists, which demonstrates the significance that nursing has given as a discipline and a profession to both science and art, and the nature of their relationship in nursing. Modern secular professional nursing since its beginnings last century has been, and continues to be, a complex set of practices that contain many anomalies and contradictions. The art and science of nursing manifests itself within a broader and changing social, cultural, and political agenda. Nursing's social mandate acknowledges the art and science of nursing. The challenge for nurses in the contemporary health care context is to exercise that mandate judiciously and creatively.

REFLECTIVE QUESTIONS

1. What do you think are the main reasons nursing has come to be viewed as an art?

2. Why has nursing made consistent attempts to align itself with science?
3. How do you think the art and science of nursing can interrelate in the current contexts of health care?

RECOMMENDED READINGS

Carper, B. (1978). Fundamental patterns of knowing in nursing. *Advances in Nursing Science, 1*(1), 13–23.
Chinn, P. L., Maeve, M. K., & Bostick, C. (1997). Aesthetic inquiry and the art of nursing. *Scholarly Inquiry for Nursing Practice, 11*(2), 83–100.
Johnson, J. L. (1994). A dialectical examination of nursing art. *Advances in Nursing Science, 17*(1), 1–14.
Peplau, H. (1988). The art and science of nursing: Similarities, differences, and relations. *Nursing Science Quarterly, 1*(1), 8–15.
Watson, J. (1985). *Nursing: Human science and human care.* Norwalk, CT: Appleton Century Crofts.

REFERENCES

Australian Nursing Council Inc. (1998). *ANCI national competency standards for the registered nurse* (2nd ed.). Dickson, Australian Capital Territory: ANCI.
Berriot-Salvadore, E. (1993). The discourse of medicine and science. In N. Z. Davis & A. Farge (Eds.), *A history of women in the West: Vol. 3, Renaissance and Enlightenment paradoxes.* Cambridge, MA: The Belknap Press of Harvard University Press.
Buchanan, T. (1999). Nightingalism: Haunting nursing history. *Collegian, 6*(2), 28–33.
Capra, F. (1982). *The turning point: Science, society and the rising culture.* New York: Simon & Schuster.
Carper, B. (1978). Fundamental patterns of knowing in nursing. *Advances in Nursing Science, 1,* 13–23.
Chinn, P. L., & Watson, J. (Eds.) (1994). *Art and aesthetics in nursing.* New York: National League for Nursing.
Chinn, P. L., Maeve, M. K., & Bostick, C. (1997). Aesthetic inquiry and the art of nursing. *Scholarly Inquiry for Nursing Practice, 11*(2), 83–100.
Cohen, J. S. (1991). Two portraits of caring: A comparison of the artists, Leininger and Watson. *Journal of Advanced Nursing, 16,* 899–909.

Darbyshire, P. (1994a). Understanding the life of illness: Learning through the art of Frida Kahlo. *Advances in Nursing Science, 17*(1), 51–59.

Darbyshire, P. (1994b). Understanding caring through arts and humanit ies: A medical/nursing humanities approach to promoting alternate experiences of thinking and learning. *Journal of Advanced Nursing, 19*(5), 856–863.

Dickens, C. (1910). *Martin Chuzzlewit.* New York: McMillan & Co.

Donahue, P. (1996). *Nursing: The finest art.* St. Louis: C. V. Mosby.

Fawcett, J. (1984). The metaparadigm of nursing: Present status and future refinements. *Image: The Journal of Nursing Scholarship, XVI*(3), 84–89.

Flaskerud, J. H., & Halloran, E. J. (1980). Areas of agreement in nursing theory development. *Advances in Nursing Science, 3*(1), 1–7.

Gortner, S. R. (1983). The history and philosophy of nursing science and research. *Advances in Nursing Science, 5*(2), 1–8.

Holden, R. J. (1991). In defence of Cartesian dualism and the hermeneutic horizon. *Journal of Advanced Nursing, 16*(11), 1375–1381.

Jennings, B. M. (1986). Nursing science: More promise than threat. *Journal of Advanced Nursing, 11*(5), 505–511.

Johnson, D. E. (1980). The behavioural system model for nursing. In J. P. Riehl & C. Roy (Eds.), *Conceptual models for nursing practice* (2nd ed.). New York: Appleton-Century-Crofts.

Johnson, J. L. (1993). *Toward a clearer understanding of the art of nursing.* Unpublished doctoral thesis, University of Alberta.

Johnson, J. L. (1994). A dialectical examination of nursing art. *Advances in Nursing Science, 1*(1), 1–14.

Johnson, J. L. (1996a). The perceptual aspect of nursing art: Sources of accord and discord. *Scholarly Inquiry for Nursing Practice: An International Journal, 10*(4), 307–327.

Johnson, J. L. (1996b). The art of nursing. *Image: Journal of Nursing Scholarship, 28,* 169–175.

Kritek, P. B. (1985). Nursing diagnosis in perspective: Response to a critique. *Image: The Journal of Nursing Scholarship, 17*(1), 3–8.

Lafferty, P. M. (1997). Balancing the curriculum: Promoting aesthetic knowledge in nursing. *Nurse Education Today, 17,* 281–286.

Levine, M. (1971). Holistic nursing. *Nursing Clinics of North America, 6*(2), 253–263.

Munhall, P. L. (1982). Nursing philosophy and nursing research: In apposition or opposition? *Nursing Research, 31*(3), 176–177, 181.

Nelson, S. (1995). Humanism in nursing: The emergence of light. *Nursing Inquiry, 2*(1), 36–43.

Parker, J. M. (1995). Searching for the body in nursing. In G. Gray & R. Pratt (Eds.), *Scholarship in the discipline of nursing*. Melbourne: Churchill Livingstone.

Parker, J. M., & Gibbs, M. (1998). Truth, virtue and beauty: Midwifery and philosophy. *Nursing Inquiry, 5*(3), 146–153.

Parker, J. M., & Rickard, G. (1999). Nursing town and nursing gown: Time space and the reinvention of nursing through collaboration. *Clinical Excellence for Nurse Practitioners, 3*(1), 36–42.

Parker, R. (1990). Nurses stories: The search for a relational ethic of care. *Advances in Nursing Science, 13*(1), 31–40.

Peplau, H. E. (1988). The art and science of nursing: Similarities, differences, and relations. *Nursing Science Quarterly, 1*(1), 8–15.

Rogers, M. E. (1970). *An introduction to the theoretical basis of nursing*. Philadelphia: F. A. Davis.

Roy, C. (1980). The Roy adaptation model. In J. P. Riehl & C. Roy (Eds.), *Conceptual models for nursing practice* (2nd ed.). New York: Appleton Century Crofts.

Smith, F. B. (1982). *Florence Nightingale, reputation and power*. London: Croom Helm.

Snow, C. P. (1964). *The two cultures: And a second look*. New York: The New American Library.

The Times (1854, November 4).

Trembath, R., & Hellier, D. (1987). *All care and responsibility: A history of nursing in Victoria, 1850–1934*. Australia: Florence Nightingale Committee.

4

Exploring Popular Images and Representations of Nurses and Nursing

Philip Darbyshire and Suzanne Gordon

LEARNING OBJECTIVES

After reading this chapter, students will be able to:

- Explain the importance of nursing's image for contemporary nursing
- Describe the prevalent stereotypes of nurses and nursing, and try to explain the persistence of these stereotypes
- Debate the issue of whether nurses really should abandon the "overworked angel" image
- Explain the difficulties involved in proposing a "realistic" portrayal of nurses and nursing
- Propose a strategy or small-scale project that could help promote alternative media representations of nurses and nursing

KEY WORDS

Images, iconography, media, stereotypes, portrayal, mythical, realism

INTRODUCTION

Since the mid-1970s, there has been a burgeoning interest in the study of popular images of nurses and nursing, and it seems that every conceivable aspect of those images has been scrutinized. Writers have focused on images of nurses and nursing on television, in cinema, in novels and short stories, in news coverage, and elsewhere. This fascination with the image of nurses is interesting. With the possible exception of doctors, there is no comparable body of inquiry regarding the image of teachers, social workers, physiotherapists, accountants, occupational therapists or other professional groups. Since most examinations of nursing's image have been produced by nurses and have been largely promoted within nursing itself, this may demonstrate the profession's discomfort with persistently stereotyped images of nurses' work—stereotypes that continue to shape public expectations of nurses and public decisions about the allocation of societal resources to nursing.In this chapter, we will explore some of the early history and iconography of nurses and nursing in order to clarify the origins of many of the issues and images which are so hotly contested and debated today. The question of relevance is important here. Why, when so many other pressing issues preoccupy nurses and the health care systems in which they work, should we worry about nursing's image? To answer this question, Delacour (1991) argues that:

Certainly it is important that we analyse the process through which dysfunctional images and discourses are maintained. Moreover, it is useful to regard reading media as a politically situated and critical activity for the nursing profession. (p. 413)

The unfortunate fact is that public beliefs of the importance of nursing are shaped by the images people see—as patients, family members, members of a community, and consumers of the media—from the journalistic to the entertainment. If nurses are silent—or visible only in particular ways—in public debates about the status and future of health care systems, the running of their institutions, and the journalistic depiction of health care work, they risk being marginalized and neglected when it comes to decisions about everything from the allocation of resources to how health care is portrayed in the morning newspaper. This will have an impact on nurses' salaries, working conditions, relationships with other members of the health care team and—most important—on their ability to protect their patients and deliver high-quality nursing care.

Developing a critical and questioning view of our historical and contemporary representations of nurses' work is thus important for every nurse's personal and professional development. Indeed, if nurses are to advocate for their patients effectively, it is a critical part of their ethical mandate. Nurses, however, should strive to move beyond the kind of "knee-jerk" or simplistic response that lauds good images of the profession while excoriating any bad coverage. They need to develop the capacity to analyze and criticize a broad range of issues and to understand both the production, meaning(s) and possible effects of popular images of the nurse and nursing.

NURSING'S EARLY ICONOGRAPHY

Representations and images of nursing are as old as nursing and healing themselves. By tracing the origins of modern nursing back to antiquity and to the earliest accounts of babies, pregnant women, family, and other members of early communities being cared for, usually by women, we can see that, "The nurse as saintly domestic is no modern invention" (Kampen, 1988, p. 36). The earliest Greco-Roman depictions were almost entirely of "baby nurses" and the image of the "modern" nurse as tender of the sick or wounded was not to appear until the fourteenth century (Kampen, 1988, p. 16).

With the emergence of religious orders and associated charitable services came a new iconography of nursing which showed women extending their care practices from the immediate household and family arena to the care of strangers. This was not always welcomed, however, and the Middle Ages in Europe especially saw the slaughter of many "wise women" who were burnt as witches (Darbyshire, 1985). Commenting on fifteenth century depictions of nurses working with the sick, Kampen (1988) makes the significant observation that:

> Several features common to scenes of nursing sisters help to define the nature of their role: they nurse patients who are most often men lying in bed; they work in a distinctive location that does not look like a house; they wear distinctive costumes; their activities are domestic and religious rather than specifically medical; and most important, they are never subordinated to patients and doctors. (p. 23)

It is salutary to think that, with the exception of the last phrase, this description would have fit any typical Victorian infirmary almost 500 years later. This depiction of nurses as tenders of the prostrate sick has been a powerful one. It was reinforced by the iconographic imagery of

Florence Nightingale wending her way through the wards of Scutari Hospital during the Crimean War. Indeed, to many members of the public, nursing is erroneously viewed as taking place in only one particular setting and centering around one particular activity. That setting is of course the hospital, and that activity is taking care of acutely ill patients. McCoppin and Gardner (1994, p. 156) noted how this one-dimensional view of nursing and nurses can occlude the view of all other forms and areas of nursing, which can somehow be deemed to be"less than or other than real nursing," which of course was deemed to be practiced exclusively at the bedsides of sick people.

The stereotypical view of nurses as working only in acute-care, high-technology areas often portrayed in the media makes it very difficult to provide the alternative view of nurses working within the community, which is more difficult to make "attention grabbing."

It is not only the various forms of community nursing which may be seen as less than "real nursing"' but also the myriad of other forms of nursings, such as working in mental health, health promotion, school nursing, working with people with learning or intellectual disabilities, and many others.

In fact, stereotypical views of nursing have a negative impact even on nurses who practice in acute care hospitals. Too few members of the public understand that the nurse is there to save patients' lives and to be what Linda Aiken and her colleagues at the University of Pennsylvania School of Nursing refer to as the "early detection and prompt intervention" system in the hospital (Aiken, Clark, Sloane, Sochalski, & Silber, 2002, p. 1992) Most members of the public view nurses as sweet, kind, honest, ethical, attentive and willing to talk, but not particularly critical to the effort to rescue them from medical errors and injuries and to make sure their treatments do not kill them. As one 65-year-old female California patient recently said (Gordon interview), "Oh, when I was in the hospital, the nurses were so nice and cheerful." Or as another 50-year-old woman commented, "When my mother was in the hospital for brain surgery, the nurses were always there; they always explained things to us." She contrasted this with the behavior of doctors who would whip in and out of the room and explain little or nothing. When Gordon pointed out that the nurse also made sure her mother did not die from the surgery and elaborated the medical and technical skill and knowledge she possessed, the woman was stunned. "I didn't know nurses did all that," she said.

This masking of what, even in 1985, was more than half of the nursing workforce (Dunn, 1985), is significant because it can help narrow and restrict students' and other nurses' perceptions of what nursing funda-mentally is. For example, in Kiger's study of student nurses in Scotland, she found that, "The picture of adult medical-surgical nursing as typical of real nursing persisted throughout (the students' concept of) 'working with people'" (Kiger, 1993). Similarly, the failure to understand the complexity of basic nursing work also pushes students away from bedside nursing and into fields like advanced practice nursing and nurse prac-titioner work. In the U.S., many students in four-year nursing schools say that they only want to work in hospitals for one or two years because they think bedside nursing is unchallenging and do not want to be perceived as "just a nurse" (i.e., just a physician's handmaiden or bed-pan emptier).

Why nursing should be such a fertile ground for image construction and manipulation is a hugely complex issue and one that has been discussed and argued over many years. One way of beginning to under-stand the heady brew of images, social constructions, myths, contradic-tions, and realities which form the image(s) of nurses and nursing is to look more carefully at the persistence and power of the major stereo-types of nurses which still exist in either blatant or more subtle forms even today.

NURSING STEREOTYPES

Stereotypes of a profession are not necessarily deleterious to the profes-sion in question. Physicians, for example, are considered to be the major players on the health care stage and are viewed as totally responsible for all the good things that happen to the patient, when in fact, it may be the nurse, nurses' aide, or another clinician who was also responsible for an excellent outcome. If the sole problem with nursing stereotypes was just that some get-well cards, tabloid newspaper stories, or X-rated films portrayed nurses as oversexualized bimbos, then perhaps we could laugh it off, but when the effects of stereotyping are more serious, then there is more at stake than nursing's collective need to lighten up.

The problem for nursing is that its major stereotypes are so unrelent-ingly negative in their connotations and so wholly untenable in their relationship to the reality of nursing. (The notion of a single nursing reality is itself contentious and we shall return to this later.)

As Delacour (1991) observes:

> even stereotypes regarded as dubious may, after a measure of expo-sure, become internalized and naturalized; they are thereby metamor-

phosed into categories of the normal, the real, and the healthy and desirable. (p. 413)

The images and perceptions of nursing, both within the profession, and in society in general, are important for several reasons. We live in an era where image and the marketing of image has never been more important. While nurses can certainly maintain that the core business of nursing is caring for the sick and assuring the health and well being of people, nurses would be foolish to ignore the importance of nursing's image.

If the public does not understand the breadth and complexity of nursing work, it cannot fight for the social and financial resources that allow nurses to do that work. If nurses do not, as Buresh and Gordon (2000) have argued, obtain the "Three Rs for RNs," that is, respect, recognition, and rewards, they will burn out and the shortage we have today will persist indefinitely. If we are to attract creative, committed, intelligent, and passionate people into nursing, then nursing needs to be seen as every bit as worthwhile, challenging, and dynamic a career as any other in the fields of health care or social service. The persistence of old, hackneyed stereotypes does nothing to enhance the attractiveness of nursing as an occupational option and hampers nurses' ability to make nursing a long-term satisfying career.

Muff (1982, p. 211) has suggested six major nursing stereotypes: angel of mercy, handmaiden to the physician, oman in white, sex symbol/idiot, battleaxe, and torturer, while Dunn (1985, p. 2) credits the average tabloid newspaper with even less imagination, being interested in only three types of nurse: angel, battleaxe, and nymphomaniac. We also have, of course, the additional image of the empty-headed nurse who is kind but dumb. This reinforces the idea that if you are a woman with a brain and want to use it in health care then your only legitimate avenue is medicine.

ANGELS WITH PRETTY FACES AND EMPTY HEADS

If nursing iconography has an enduring stereotypic image, it must surely be the nurse as angel. While much of the earliest artwork and imagery of nurses showed nurses ministering to the sick in various quasi-religious ways and settings, nurses in Australia, even in the late 1800s, were "redefining the image of nurses as motivated primarily by self-sacrifice"

(Bashford, 1997). However, it was Florence Nightingale's story that captured the public imagination and stimulated a swathe of hagio- graphic accounts, which critic Leslie Fiedler (1988, p. 103) called "shameless schlock." The "saccharinizing" of Nightingale's image began almost as soon as she moved into public view. Nightingale was, to say the least, a difficult woman who drove her colleagues and used whatever means she felt necessary to pursue her goals. Yet, the public and media quickly sugarcoated her image. She became—and has remained—the "angel of the Crimea," and the "lady with the lamp." Not just a coura- geous heroine, she became a secular saint (a reputation that was cer- tainly reinforced by her more than fifty-year retreat from the world, although not from public life). For example, in 1857 the American poet Henry Wadsworth Longfellow wrote an ode to Nightingale entitled Santa Filomena that morphed Nightingale into the image so persistent to this day:

The wounded from the battle-plain,
In dreary hospitals of pain,
The cheerless corridors,
The cold and stony floors.
Lo! In that house of misery
A lady with a lamp I see
Pass through the glimmering gloom,
And flit from room to room.
And slow, as in a dream of bliss,
The speechless sufferer turns to kiss
Her shadow, as it falls,
Upon the darkening walls.
(Donahue & Donahue, 1996, pp. 203–204)

Twentieth century movies such as *The White Angel* and *The Lady with the Lamp* (Jones, 1988; Kalisch & Kalisch, 1983b) did not update Nightin- gale's image but simply repackaged it. So powerful were these images of the angelic presence which lit up the wards of Scutari with her lamp, that Florence Nightingale has become easily identified as the soul or spirit of nursing and as the embodiment of selfless, devoted, compassion- ate care which borders on the saintly. In some cases, Nightingale's very name has come to symbolize the precise opposite of what she actually was, and is used to suggest that a person is a naïve, do-gooder. Thus people may say to you, if they believe you are misguidedly altruistic, "Oh don't be such a Florence Nightingale."

Despite some of the more recent, critical, and balanced scholarship concerning the life and work of Florence Nightingale (e.g., Hektor, 1994), the stereotype of the nurse as selfless angel is still prevalent, especially in the public imagination. At first glance, some nurses may believe that the angel image actually gives them credit, credence, and legitimacy. "What's so bad about people thinking we're angels?" a fourth-year nursing student in a prestigious Northeastern nursing school recently asked. Perhaps she had seen too many episodes of the American television show *Touched by an Angel.* If angels accomplish miracles, who would not like to be thought of in such a positive light? Which nurse would not like to think that she was capable of such profound caring that could earn such adoration? Is this not just being held in high regard by society? Don't we feel good when opinion polls put nurses near the top of the list for perceived honesty, trustworthiness, and hard work?

But consider for a moment what an angel really is. In Catholic theology, for example, angels are said to be "pure, bodiless spirits" created by God to uncritically help Him execute his divine plan" (www.catholic.org/saints/angel.shtml). Like saints, they uncritically accept religious dogma and do what they are told. Jane Salvage (1983) perceptively pointed out that nurses often collude in sustaining the selfless angel stereotype while professing to scorn it. As she noted, "The trouble is we are secretly flattered by the myths, especially those emphasizing dedication and high-minded self-sacrifice" (p. 14).

However, buying into the "angel" stereotype may be a Faustian bargain, for there is a price to pay. Angels may be saintly, but such perfection is impossible for mere mortal nurses to achieve or maintain; nurses are, after all, only human. Because they were created by God, angels do not require any education or experience. Their sanctity is a divine gift and entails self-sacrifice and devotion. Angels do not, therefore, get paid for their work. Virtue is, after all, its own reward, and for the angel nurse, there can be no such person as the patient from Hell.

Real people may be born with particular dispositions and talents (although some would dispute even this), but they cannot be born nurses. Real nurses are educated, not born, and the path to becoming skilled and competent is a long and hard one that requires not divine, but human, intervention. Real nurses are educated in school, through on the job experience, and by continuing education throughout their career. Whatever shafts of grace real nurses achieve are often hard won through their sustained engagement in the lives of those people who place their trust in them.

DOCTORS' HANDMAIDENS

If the "angel" myth is a remnant of nursing's religious order origins, then the unquestioning obedience of the doctor's handmaiden owes much to nursing's military origins and to its origins in Christian religion (Nelson, 2001). This stereotype is grounded in the image of the nurse as a kind of lady in waiting or doctor's right-hand woman. This image was born in the nineteenth century, when medicine insisted that nursing have no other purpose than to serve the physician, not the patient. As one English physician put it in the late 1800s:

> In fact, there is no proper duty which the nurse has to perform, even to the placing of a pillow, which does not or may not involve a principle, and a principle which can only properly be met by one who has had the advantage of medical instruction. It is a fundamental and dangerous error to maintain that any system of nursing has sources of knowledge not derived from the profession. (Gull, cited in Peterson, 1978, p. 183)

The view of the nurse as someone with no knowledge and judgment of her own has shaped the media view of nursing. In this handmaiden role, the nurse is essentially an empty head who borrows the doctor's knowledge, skill, and judgment, and acts as his agent, or "eyes and ears" (a medicalized version of the angel nurse who is God's agent).

We see this image in many television shows and other media depictions of nursing. In the recent TV prime-time show *Chicago Hope*, the main nursing character did little but service the doctor inside and outside of the examining room. The ex-wife of one of the physician characters, she made her rounds with patients reluctantly because she was so busy charting her ex-husband's love life. In countless media reports of health care, doctors are presented as the main players on the stage, while nurses appear in the background mainly to provide color and set the scene. In some movies, nurses are utterly ditzy. Neil La Bute's 2000 movie *Nurse Betty* is a case in point. The main character, played by Renee Zellweger, is a frustrated housewife who once wanted to be a nurse. Traumatized by seeing her husband's murder, she believes that she has become the nurse heroine in a TV soap opera. Madly in love with the physician character in the show, she goes to find him in Los Angeles and actually gets a job as a nursing assistant in a hospital. Why? Because, after seeing so many episodes of the show, she was able to perform a life saving procedure on a patient in an ambulance. The message? Nursing is so simple, you can learn to do it by watching the afternoon soaps.

The flip side of this empty-headed image is the idea that the nurse with brains and ambition can prove herself only by becoming a doctor. In the 1998 movie *Living Out Loud*, Holly Hunter plays a nurse who has been deserted by her cad husband, a doctor. After falling to pieces alone in her apartment, seeking the services of a male prostitute (if guys can do it, why shouldn't women?), she finally pulls herself together and goes back to school—not to get an advanced degree in nursing, but to become a pediatrician.

Like the "angel" myth, this view has often been sustained by nurses themselves. One sometimes hears nurses today who refer to themselves as the doctor's eyes and ears. We hear far fewer nurses who believe that they are the doctor's brains as well (Gordon, 1999). Some seem to be flattered by the idea that their doctor or their specialist says that he/she could not manage without them. Conveying the image of hand-maiden to patients, they will introduce themselves as "doctor so and so's nurse."

In her analysis of nurses' image in post-war Britain, Hallam (1998, p. 37) noted also that "Within the broadcasting environment, nursing's professional discourse of 'service' was interpreted as service to medicine; nurses themselves did little to challenge the picture." In this sense, the handmaiden stereotype may be less mythical than nursing would like to acknowledge. While nationally and internationally particular nurses and nursing projects/initiatives have led health care advances (often in collaboration with medical colleagues), there are still many nurses who work with doctors who seem not to recognize nurses' ability and responsibility to make an equal contribution to care. They have accepted the medical view that the nurse's role is to make coffee, or change the bedpan, not make decisions. Despite claims of teamwork and multidisci-plinary cooperation, some nurses do not protest the definition of a team in which a lot of people are doing what one person says—that one person being the doctor.

THE BATTLEAXE OR MONSTROUS FIGURE

For images to be powerful and long lasting, they must be capable of being both sustained and subverted. The battleaxe figure is in many ways a magnificent subversion of other stereotypes of the nurse, what Hunter (1988) calls in a slightly different context the "translocated ideal." Whereas the angel is often portrayed as pretty, feminine, Caucasian, slim, caring, white-clad for purity, fun, deferential, and loved by patients, the battleaxe or matron figure was almost the exact opposite—tyrannical, fearsome, asexual, cruel, monstrously large, dark-clad, and set on crushing all fun and individuality. On a BBC radio program that Darbyshire compiled several years ago, he listened to a recording of a 1960s radio quiz show where one of the male panelists joked that the tragedy of nurses is that they were one day destined to become matrons or managers. Nurse managers, like other nurses who refuse to fit the accepted stereotype of the pretty, kind, compliant nurse, are banished to the moral margins of societal acceptance where they become objects of fear or ridicule. Think here of "bad" nurses like Charles Dickens' Sairey Gamp (Summers, 1997), Ken Kesey's "Big Nurse/Nurse Ratched" from *One Flew Over the Cuckoo's Nest* (Darbyshire, 1995), Annie Wilkes from Stephen King's *Misery*, and the more comic figures of Hattie Jacques from the *Carry On* film series, or Matron Dorothy from Australia's 1990 television series, *Let the Blood Run Free* (Delacour, 1991).

The battleaxe stereotype cries out for a feminist analysis which would reveal the fate of any nurse who does not comply with the mythical norms of the ideal nurse and who challenges male power (usually patients and doctors). Worse than this, perhaps, is that the battleaxe figure is a powerful woman who is not attracted to men or medicine (Darbyshire, 1995). This proves that she cannot be a real nurse, as one of the most prevalent and damaging stereotypes is the nurse as an easily available sex bomb.

Like the angel nurse and physician handmaiden, this image is also perpetuated by nursing. In their book *Silence to Voice*, Gordon and Buresh argue that American nurses should introduce themselves as "Nurse Smith" rather than with "Hi, I'm Joanie." Although nurses often reject the suggestion that they use the term "nurse" coupled with their last name as a form of introduction because it is too formal, hundreds insist that to do so would remind patients of "Nurse Ratched." When Gordon interviewed dozens of patients to ask them how they would respond to a nurse who attached the word nurse to her or his surname, not a single one thought of the monster nurse. Most liked the idea—"Thank God, we know who we're dealing with; most of the time we can't figure out who's the nurse." one former patient recapitulated the majority opinion. Few people under fifty—or not in the upper middle class—had ever heard of Nurse Ratched. Very few students in nursing school had heard of her, until that is, their nursing professors told them. Like the angel, it seems that some nurses are determined to keep Nurse Ratched alive and to wield her image as a shield to justify what could be positive changes in their own personal self-presentation.

NAUGHTY NURSES AND NYMPHOMANIACS

When Darbyshire was a lecturer in Scotland, he would discuss the question of nurses' image with the first-year students who had just begun their course. He asked them what a common reaction would be at a party if they happened to mention that they were nurses. After the laughter and ribaldry had settled, it was clear that a common, if not thankfully universal, reaction from some men was a "knowing grin" and some suggestion that a night of unbridled sexual abandon might lie ahead. For this reason, many of the students said that they would make up an occupation rather than "admit" to being a nurse.

Why is the naughty nurse stereotype so prevalent? Why are there no naughty lawyer sexual stereotypes? Why are there no pornographic films made about the adventures of a group of occupational therapy students? Why do sex shops not sell physiotherapist uniforms? What is it about nurses that makes them such a target? This is a deep and complex issue but consider the following points in relation to Hunter's (1988) notion of a "translocated ideal." Nursing is utterly implicated in social power relations, between nurses and doctors, nurses and other nurses, nurses and patients, nurses and relatives, and more. When patients enter a hospital, the traditional power relations are reversed and they find themselves vulnerable and dependent rather than strong and in control. At a societal level (for not every male patient will see his situation in this way), one way of redressing this balance is to metaphorically (or perhaps even practically) sexualize the encounters between nurses and patients. This gives men power over women who have power over them. The man in question may not be able to walk, or pee, or feed himself. He may be frightened, anxious and vulnerable. But he can pat butt or dream about it and turn the nurse who has power over him into someone he can dominate, if not in reality, then in his fantasy.

We also know that nurses' practices in relation to patients' bodies is part of this process. Nurses are exceptionally privileged in that we are intimate body workers. Nurses have access to people's most private body areas and bodily functions (Lawler, 1991). One of the most important practices that a nurse develops is the ability to work with patients' intimate body parts without sexualizing the encounter. (Gordon, 1996) If the nurse transgresses this boundary, it would be both embarrassing and dangerous. In an almost-too-painful-to-watch scene in Dennis Potter's television play, *The Singing Detective*, a nurse has to anoint with cream the genital areas of hero Philip Marlowe, as he has extremely debilitating psoriasis and cannot do this for himself. As the nurse applies his cream, he becomes sexually aroused and, despite trying desperately to divert his thoughts, he develops an erection. The nurse, however, wants to get the procedure done and continues creaming, causing him to ejaculate and suffer an agony of humiliation.

If the patient does it in his fantasies, it may make him feel less vulnerable. In the 1989 movie *War of the Roses*, Michael Douglas and Kathleen Turner play a couple going through a vicious divorce. Danny DeVito plays Douglas' friend. In one of the movie's more memorable scenes—from the point of view of nursing that is—Douglas sits alone in a darkened hospital room with a suspected heart attack that turns out to be esophagitis. A nurse comes in to speak with him. As she walks out the door, De Vito walks in. He takes a seat and, after asking Douglas how he is, says crudely, "Think we can get that nurse to come back here with a bottle of musk oil?" It is a perfect example of this kind of power dynamic.

Fagin and Diers (1983) are clear on the damaging implications of conflating equalization and intimate body work, "Thanks to the worst of this kind of thinking, nursing is a metaphor for sex. Having seen and touched the bodies of strangers, nurses are perceived as willing and able sexual partners" (p. 117). The naughty nurse stereotype also encourages the subversion of another ideal, that of the saintly purity of the nurse as angel. Beneath the pristine white uniform, tightly bunched and restrained hair, and sheepish obedience to authority lies the pornographer's win-win scenario. Either the nurse is really a sex-bomb being barely held in check by the rules and regulations of the institution and awaiting the slightest excuse to release all of this pent-up passion, or she really is completely subservient to (male) authority, in which case she will willingly agree to every sexual demand.

If you think that these scenarios are farfetched, consider a feature that ran several years ago in the U.K. tabloid newspaper, *The Sun*, which aroused furious opposition, and not only from nurses and their organizations. The feature had the headline, "Calling All You Naughty Nurses" and read:

Yes, we know you're out there. Lots and lots of people tell stories about those saucy times when temperatures soared in the wards. Who hasn't heard about the time the young nurse turned a bed bath into a saucy romp? And delighted male patients are always revealing how they got some very special medicine from the attractive sister when the screens were drawn. So come on folks. Let's hear from the naughty night nurses—and their happy patients—about the fun times in Britain's hospitals. We're opening our own special phone line between 10 am and 6 pm today. Ring the number below and tell us your stories.

Such was the wave of protest from nursing organizations and others that the feature was withdrawn within days.

In the United States, a TV prime-time show, *Nightingales,* provoked similar outrage. The show—about student nurses—aired its pilot episode in June of 1988. It ran from January 1989 till April of 1989, when it was cancelled. Portraying nurses as sexpots who spent more time in exercise class or dating than cracking books or in school, it received similar protests from nurses and nursing organizations who tried first to work with the producers to change the focus and when that did not succeed, managed to get the show cancelled.

NURSING'S IMAGE: BLAME THE MEDIA?

Many nurses blame the media for everything that is wrong with nursing's image. The media is an easy target of scorn. In fact, the issue of nursing's image is very complex. According to a 1997 study cosponsored by the National Health Council and PBS's Health Week, most Americans get most of their information about health care from the media. "More people turn to television (40 percent) as their primary source of health care information than they do to physicians (36 percent)" (Starch, 1997, cited in Buresh & Gordon, 2000).

A study conducted last year by the Kaiser Family Foundation found that regular *ER* viewers learn about health-related subjects from the show and some consult their doctors because of what they have seen. An earlier study found that children's strongest impressions of various medical professions were primarily derived from *ER* and other television dramas (Boodman, 2003, p. HE01).

Delacour (1991) makes the important point that often it is not only the ways in which nursing is portrayed but, more than that, it is that nursing is "symbolically annihilated by the mass media" (p. 418) and virtually ignored. To test this claim, it would be interesting to keep a local and a national newspaper for a month or two with a view to checking how many health stories included authoritative comments from nurses as compared with doctors. Many nurses would say that they could confidently predict the results of such a survey well in advance. When Buresh, Gordon, and Bell conducted such a survey in 1990, they found that nurses were used less as sources of health care news than any other group in the industry. Considerable research has been undertaken into the role of the media in constructing and shaping nursing's image. In the U.S. in particular, Philip and Beatrice Kalisch in the 1980s produced numerous books and papers on many different aspects of this question (Kalisch, Kalisch, & McHugh, 1982; Kalisch & Kalisch, 1983a, 1983b, 1984, 1987; Kalisch, Kalisch, & Scoby, 1983). Criticism of the media in general continues to this day. Holmes (1997), for example, advises that we should (perhaps) give up watching medical soap operas on television as they are "anodyne and legitimating rather than transformative and critical" (p. 137). While soaps may well be anodyne, there are probably few viewers of *ER* or other shows of this genre, who complain that the show is no longer as "transformative and critical" as it used to be. Blaming genres for not being what we would wish them to be is surely tilting at windmills. To simply stop watching soaps because we disagree with aspects of their portrayal of nurses and nursing is scarcely a mode of engagement. Nor is it particularly astute to imagine that the media exist to accurately (or should we say positively/flatteringly?) depict nurses and their work. Much as we may dislike the notion, the mass media exists primarily as a profit-making business. It is not nursing's public relations machine.

The authors disagree on an interesting point here regarding genre and representation. Philip suggests that criticisms of the portrayals of nurses often seem to misunderstand the different genres of representation, especially comedy. Philip argues that criticizing a film like *Carry On Nurse* for giving a false image of nurses and nursing makes little sense as these are not documentaries and their purpose was never to represent the reality of nursing. They are comedies, and they work by upsetting—and yes, even ridiculing—our understandings and expectations of nursing. Condemning a film like *Carry On Nurse* for not being a true-to-life account of nursing is like criticizing Thursday for not being the Rocky Mountains. Suzanne takes a different view and argues that nurses should criticize these shows regardless of their genre or intention. She advocates that nurses should criticize blatantly incorrect portrayals of nursing wherever they appear, but only if they are willing to work with the media to achieve a more accurate picture of their work.

Working with the media in order to help create more realistic portrayals of nursing's work can help create a more balanced view of health care (Buresh & Gordon, 1995). In the early days of the filming of the medical soap *ER*, there was virtually no consultation with nurses or ER departments. U.S. emergency room nurses, however, did more than complain or stop watching—they became active and contacted the producers regularly with comments and criticisms, but also with offers of help, story line ideas, and the names of subspecialty ER nurses who were willing to help the show "get it right." Unfortunately, *ER*'s producers and writers keep slipping back into negative nursing images. In the fall of 2003, the show painted nursing in a negative light. Doctors were routinely doing nursing work and the show's main nursing character abandoned nursing to go to medical school. Nurses, however, did not just stand by and watch this happen without comment. The two-year-old Center for Nursing Advocacy, started by nurse Sandy Summers, launched a protest campaign that attracted the attention of the Washington Post. If nurses remain vigilant, *ER* may have to change or go the way of *Nightingales*.

NURSING'S IMAGE: DEPICTING REALITY?

Joanne Rule, former head of the RCN (UK) Public Relations office, once commented that "if nursing were to succeed finally in shaking off the 'angel' image it so professes to hate, it might be replaced by an image that it hated even more" (Rule, 1995). In challenging potentially damaging images of nursing, what seems to be the most difficult thing for nurses is to agree upon an account of what a "good portrayal" of the profession would be. As Bashford (1997) noted in her study of how early Australian nurses challenged their systems:

> resistance was never straightforward. Often, rather than new discourses offering empowering new subject positions, they produced confusion, contradiction and insecurity. Women were asked to think about their work in religious terms in one moment and in one context, in scientific terms in another, and as a type of professionalism in another. (p. 74)

This historical dilemma will seem blindingly contemporary to today's nurses who are struggling with very similar issues. Everyone wants a new image. But who is the new nurse one should promote? Is she a staff nurse who, studies now confirm, is critical in preventing complications, tragedies, medical errors and injuries? Is she the advanced practice nurse, or the nurse practitioner? Is she a researcher or so-called nurse leader. Is she a he?

Similarly, in looking for a realistic image of nurses, many nurses seem to believe that only the most positive images are acceptable. But acceptable to whom? To me personally? To nurses at my hospital? To nursing in general? Medicine certainly does not ask for bad publicity. But doctors understand that media coverage of medicine's problems is a sign that the public takes medicine so seriously that even its flaws must be examined. Gordon and Buresh argue that "bad coverage implies that what doctors do matters. They are indispensable. They are so important that their mistakes, as well as their successes, are a public issue deserving the most serious scrutiny (Buresh & Gordon, 2000). Doctors all can rest assured that coverage of these flaws will be balanced by coverage of medical innovations and accomplishments. Thus they do not run for cover from journalists because newspapers and TV misquote them, get it wrong, or sensationalize medical missteps.

Nursing and nurses tend to be extremely thin skinned about the slightest hint of critical coverage. Nurses tend not to respond expeditiously to journalists' inquiries and often flee even positive depictions of their work. If a nurse is misquoted, quoted out of context, or a story is not positive, nurses tend to want to avoid the media altogether. This puts nurses in the paradoxical position of seeking a better media image while failing to take advantages of the opportunities that might rectify public misinformation about the profession.

Hallam (1998) questioned this quest for a 'positive' portrayal of nursing by arguing that

> This search for a positive image of nursing identity poses two crucial problems. On the one hand, it tends to presume a professional consensus in terms of what this image is or could be . . . the positive image approach can also be critiqued from the viewpoint of media reception; it conceptualizes readers and viewers as uncritical receivers of messages who unquestioningly digest the authority of the image. (p. 33)

Similarly, Cheek (1995) has observed that "the task is not to look for real and authentic representations of nursing, but rather to look for the speaking and representation that is done about nursing" (p. 239).

Perhaps nurses would be more emboldened if they focused on some of the truly positive images and accounts of nurses and nursing that can be found. For example, in his account of his serious injury and recovery, surgeon and rehabilitation specialist Tony Moore (1991) describes the artistic and technical expertise of the intensive care nurses who gave him a blanket bath:

> They worked like a ballet corps in slow motion, softly moving me forwards, to the side, sponging, touching, toweling with clean tenderness, and when one gently washed my genitals I felt nothing but the compassion of her care. (p. 11)

Richard Selzer (1993) was another surgeon who found himself a patient in intensive care following Legionnaire's Disease. He is hugely embarrassed by his dependency and incontinence, but again, his nurses were memorably skilled in what he calls "the forgiveness of the flesh" (p. 56). Unlike the unfortunate Philip Marlowe in *The Singing Detective*, nurses spare Selzer the embarrassment and pain that could so easily become part of his intimate body care. One nurse who makes such a profound difference to Selzer's care and recovery is Patrick, whom Selzer describes as being "the sort of nurse who can draw the pus out of a carbuncle with his gaze alone, and turn it into a jewel" (p. 56). Selzer is quite emphatic that the power of skilled nursing care is not merely "nice to get" but that it is actually transformative. He describes his being carried back to bed by Patrick following a tub bath as the moment when his "molecules rearranged themselves." "It is the true moment of cure," he says (p. 93).

Read these authors' accounts of their care and then consider that some patients deem bathing patients to be "basic" nursing care. By this they do not mean trivial activities that anyone could perform, but important actions that require skill and experience. There are many other positive accounts in literature and popular culture of nurses and nursing in which nurses are valued, appreciated, and have a markedly beneficial effect on the recipient. However, we should be careful not to fall into the trap of collecting these accounts as a kind of trophy for nursing. If we are to cultivate and develop our questioning and critical powers, then the positive accounts also need to be questioned and discussed.

CONCLUSION: FROM AFFRONT TO ACTION

During the past two decades, there has been a plethora of research and discussion regarding nursing's image and the portrayals of nursing.

We are now much more aware of the forces that shape and maintain many of popular culture's images of nurses and nursing. Perhaps the next two decades will see nurses moving from a position of greater awareness to one of more positive action. By this we mean that nurses will move beyond their outrage at the negative stereotypes that they encounter, that they will talk more with the media and the political community—as well as friends, neighbors, and family members—and that they will encourage their hospitals to promote their work.

Indignation and refusing to watch are not strategies for change. Nor will it be enough to merely call for negative images of nurses to be withdrawn or banned. The most difficult task ahead is for nurses and nursing to use the media in a much more streetwise way than they have in the past. If nurses do not like the images that are being presented, then they have a responsibility to make their criticisms clear and provide alternative accounts of their own work that move beyond the stereotypes we have analyzed. If nurses think that media reports and stories about nursing are inaccurate or inadequate, then they need to interest the media in alternatives. If they feel that the media completely ignore a particularly important program, service, or aspect of nursing, then why not alert them to this and highlight the importance of what it is that they are missing? None of the media like to feel that they are missing something interesting or important, especially in their local area. Nurses, like women and minorities, also have to be willing to persist in the face of rejection. Today, too many nurses retreat when the media give them the cold shoulder. This is an ineffective way to change their image and gain the legitimacy they desire.

Delacour (1991) lists excellent questions that we should ask about the images and representations of nurses and nursing:

> Who has speaking rights? Who says what? Which position? On behalf of whom? Who is silenced? What are the assumptions? What is privileged in the text? What is ignored, glossed over or marginalised? What is the target audience and how is the reading/viewing position constructed to promote a 'preferred' reading? Which genre and its codes and effects? What type of publication/program and resultant status of discourse? How are power and knowledge articulated? How are gender, sexuality, roles and relationship, race, class, deviance and normality constructed? Which rhetorical devices? Which linguistic features? (p. 419)

These are questions which do not naively assume that there is a right or wrong image, but that begin the task of unpacking and exploring this complex yet highly revealing area wherein nurses can learn so much about both themselves, their society and those whom they care for. To these questions we should add some others that will help nurses be more active in redressing the profession's image. Questions such as: What images would nurses want to see in the media? How can nurses show the positive power of nursing to local and national media? Why would/should the media be interested in this program/innovation/ nursing development? How can nurses present this idea or story to them in such a way that they cannot ignore it? Whose expertise and support could nurses call upon to help them do this? (Clarke, 1989; Monahan, 1996; Strasen, 1992).

We now know a great deal about representations of nurses and nursing in the various media and popular culture. As nurses, our task now is not simply to adapt to, or merely observe and comment on, future changes, but to get out there and make the changes happen.

REFLECTIVE QUESTIONS

1. Discuss with a group of your peers the reactions that you have encountered, both favorable and unfavorable, when you have told people that you are a nurse/student nurse and how you feel about such reactions.
2. Use Delacour's list of questions to assess and question some selected images of nurses/nursing, e.g., a film, documentary, novel, soap opera, etc.
3. Plan how you would go about creating your own media story about nurses or nursing? What would you choose as the issue? Would it be a nurse-led clinical initiative, an ethical dilemma, a particularly successful patient outcome, an exciting new approach in nursing education, or a particular nurse who is doing something really special in a particular area? How would you go about get the media interested in the story and how would you present it?

RECOMMENDED READINGS

Abrams, P. (2001). Perspectives in leadership: Improving nursing's professional image. *Nursing Spectrum, 11*(2), 9.

Belcher, D. (2003). Nurses making a difference. Bridging the gap between nurses and the media: The grassroots Center for Nursing Advocacy. *American Journal of Nursing, 103*(5), 130.

Boivin, J. (2001). Real nurses bring media campaign to life . . . television commercial to promote the nursing profession. *Nursing Spectrum, 14*(10), 16–17.

Davis, C., & Schafer, J. (Eds.) (2003). *Intensive care: More poetry and prose by nurses.* Iowa City: University of Iowa Press.

Davis, C., & Schaefer, J. (1995). *Between the heartbeats: Poetry and prose by nurses.* Iowa City: University of Iowa Press.

Jecker, N. S. S., & Donnie, J. (1991). Separating care and cure: An analysis of historical and contemporary images of nursing and medicine. *The Journal of Medicine and Philosophy, 16*(3), 285–306.

Lenzer, J. (2003). *ER* blamed for nursing shortage. *British Medical Journal, 327*(7426), 1294.

Mason, D. J. (2002). Invisible nurses: Media neglect is one cause of the nursing shortage. *American Journal of Nursing, 102*(8), 7.

Meier, E. (1999). The image of a nurse—Myth vs. reality. *Nursing Economics, 17*(5), 273–276.

Peterson, M. J. (1978). *The medical profession in mid-Victorian London.* Berkeley: University of California Press.

Pinkerton, S. (2002). K–12: Encourage children to consider careers in nursing. *Nursing Economics, 20*(4), 198–200.

Sadaniantz, B. T. (2002). Mirror, mirror . . . nurse leaders reflect on nursing's image. *Nursing Spectrum, 6*(6), 6–7.

Scannell-Desch, E. (1999). Images & relationships forged in war: A study of women nurses who served in Vietnam. *Journal of Psychosocial Nursing & Mental Health Services, 37*(8), 32–42.

Schmidt, K. (2001). A sharper image: Nurses strive to garner more—and more accurate—media coverage. *NurseWeek, 6*(25), 19–21.

Takase, M., Kershaw, E., & Burt, L. (2002). Does public image of nurses matter? *Journal of Professional Nursing, 18*(4), 196–205.

REFERENCES

Aiken, L. H., Clarke S. P., Sloane, D. M., Sochalski, J., & Silber J. H. (2002). Hospital nurse staffing and patient mortality, nurse burnout, and job dissatisfaction. *Journal of the American Medical Association, 288*(16), 1987–1993.

Bashford, A. (1997). Starch on the collar and sweat on the brow: Self-sacrifice and the status of work for nurses. *Journal of Australian Studies, 67,* 74.

Begany, T. (1994). Your image is brighter than ever. *RN, 57,* 28.

Boodman, S. G. (2003, November 18). Nursing a lousy image. RNs blame crisis on TV's *ER. The Washington Post,* p. HE01.

Buresh, B., & Gordon, S. (1995). Taking on the TV shows. *American Journal of Nursing, 95*(11), 18–20.

Buresh, B., & Gordon, S. (2000). *From silence to voice: What nurses know and must communicate to the public.* Ithaca, NY: Cornell University Press.

Cheek, J. (1995). Nurses, nursing and representations: An exploration of the effect of viewing positions on the textual portrayal of nursing. *Nursing Inquiry, 2,* 235–240.

Clark, G. (1989). To be or not to be—it's time to market nursing's image. In G. Gray & R. Pratt (Eds.), *Issues in Australian Nursing 2.* Melbourne: Churchill Livingstone.

Darbyshire, P. (1985). Bedpans or broomsticks? *Nursing Times, 81,* 44–45.

Darbyshire, P. (1995). Reclaiming 'Big Nurse': A feminist critique of Ken Kesey's portrayal of Nurse Ratched in "One Flew Over the Cuckoo's Nest." *Nursing Inquiry, 2,* 198–202.

Delacour, S. (1991). The construction of nursing: Ideology, discourse and representation. In G. Gray. & R. Pratt (Eds.), *Towards a discipline of nursing.* Melbourne: Churchill Livingstone.

Donahue, M. P., & Donahue, P. M. (1996). *Nursing: The finest art.* St. Louis: Mosby-Year Book.

Dunn, A. (1985). Images of nursing in the nursing and popular press. *Bulletin of the Royal College of Nursing (UK) History of Nursing Group, 6,* 2–8.

Fagin, C., & Diers, D. (1983). Nursing as a metaphor. *The New England Journal of Medicine, 309,* 116–117.

Fiedler, L. (1988). Images of the nurse in fiction and popular cultures. In A. Jones (Ed.), *Images of nurses: Perspectives from history, art and literature.* Pennsylvania: University of Pennsylvania Press.

Gordon, S. (1996). *Life support: Three nurses on the front lines.* New York: Little, Brown and Co.

Gordon, S. (1999). Doctor's Brains. *The Nation, July 26,* 32–33.

Hallam, J. (1998). From angels to handmaidens: Changing constructions of nursing's public image in post-war Britain. *Nursing Inquiry, 5,* 32–42.

Hektor, L. (1994). Florence Nightingale and the women's movement: Friend or foe? *Nursing Inquiry, 1,* 38–45.

Holmes, C. (1997). Why we should wash our hands of medical soaps. *Nursing Inquiry, 4,* 135–137.

Hunter, K. (1988). Nurses: The satiric image and the translocated ideal. In A. Jones (Ed.), *Images of nurses: Perspectives from history, art and literature.* PA: University of Pennsylvania Press.

Jones, A. (1988). *Images of nurses: Perspectives from history, art and literature.* PA: University of Pennsylvania Press.

Kalisch, B., & Kalisch, P. (1983a). An analysis of the impact of authorship on the image of the nurse presented in novels. *Research in Nursing and Health, 6,* 17–24.

Kalisch, B., & Kalisch, P. (1983b). Heroine out of focus: Media images of Florence Nightingale, Part 1: Popular biographies and stage productions. *Nursing & Healthcare, 4,* 181–187.

Kalisch, B., & Kalisch, P. (1984). An analysis of news coverage of maternal-child nurses. *Maternal-Child Nursing Journal, 13,* 77–90.

Kalisch, B., Kalisch, P., & McHugh, M. (1982). The nurse as a sex object in motion pictures. *Research in Nursing & Health, 5,* 147–154.

Kalisch, P., & Kalisch, B. (1987). *The changing image of the nurse.* Menlo Park, CA: Addison Wesley.

Kalisch, P., Kalisch, B., & Scobey, M. (1983). *Images of nurses on television.* New York: Springer Publishing.

Kampen, N. (1988). Before Florence Nightingale: A prehistory of nursing in painting and sculpture. In A. Jones (Ed.), *Images of nurses: Perspectives from history, art and literature.* PA: University of Pennsylvania Press.

Kiger, A. (1993). Accord and discord in students' images of nursing. *Journal of Nursing Education, 32,* 309–317.

Lawler, J. (1991). *Behind the screens: Nursing, somology and the problem of the body.* Melbourne: Churchill Livingstone.

McCoppin, B., & Gardner, H. (1994). *Tradition & reality: Nursing and politics in Australia.* Melbourne: Churchill Livingstone.

Monahan, B. B. (1996). The nurses' media handbook: A reference for nurses planning to meet the media. *Massachusetts Nurse, 66*(5), 2, 6, 12.

Moore, T. (1991). *Cry of the damaged man.* Sydney: Picador.

Muff, J. (1982). Battle-axe, whore: An explanation into the fantasies, myths and stereotypes about nurses. In J. Muff (Ed.), *Socialization, sexism and stereotyping: Women's issues in nursing.* St Louis: CV Mosby.

Nelson, S. (2001). *Say little, do much: Nursing, nuns and hospitals in the 19th century.* Philadelphia: University of Pennsylvania Press.

Peterson, M. J. (1978). *The medical profession in mid-Victorian London.* Berkeley: University of California Press, p. 182.

Rule, J. (1995). Nurses may live to regret the 'angel' image era has ended. *Nursing Management, 2*(6), 5.

Salvage, J. (1983). Distorted images. *Nursing Times, 79,* 13–15.

Selzer, R. (1993). *Raising the dead: A doctor's encounter with his own mortality.* Harmondsworth: Penguin.

Strasen, L. (1992). *The image of professional nursing: Strategies for action.* Philadelphia: Lippincott.

Summers, A. Sairy Gamp: Generating fact from fiction. *Nursing Inquiry, 4*(1), 14–18 (24 ref).

5

Nursing, Philosophy, and Knowledge: A Commitment to Know Oneself and Others

Gail J. Mitchell

LEARNING OBJECTIVES

After reading this chapter, students will be able to:

- Describe at least two philosophical streams of thinking that have had an important impact on the development of nursing knowledge.
- Synthesize philosophical beliefs with personal views and identify a rationale for a personal preference of one philosophical paradigm over another
- Defend, with literature and personal reflection, a position on the matter of a unifying focus for the discipline of nursing
- Articulate anticipated outcomes for persons in society if nurses fulfill the commitment to know self and others

KEY WORDS

Nursing, philosophy, theory, knowledge, knowing the person, values

WALK WITH ME A WHILE

Have you ever walked gingerly into a pond or bog that was dark and mysterious, where with the first hesitant step you felt a swathe of snake-like tendrils swish against your skin? Have you ever walked in this mysterious bog and felt the mushy, grainy earth ooze between your toes as your feet sank deeper into the dark and porous mire? Have you been in a place like this bog and felt your stomach muscles contract and your arms rise in an attempt to keep your courage from sinking along with your feet? Well, in this chapter, I am inviting you to walk with me into this place of shifting earth and snake-like tendrils of unseen things that might grab your thinking and change your life. This dark and mysterious place is the most enticing way I could think of to describe what it can be like to engage the literature on nursing, philosophy, and knowledge. Perhaps that is why some philosophers like Berlin (1997) and Masters (1993), to name just two, have turned to art, language, and values to better understand the relationships among human life, philosophy, and knowledge. But I digress.

To get back to the walk, one of the few things I feel certain about is that nurses, and ultimately persons, families, groups, and societies, will benefit by engaging the unknown things in the bog. Nurses require understanding about knowledge, so they can choose their actions with care. Nurses also require an understanding of philosophy because philosophical assumptions and values form the substance of the shifting sands of knowledge (i.e., the substance that informs every thought and action chosen and expressed in nursing education, practice and research) (Cooper, 2000).

In my experience, there are diverse perspectives among nurse scholars about what philosophical assumptions, values, and beliefs are best for the discipline of nursing (see, for example, Bunkers, Clarke, & Frederickson, 2002; Cody, 2003; Cody & Mitchell, 2002; Cull-Wilby & Pepin, 1987; Kidd & Morrison, 1988; Kim, 2000; Mitchell & Cody, 1992, 1999; Polifroni & Welch, 1999; Rawnsley, 2003; Reed, Shearer, & Nicoll, 2003; Schlotfeldt, 1988; Thorne & Hayes, 1997). Diverse views are to be celebrated because they serve to provide for debate, reflection, and exploration of ideas. Further, the disagreements and differences currently being debated are contributing to a dialogue that may turn out to be more meaningful to nurses who are not yet in the dialogue. Sometimes meaning is not obvious, but slow to surface. Maybe students reading this chapter will have new understandings not yet evident to those of us who are walking among the tendrils of philosophical and theoretical alternatives. My engagement with the literature on nursing knowledge leaves me somewhat perplexed and somewhat amazed with the diversity of assumptions, ideas, definitions, misunderstandings, and perspectives. At the end of the day, I believe the ambiguity is a gift because it makes room for me, and for you, the reader, to ponder the possibilities and to choose our direction through the bog.

In the words below, I hope you find some ideas that give you pause, others that inspire you and, perhaps, even a few that excite you because of their potential to help you think about and choose the kind of nurse you want to become. That is what philosophy is really all about—discovering what you need, thought-wise and possibility-wise, to become the kind of nurse you want to be, and to contribute to the kind of nursing knowledge you want to see grow and expand. The view offered here is a personal one, and I state clearly that I have just scratched the surface of this very deep and important area of study—the interplay of philosophy, nursing knowledge, and nurses' actions. My own perspective has been mightily influenced by the nurse theorist, Rosemarie Rizzo Parse (1981, 1987, 1995, 1998), and by human science and existential philosophers and scholars. If I can assist colleagues in their struggle with discovery, I will have met my goal as the author of this chapter. Before examining nursing philosophy and nursing knowledge, a look at philosophy, in a more general way, may help enhance understanding about the layers of meaning and recent history that have contributed to where we are today.

WHY IS PHILOSOPHY IMPORTANT?

Philosophy and philosophical beliefs expand options for thinking about things in different ways. O'Connor (1993) identifies some of these different ways in the following presentation of contrasting beliefs:

- the specific and unique versus the repetitive and the universal
- the concrete versus the abstract
- perpetual movement versus rest
- the inner versus the outer
- quality versus quantity
- culture-bound versus timeless principles
- mental strife and self-transformation versus the possibility (and desirability) of peace, order, and final harmony (p. 109)

Some contrasts present in nursing include:

- unitary versus holistic
- simultaneity versus totality
- subjective/objective versus intersubjective/interpretive
- linear process versus mutual process
- the nursing process versus the process of nursing
- order and stability versus pattern and change

Each line of thinking in these concept comparisons is like a doorway for generating understanding of human beings and their experiences of health and illness, as well as the work and intent of nursing. Some nurse scholars think the contrasting ways of thinking are helpful for sorting through options and choices, while others believe the contrasts are divisive and distracting (for discussion, see Reed, 1995). One thing I have learned is that every scholar has a different understanding of philosophy, of the role of philosophy in nursing, of the assumptions of different philosophical paradigms, and of the interplay of philosophy and nursing practice and research. Even the same words can be, and often are, defined and understood differently by individual authors. I am in agreement here with Cooper (2000) who proposed:

> Whether we are concerned with stones, volcanoes or people, it is we who connect, relate, structure, order, assimilate, differentiate, exemplify, detail, and emphasize. The manner in which we perform such intellectual actions is a matter for our choice and we find reasons for our choices in our experience of the physical world and of our fellow human beings. In this way, we come to understand and appreciate the significance of what we know.... Hence, every agent needs a conceptual framework adequate to label, interpret, and appraise practical situations.... Understanding *anything* involves appreciating and appraising significance. (pp. 384–385)

A place to begin with all the myriad possibilities and different ways of thinking is to appraise where your own thinking aligns, make choices about what is important to you, and then offer your views to others in discussions and publications. In other words, identify and read authors who present ideas that seem to fit with your thinking. Start speaking, writing, and reflecting to continue developing your own ideas and views, and to contribute to the community of nurse scholars. It also can be helpful to read authors whose views do not align with your thinking.

Contrasting views can help clarify ideas that are inconsistent or incongruent with your assumptions and beliefs about reality. The philosopher Bloom (1987) proposed that philosophy creates different worlds of understanding. The notion of different worlds helps persons to appreciate how different nurses can think very differently about the knowledge and discipline of nursing.

Personal Reflection

When you think about the nursing literature, who are the authors you like to read? What is it about the authors' writings that you like? What ideas do you find attractive and inviting? Who are the authors you do not like to read? What ideas do you disagree with?

As noted above, Bloom (1987) suggests that philosophy makes worlds. The clockwork universe is a good example of how philosophy makes worlds. Philosophical assumptions and beliefs were crafted together to create an image of a perfect, mechanistic (machine-like) world/universe. In such a universe, order, precision, dependability, and the predictability of interacting parts create an environment/world/universe where humans, through observation and reason, generate truth or probability statements and predictions about what will happen, given certain conditions. This mechanistic model gave nursing systematic approaches to practice and research. The traditional nursing process consisting of specific steps (assess, plan, implement, evaluate) that constituted a method consistent with the clockwork paradigm thinking. The way I see it, the clockwork method—and the nursing process—were, and still are, helpful for engaging technology and machines. For instance, nurses can assess the functioning of an intravenous line solve the problem if a malfunction occurs. Technical competence is essential for nurses working in settings where they are expected to work with technology, clinical protocols, and procedures. But, according to some authors, and I concur, the nursing process of assess, plan, implement, and evaluate does not provide best practice for the nurse-person relationship (Hagey & McDonough, 1984; McHugh, 1987; Mitchell, 1991, 1995; Shamansky & Yanni, 1983; Takemura & Kanda, 2003; Yeo, 1989). One concern about the traditional nursing process is that it encourages the division of people into identifiable parts.

Holism is the concept that represents how professionals can think of people as a body-mind-spirit unit. It is a concept created to advance understanding of whole human beings and their complex interactions in light of a belief in an orderly, predictable, manageable view of human beings and their environments. The concept of holism created a world of opportunity for thinkers and researchers who saw and dreamed about the potential discoveries that could enlighten and liberate humankind. There were many important discoveries and advancements made within the clockwork view of reality. But for some scholars, it also became clear that the clockwork model and its related concept of holism could not fulfill dreams in all of the life sciences such as biology (Cooper, 1996) and nursing (Parse, 1981, 1987, 1998; Rogers, 1970, 1990). In nursing, some authors propose that dividing people into bio-psycho-socio-spiritual or body-mind-spirit parts, in order to define and assess how the parts function and contribute to the working of the whole human, has detracted from practices concerned with irreducible persons and their experiences of health (Hagey & McDonough, 1984; McHugh, 1987; Mitchell, 1991, 1995; Takemura & Kanda, 2003). The dissatisfaction with holism and the mechanistic paradigm helped fuel the desire for new ways of thinking about human beings and their relationships in the world. The twentieth century was a time of accelerated, out-of-the-box thinking. Many scholars in various disciplines searched for more "unitary accounts of reality into which human existence is integrated" (Cooper, 1996, p. 410), and which is known for its continuous growth, change, and unpredictability. The later twentieth century scholars were not the first to ponder the possibilities of a more unified and dynamic world view.

For instance, Cooper (1996) wrote about Henri Bergson (1859–1941), a celebrated philosopher, who spoke of a seamless flux of experience, a conscious force that gallops through time, and of a unified consciousness that could not be contained in a clockwork universe. Cooper quotes Bergson who stated, "Science and intellect carve up the world for our convenience and then promptly forget that they have done so" (p. 412). Bergson proposed that science can show how to make things and how to act on things to achieve goals. However, science does not disclose the nature of reality or the nature of human life, which he thought was "a continuity in which memories, moods, perceptions flow into and give shape to one another" (Cooper, 1996, p. 413).

Bergson's contemporaries, Alfred North Whitehead (1861–1947) and Wilhelm Dilthey (1833–1911), also worked to develop different philosophies of science that were more human, coherent, meaningful, and unified (Dilthey, 1988; Ermarth, 1978). Whitehead wanted a world view that could provide meaning for the aesthetic and the moral, as well as the empirical and mathematical. Cooper (1996) suggests that Whitehead was encouraged by new physics and its reliance on process as the ultimate route to understanding. He, too, saw life as vibrant and pulsating, full of emotion and enjoyment. Dilthey (1988), known by some as the thinker that coined the term human science, worked to create a philosophical system of thought that elevated human life out of the objective, sterile world of the mechanistic universe. Phenomenological philosophers proposed that the essences of life could be studied in systematic and rigorous ways such that the unity of lived experience could be preserved, and meaningful knowledge generated, that could add to the betterment of humankind. Gradually, ideas about meanings, values, understanding, history, experience, essence, the arts, and unity began to shape and give form to a different view of the human-world-universe. This new view has various streams of thinking in nursing including simultaneity (Parse, 1987) and the unitary-transformative (Newman, 1992). Such is the purpose of philosophy: to create worlds of meaning and space for new worlds to emerge.

Other worlds of meaning and possibility grew, and contribute to the current cornucopia of coexisting philosophical and theoretical frames that inform nursing. We have the critical social theorists, the postmodern feminists, the caring theorists, the simultaneity and totality theorists, and the behavioral and cognitive theorists. We have medical science, nursing science, human science, and unitary science. The tendrils of theory and science gently, but securely, wrap around tentative thoughts and sometimes bog one down while trying to consider and clarify the various possibilities for thinking. So, how does a nurse figure things out in a way that makes sense, in light of notions of integrity and coherence, and that also (most important) contributes to the betterment of humankind? It is time now to consider, in more depth, some notions important to nursing, philosophy, and knowledge.

PHILOSOPHY AND KNOWLEDGE FOR NURSES

As noted above, philosophy presents different mythologies, or stories, that capture the imagination and entwine us in intricate patterns of thinking, speaking, and acting. These philosophical stories are not merely interesting, they are essential. Philosophy sets up rules for thinking, seeing, speaking, and acting. According to Cooper (1996, p. 450),

"Philosophical paradigms shape scientists' outlooks so that they do not see the same evidence—they are working in different worlds—thinking with different words and no data can confirm or decide between competing paradigms." I agree with Cooper. Nurses, too, are showing in their thinking, speaking, writing, and actions, that philosophy matters because it offers different worlds of understanding, speaking and acting.

Philosophical assumptions and beliefs about reality form the *ontology* or world view of a paradigm. Different paradigms are built on different assumptions and beliefs. *Epistemology* is about knowledge (Cooper, 1999) and how concepts like belief, doubt and knowledge can be understood within a certain view of reality (ontology). *Methodology* is tied with ontology and epistemology in that, given the nature of reality and beliefs about knowledge of that reality, it shows how to generate new knowledge that is consistent with the epistemology and ontology. Methodology is about the how. Given one's belief system (ontology) and beliefs about what will constitute knowledge in that ontology (epistemology), what is the best methodology to identify, gather, and interpret the information identified? Figure 5.1 shows how ideas flow from ontology (the most general and abstract notions) to epistemology, on to methodology, and finally on to specific theories of nursing.

Questions for nurses reflecting on links between philosophy and nursing knowledge

Consider the two streams of thinking in Figure 5.1 and imagine working as a nurse in each one. What thoughts interest you? What ideas are you comfortable with? What ideas perplex or disturb you? What is one possible explanation for your preferences and for your discomfort with certain ideas? What kind of nurse do you want to become? What kind of knowledge do you think is worth pursuing? What are the key messages you want to give to the persons, families, and groups you work with?

It is interesting that postmodernists are said to have abandoned belief of universal truths or essences of human beings and their realities. Reed (1995) suggests that postmodernists concluded that philosophy is of little use since there is nothing except culture that imposes beliefs on subjects. This is an interesting notion, but one that I personally do not believe is sustainable. In my world there are universal essences of human life (such as grieving or hope). In my reality, most, if not all, nurses and other scholars act as if they believe the realties represented in one

Ontology	Totality (Interactive) Paradigm	Simultaneity (Unitary/ Transformative) Paradigm
	There is an inherent logic and predictable sense about the universe and all things in it.	There is inherent mystery and process in the universe and in the human beings that inhabit it.
	There are laws and rules in the universe that govern human behavior and the functioning of all organisms and matter.	The world is ever-changing and evolving, as are humans who themselves change and are changed in the world.
	Human beings are complex systems that interact with other complex systems in predictable patterns.	Human beings exist within a culture, language, and history, and all these forces shape human experience.
Epistemology	Human beings are holistic entities comprising identifiable parts.	Human beings are irreducible/ unitary and live with situated freedom.
	Human beings strive for balance, harmony, and adaptation.	Intersubjectivity, meaning always in the world with others creating and interpreting.
	There are objective and subjective ways of thinking, knowing, and informing.	Every human being is unique and has a personal view of life, quality, and health.
	Knowledge of relationships among variables helps to predict human behavior.	Specifying patterns of lived experiences of health and illness builds knowledge for the discipline of nursing.
Methodology	Categorizing and standardizing human responses will build the knowledge of nursing.	
	Nursing happens in relationships that focus on identifying and solving problems with clients.	Nursing happens in relationship with persons and requires individualized plans of care informed by knowledge of patterns of unitary humans.
	Desired nursing outcomes include therapeutic relationships, integration of bio-psycho-social functioning, coping, adaptation, and harmony.	Desired nursing outcomes include meaningful relationships, changing health patterns, quality of life, and patient satisfaction.
Examples of Consistent Nursing Theories	Neuman's Systems Model (Neuman, 1995, 1996)	Human Becoming School of Thought (Parse, 1981, 1998)
	Roy's Adaptation Model (Roy & Andrews, 1999)	Health as Expanding Consciousness (Newman, 1994, 1997)
	Orem's Self-Care Deficit Theory (Orem, 1995)	Science of Unitary Human Beings (Rogers, 1970, 1990)

FIGURE 5.1   Contrasting streams of philosophical thinking for nurses.

or the other of the two major streams of philosophical thought identified in Figure 5.1. If everyone acts as if there are different realities, the postmodernists may well feel dread and despair. However, there are other ways to think. There are still truths about unrelenting values to inform the knowledge of nursing. The question that comes to mind here is: What theories are required to develop knowledge that advances particular values in particular disciplines? It is nursing theory that currently houses different values in nursing. It is theory that guides practice (Parse, 1999). This view is in contrast to those who propose that theory emerges from the study of practice. As noted by Reed (1995, p. 75), "Data alone do not yield up theory any more than brushes and paint produce a painting." Not all nurses are comfortable with this notion, and many nurses are still searching for truths independent of nursing theory. My view parallels that of Reed (1995), who suggests that nurses are in a neomodernist time when, "Nursing knowledge development need not abandon completely modernist views about high theory or universal ideas. Rather than capitulate entirely to postmodernism, nurses can knowingly involve in their science the realm of perspectives and values, initially put forth by modernist nurses, that distinguish nursing knowledge" (p. 76). From my viewpoint, modernist nurses include theorists like Rogers (1970, 1990), Parse (1981, 1998), Roy (1988), Roy and Andrews (1999), and Newman (1994, 1997). These theorists have given nurses different ways of knowing.

KINDS AND WAYS OF KNOWING

There are many views about nursing knowledge, too many to cover in this chapter. There are those who define different ways of knowing in nursing, including moral/ethical, technical, practical, empirical, aesthetic, and personal (see, for example, Carper, 1978; Chinn, 1989; Johns, 1995; Liaschenko, 1997; Moch, 1990; Munhall, 1993; Van der Zalm & Bergum, 2000; White, 1995). In contrast, there are other scholars who propose that every individual has personal knowledge that is continuously changing as persons live and choose to go forward in life, and that personal knowing can be examined for its ethical, practical, and aesthetic expressions in the world (Mitchell & Cody, 1992; Parse, 1981, 1998; Polyani & Prosch, 1975). Whether viewed as separate, distinct ways of knowing, or as a personal way of knowing with various expressions, the persisting call is for nurses to gain knowledge and to continuously reflect on knowledge so that expressions and consequences enhance quality of care and quality of life for clients. Nursing is a service, the quality of which always should be examined in light of person/client experience and satisfaction.

IS NURSING A KNOWLEDGE-BASED PROFESSION?

If nurses are to be trusted as professionals who are helpful, caring, compassionate, loving, and skillful, then nurses must use and develop knowledge. Popper is credited by Reed (1995) as the philosopher who helped scholars see that all knowledge is value-based and embedded in theory. Nurses bear the responsibility of choosing the best strands of knowledge—the best values—that enable them to weave an understanding and a way of acting so that particular values are disclosed. If nurses do not choose their own knowledge they risk becoming practitioners of other professions. Some nurse practitioners have expressed concerns to me about expectations that they are to practice according to the knowledge and values of medicine. Or consider the psychologist who, as a member of a multidisciplinary team, directs nurses to use principles of behavior modification (a system of punishments and rewards) in order to get mental health patients to comply with the treatment regime. Nurses may not be comfortable using the punishments and rewards of behaviorism. Perhaps they comply with behavior modification because they have never learned about unique nursing knowledge, philosophy, autonomy, and the professional responsibility to choose from existing nursing paradigms. Nursing is a self-regulating profession, and this means that nurses bear responsibility to knowingly guide practice with theory that matches their public mandate to serve and be helpful to persons experiencing changes in health and quality of life.

NURSING KNOWLEDGE

I, like others, contend that the unique knowledge base of nursing lies in the extant nursing theories (Parse, 1987, 1999). It is not possible to review all the nursing theories in this chapter, and, in addition to the theorists themselves, there are many excellent sources that offer overviews of nursing theories for nurses looking for direction (Alligood & Tomey, 2002; Fawcett, 2000; Parker, 2001). It is also important to state that there is no agreement about what constitutes nursing knowledge or how best to build nursing knowledge (see, for example, Hall, 1981; Kidd & Morrison, 1988; Packard & Polifroni, 1991; Reed, 1995; Van der Zalm & Bergum, 2000). As nursing theories develop, they will introduce new language to nurses. This is a good thing for, as noted by Bloom, "A new language always reflects a new point of view" (1987, p. 141). I believe that nurses need points of view that advance specific values of the nursing discipline. Maybe nurse scholars, who have been looking for a unifying phenomenon of concern, have helped us come to this place of asking if there is a value that might unify the discipline.

It may be that amid all the mystery surrounding nursing knowledge and nursing theory development, there is now a value surfacing and it is appearing in different paradigms. That value is *the commitment to know the person/family who is engaging nurses for care and service.* A closer look at the literature surrounding the topic may be helpful.

THE COMMITMENT TO KNOW THE PERSON

Nurses show in many ways that they have knowledge about many different things. There are the technical and procedural things, the practical things, the physiological and disease things, the things called cases and the ethical things that can happen within cases, and of course there are the empirical, the social, and the political things that influence day to day life. Knowledge about *things* is, I propose, quite different from knowledge about *persons.*

Personal/group reflection

What do you think is different about the knowledge of things and the knowledge of persons? How do nurses gain each kind of knowledge? How do teaching and learning about each vary and how are they similar? How is knowledge of things and knowledge of persons built and enhanced?

The things nurses know direct their attention, and shape the nature and quality of the nurse-person process. It seems to me that what a nurse knows is, as it should be, a matter of personal choice. I would add that it is also a matter of public interest and concern. The public interest is the single most important reason for nurses to give serious thought to the knowledge and values they choose to live out in practice and research. Nurses provide services to people, and, from my perspective, there should be no hesitancy in identifying unifying values for what knowledge nurses will develop. But nurses do not yet have a unifying focus, or is it only now showing up in the discourse about knowing the person? Bournes (2002) called for nurses to commit to a set of universal values that included "(a) being accountable to the people served by nursing; (b) listening to what people say is important for their health; (c) honoring people's opinions about issues related to their health; and (d) respecting people's right to self-determination" (p. 194). These proposed universal values connect with the commitment to know the person.

Interestingly, the commitment to know the person is showing up in the literature from a variety of different philosophical paradigms and theoretical perspectives. Patients are asking to be known as persons (for instance, see Deegan, 1993; Fisher & Mitchell, 1998; Macurdy, 1997), and professionals such as Bournes (2002), are asking what values should guide practice in order to ensure patients are treated as persons. I believe that nurses have a moral commitment to know the person, family, or groups with which they work. In order to know persons, you must listen to their meanings, concerns, fears, questions, hopes, plans, and issues linked to their health and quality of life. The commitment to know the person surfaces in the stories nurses tell about their relationships with patients and families. The commitment to know the person shows itself in nursing's theoretical frameworks (see, for example, Boykin & Schoenhofer, 2001; Newman, 1994, 1999; Parse, 1981, 1995, 1998; Watson, 1990, 1997). The commitment to know the person is showing up in the literature from practicing nurses and it is clearly evident in research studies from scholars with different backgrounds (see, for example, Evans, 1996; Henderson, 1997; Jenny & Logan, 1992; Luker, Austin, Caress, & Hallett, 2000; Radwin, 1995a, 1995b, 1996; Takemura & Kanda, 2003; Whittemore, 2000).

Perhaps knowing persons and their experiences of health, illness, and quality of life is one commitment all nurses could stand for and even promise to the persons who look to them for care and service. I believe that if nurses make the commitment to be open to know the person they avoid the legitimate danger raised by Liaschenko (1997), that knowing the person should not become a nursing intervention—is not something the nurse *does to* others. Imagine a nurse entering a patient's room and saying, "Now I have to get to know you." Some people do not want to disclose to nurses and that is fine. However, nurses could still have the commitment to be open to know the person and family to the extent that they choose to disclose. I wonder if the intent to be open to knowing the person could unify the discipline of nursing or if this intent would also be interpreted from different philosophical perspectives that lead to different thoughts, actions, and consequences.

It is quite remarkable that nursing has not yet defined a simple and unifying focus. As noted by Packard and Polifroni (1991), "If you do not know where you are going, how can you best judge the means to get there?" (p. 12). Schlotfeldt (1988) was in line with this thinking when she claimed that "there is little agreement among nurses concerning the human phenomena that are of concern to nurses and how they should be characterized and classified and how knowledge of them should be advanced" (p. 370). Volker (2003) proposed that nursing does not even have a unifying ethic. She cautions readers to resist thinking that caring can provide a unifying focus for the discipline of nursing. Nurses have been trying to figure out what beliefs and what values are essential to their discipline, but it is clear that they continue to walk in the mystery of figuring out what direction or directions to take.

I agree that as long as nurses have not named the central phenomenon that defines the borders of our science and our art, we will continue to struggle and go in diverging directions. I suggest, as Bournes (2002) and others have done in the past, that it might be worth trying to name the central values, such as openness to knowing the person. One comment worth noting is that *knowing the person* is not about being nice and proceeding to assess people from an external reference point without listening and acting according to their meanings, concerns, fears, and hopes. In the literature an expanding understanding exists about the consequences of knowing and not knowing the person in the nurse-person relationship. Some specific points worth noting are as follows:

- Knowing the person promotes individualized care planning and teaching (Evans, 1996; Henderson, 1997; Radwin, 1995a, 1995b, 1996; Takemura & Kanda, 2003; Whittemore, 2000)
- Knowing the person helps to decrease risk and increase patient safety (Whittemore, 2000)

- Knowing the person helps staff to interpret what is happening and what needs attention (Luker, Austin, Caress, & Hallett, 2000; Tyndall 1994)
- Knowing the person helps staff to make better clinical decisions (Jenny & Logan, 1992; Tyndall, 1994)
- Knowing the person improves communication and trust among staff and patients/families (Luker, Austin, Caress, & Hallett, 2001)
- Knowing the person leads to fewer complications and to earlier identification of risks/threats to patients (Whittemore 2000)
- Knowing the person shows respect and enhances the potential for being helpful to others (Bournes, 2002; Macurdy, 1997; Takemura & Kanda, 2003)
- Knowing the person changes quality of life, living, and dying (Bournes, 2002)

I wonder if the commitment to being open to know the person is meaningful to new nurses. Is the idea meaningful to students? Will the idea continue to be important to the public we serve?

TO KNOW OR NOT TO KNOW?: THAT IS THE QUESTION

I started the chapter by asking you to walk with me in mystery surrounding nursing, philosophy, and knowledge. My intent was to present some ideas that give you pause, some that inspire, and others that might even excite you because of their potential to help you think about and choose the kind of nurse you want to be. I hope I have achieved some of this intent. Philosophy and nursing knowledge can help you discover the thinking and being that are required to become the kind of nurse you want to be. This is what happened for me. Both philosophy and the "theory of human becoming" (Parse, 1981, 1995, 1998) continue to provide inspiration and insight for my day to day thinking about practice and research. I hope you choose to walk in the bog, and I hope that your journey is made with an unwavering courage to clarify your own philosophical beliefs and preferences. I also hope that you will consider the commitment to know the person as a value worthy of your effort. Nursing theories have the potential to help you know how to be the nurse you want to become. The choice and commitment to knowledge must be yours.

RECOMMENDED READINGS

Bunkers, S. S., Clarke, P. N., & Frederickson, K. (2002). Analysis and evaluation of contemporary nursing knowledge: Nursing models and theories. *Nursing Science Quarterly, 15,* 172–177.

Cody, W. K., & Mitchell, G. J. (2002). Nursing knowledge and human science revisited: Practical and political considerations. *Nursing Science Quarterly, 15,* 4–13.

Parse, R. R. (Ed.) (1995). *Illuminations: The human becoming theory in practice and research.* New York: The National League for Nursing.

Radwin, L. E. (1995b). Knowing the patient: A process model for individualized interventions. *Nursing Research, 44*(6), 364–370.

Radwin, L. E. (1996). 'Knowing the patient': A review of research on an emerging concept. *Journal of Advanced Nursing, 23,* 1142–1146.

REFERENCES

Alligood, M. R., & Tomey, A. M. (2002). *Nursing theory: Utilization & application* (2nd ed.). St. Louis: Mosby.

Berlin, I. (1997). *Against the current: Essays in the history of ideas.* London: Pimlico.

Bloom, A. (1987). *The closing of the American mind.* New York: Simon & Schuster.

Bournes, D. (2002). Research evaluating human becoming in practice. *Nursing Science Quarterly, 15,* 190–195.

Boykin, A., & Schoenhofer, S. (2001). *Nursing as caring: A model for transforming practice.* Sudbury, MA: Jones & Bartlett.

Bunkers, S. S., Clarke, P. N., & Frederickson, K. (2002). Analysis and evaluation of contemporary nursing knowledge: Nursing models and theories. *Nursing Science Quarterly, 15,* 172–177.

Carper, B. A. (1978). Fundamental patterns of knowing in nursing. *Advances in Nursing Science, 1,* 13–23.

Chinn, P. L. (1989). Nursing patterns of knowing and feminist thought. *Nursing & Health Care, 10,* 71–75.

Cody, W. K. (2003). Response to Rawnsley's column: A theoretician's perspective. *Nursing Science Quarterly, 16,* 14–15.

Cody, W. K., & Mitchell, G. J. (2002). Nursing knowledge and human science revisited: Practical and political considerations. *Nursing Science Quarterly, 15,* 4–13.

Cooper, D. E. (1996). *World philosophies. An historical introduction.* Oxford: Blackwell.

Cooper, D. E. (Ed.) (1999). *Epistemology: The classic readings.* Oxford: Blackwell.

Cooper, N. (2000). Understanding people. *Philosophy, 75,* 383–400.

Cull-Wilby, B. L., & Pepin, J. L. (1987). Towards a coexistence of paradigms in nursing knowledge development. *Journal of Advanced Nursing, 12,* 515–521.

Deegan, E. (1993). Recovering our sense of value after being labelled mentally ill. *Journal of Psychosocial Nursing & Mental Health, 31,* 7–11.

Dilthey, W. (1988). Introduction to the human sciences. (R. J. Bentanzos, Translator; Original published in 1883). Detroit, MI: Wayne State University Press.

Ermarth, M. (1978). *Wilhelm Dilthey: The critique of historical reason.* Chicago, IL: The University of Chicago Press.

Evans, L. K. (1996). Knowing the patient: The route to individualized care. *Journal of Gerontological Nursing, 22,* 15–19.

Fawcett, J. (2000). *Analysis and evaluation of contemporary nursing knowledge: Nursing models and theories.* Philadelphia: F. A. Davis.

Fisher, M. A., & Mitchell, G. J. (1998). Patients' views of quality of life: Transforming the knowledge base of nursing. *Clinical Nurse Specialist, 12*(3), 99–105.

Hagey, R. S., & McDonough, P. (1984). The problem of professional labeling. *Nursing Outlook, 32,* 151–157.

Hall, B. A. (1981). The change paradigm in nursing: Growth versus persistence. *Advances in Nursing Science, 3*(4), 1–6.

Henderson, S. (1997). Knowing the patient and the impact on patient participation: A grounded theory study. *International Journal of Nursing Practice, 3,* 111–118.

Jenny, J., & Logan, J. (1992). Knowing the patient: One aspect of clinical knowledge. *IMAGE: Journal of Nursing Scholarhip, 24*(4), 254–280.

Johns, C. (1995). Framing learning through reflection within Carper's fundamental ways of knowing in nursing. *Journal of Advanced Nursing, 22,* 226–234.

Kidd, P., & Morrison, E. F. (1988). The progression of knowledge in nursing: A search for meaning. *IMAGE: Journal of Nursing Scholarship, 20*(4), 222–224.

Kim, H. S. (2000). *The nature of theoretical thinking in nursing* (2nd ed.). New York: Springer Publishing.

Liaschenko, J. (1997). Knowing the patient? In S. E. Thorne & V. E. Hayes (Eds.), *Nursing praxis: Knowledge and action.* Thousand Oaks, CA: Sage.

Luker, K. A., Austin, L., Caress, A., & Hallett, C. E. (2000). The importance of 'knowing the patient': Community nurses' constructions of quality in providing palliative care. *Journal of Advanced Nursing, 31,* 775–782.

Macurdy, A. H. (1997). Mastery of life. In J. Young-Mason (Ed.), *The patient's voice: Experiences of illness.* Philadelphia, PA: F. A. Davis.

Masters, R. D. (1993). *Beyond relativism. Science and human values.* Hanover, NH: University Press of New England.

McHugh, M. K. (1987). Has nursing outgrown the nursing process? *Nursing 87, 9,* 50–51.

Mitchell, G. J. (1991). Nursing diagnosis: An ethical analysis. *IMAGE: International Journal of Nursing Scholarship, 23,* 99–103.

Mitchell, G. J. (1995). Nursing diagnosis: An obstacle to caring ways. In A. Boykin (Ed.), *Power, politics and public policy: A matter of caring* (pp. 11–23). New York: National League for Nursing.

Mitchell, G. J., & Cody, W. K. (1992). Nursing knowledge and human science: Ontological and epistemological considerations. *Nursing Science Quarterly, 5,* 54–61.

Mitchell, G. J., & Cody, W. K. (1999). Human becoming theory: A complement to medical science. *Nursing Science Quarterly, 12,* 304–310.

Moch, S. D. (1990). Personal knowing: Evolving research and practice. *Scholarly inquiry for nursing practice: An international journal, 4*(2), 155–165.

Munhall, P. L. (1993). 'Unknowing': Toward another pattern of knowing in nursing. *Nursing Outlook, 41,* 125–128.

Neuman, B. (1995). *The Neuman systems model* (3rd ed.). Norwalk, CT: Appleton & Lange.

Neuman, B. (1996). The Neuman systems model in research and practice. *Nursing Science Quarterly, 9,* 67–70.

Newman, M. A. (1992). Prevailing paradigms in nursing. *Nursing Outlook, 40,* 10–13.

Newman, M. A. (1994). *Health as expanding consciousness* (2nd ed.). Sudbury, MA: James & Bartlett.

Newman, M. A. (1997). Evolution of theory of health as expanding consciousness. *Nursing Science Quarterly, 10,* 22–25.

Newman, M. A. (1999). The rhythm of relating in a paradigm of wholeness. *IMAGE, the Journal of Nursing Scholarship, 31,* 227–230.

O'Connor, T. (1993). Intentionality, ontology, and empirical thought. In H. J. Silverman (Ed.), *Questioning foundations: Truth/Subjectivity/Culture* (pp. 98–109). New York: Routledge.

Orem, D. E. (1995). *Nursing: Concepts of practice* (5th ed.). St. Louis: Mosby.

Packard, S. A., & Polifroni, E. C. (1991). The dilemma of nursing science: Current quandaries and lack of direction. *Nursing Science Quarterly, 4,* 7–13.

Parker, M. (Ed.) (2001). *Nursing theories and nursing practice.* Philadelphia: F. A. Davis.

Parse, R. R. (1981). *Man-living-health: A theory of nursing.* New York: Wiley.

Parse, R. R. (1987). *Nursing science: Major paradigms, theories, and critiques.* Philadelphia: W. B. Saunders.

Parse, R. R. (Ed.) (1995). *Illuminations. The human becoming theory in practice and research.* New York: The National League for Nursing.

Parse, R. R. (1998). *The human becoming school of thought: A perspective for nurses and other health professionals.* Thousand Oaks, CA: Sage.

Parse, R. R. (1999). Nursing: The discipline and the profession. *Nursing Science Quarterly, 12,* 275–276.

Polifroni, E. C., & Welch, M. (Eds.) (1999). *Perspectives on philosophy of science in nursing: An historical and contemporary anthology.* Philadelphia: Lippincott.

Polyani, M., & Prosch, H. (1975). *Meaning.* Chicago, IL: The University of Chicago Press.

Radwin, L. E. (1995a). Conceptualizations of decision making in nursing: Analytic models and "knowing the patient." *Nursing Diagnosis, 6*(1), 16–22.

Radwin, L. E. (1995b). Knowing the patient: A process model for individualized interventions. *Nursing Research, 44*(6), 364–370.

Radwin, L. E. (1996). 'Knowing the patient': A review of research on an emerging concept. *Journal of Advanced Nursing, 23,* 1142–1146.

Rawnsley, M. M. (2003). Dimensions of scholarship and the advancement of nursing science: Articulating a vision. *Nursing Science Quarterly, 16,* 6–15.

Reed, P. G. (1995). A treatise on nursing knowledge development for the 21st century: Beyond postmodernism. *Advances in Nursing Science, 17*(3), 70–84.

Reed, P. G., Shearer, N. B., & Nicoll, L. H. (Eds.) (2003). *Perspectives on nursing theory.* Philadelphia: Lippincott Williams & Wilkins.

Rogers, M. E. (1970). *An introduction to the theoretical basis of nursing.* Philadelphia: F. A. Davis.

Rogers, M. E. (1990). Nursing science of unitary, irreducible, human beings: Update 1990. In E. Barrett (Ed.), *Visions of Rogers' science-based nursing.* New York: National League for Nursing.

Roy, Sr., C. (1988). An explication of the philosophical assumptions of the Roy Adaptation model. *Nursing Science Quarterly, 1,* 26–34.

Roy, Sr., C., & Andrews, H. A. (1999). *The Roy adaptation model* (2nd ed.). Stamford, CT: Appleton & Lange.

Schlotfeldt, R. M. (1988). Structuring nursing knowledge: A priority for creating nursing's future. *Nursing Science Quarterly, 1,* 35–38.

Shamansky, S. L., & Yanni, C. R. (1983). In opposition to nursing diagnosis: A minority opinion. *IMAGE: The Journal of Nursing Scholarship, 15,* 47–50.

Takemura, Y., & Kanda, K. (2003). How Japanese nurses provide care: A practice based on continuously knowing the patient. *Journal of Advanced Nursing, 42,* 252–259.

Thorne, S. E., & Hayes, V. E. (Eds.) (1997). *Nursing praxis: Knowledge and action.* Thousand Oaks, CA: Sage.

Tyndall, A. V. (1994). [Commentary on] The phenomenology of knowing the patient. *AACN Nursing Scan in Critical Care, 4*(3), 1–2.

Van der Zalm, J. E., & Bergum, V. (2000). Hermeneutic-phenomenology: Providing living knowledge for nursing practice. *Journal of Advanced Nursing, 31,* 211–218.

Volker, D. L. (2003). Is there a unique nursing ethic? *Nursing Science Quarterly, 16,* 207–211.

Watson, J. (1990). Caring knowledge and informed moral passion. *Advances in Nursing Science, 13*(1), 15–24.

Watson, J. (1997). The theory of human caring: Retrospective and prospective. *Nursing Science Quarterly, 10,* 49–52.

White, J. (1995). Patterns of knowing: Review, critique, and update. *Advances in Nursing Science, 17*(4), 73–86.

Whittemore, R. (2000). Consequences of not "knowing the patient." *Clinical Nurse Specialist, 14*(2), 75–81.

Yeo, M. (1989). Integration of nursing theory and nursing ethics. *Advances in Nursing Science, 11*(3), 33–42.

6

Tracing Nurse Caring: Issues, Concerns, Debates

Jean Watson, Debra Jackson, and Sally Borbasi

LEARNING OBJECTIVES

At the completion of this chapter, the reader will be able to:

- Define caring as a professional concept
- Differentiate professional and informal caring
- Delineate issues related to care and cure
- Discuss perceptions of nurse caring behaviors from the perspective of patients and nurses
- Describe some problems that might occur if caring formed the basis of the discipline of nursing
- Identify threats to nurse caring

KEY WORDS

Care, care-cure debate, nursing work, power, altruism

INTRODUCTION

In this chapter we introduce you to some of the issues and debates surrounding the concept of caring in nursing. As you engage with this chapter, you will note from the range of literature we draw on that many of these debates and issues are not new. Rather, they have confounded and captivated nurses for years—even decades—and continue to do so. The discussion on caring remains one of the great philosophical debates in nursing, and in this chapter we trace some of the recent developments that have informed nurse caring to date. You will also notice that the discourse is international, making these issues, concerns, and debates global in nature. So, regardless of whether you study or practice nursing in Cincinnati or Sydney, Wichita or Washington, Amarillo or Amsterdam, Honolulu or Hamburg, Lexington or London, the issues we raise in this chapter are fundamental to nursing, and affect nursing and nurses, as well as clients and communities across continents and across the globe.

NURSE CARING

Caring is positioned as essential to the theory and practice of nursing. It occupies a prominent position in nursing scholarship, has high visibility in key nursing documents, is acknowledged and addressed by professional bodies such as the American Nurses Association (ANA) and the National League for Nursing (NLN), and is featured among the major recommendations from national think tanks (Sigma Theta Tau, 1989 Wingspread Conference). In addition, there have been journal issues, special monographs, conferences, and ethical positions devoted to caring in nursing, and the desire to "care for" or help people remains a motivation for choosing a nursing career (Woodward, 2003).

Though it may be argued that a caring perspective is not unique to nursing, it is almost universally accepted within the discipline, that nursing has an imperative to care for the health of individuals, families and communities, and many believe the care given by nurses has the potential to restore health (Benner, Hooper-Kyriakidis, & Stannard, 1999; Williams, 1997). Indeed, the caring imperative of nursing is reflected in the many definitions and perspectives of nursing which proclaim caring as inherent and central to the nursing role (see, for example, Benner, 1984; Leininger, 1984; Watson, 1988).

Though the words "care" and "caring" are in common usage, and despite their centrality to nursing, caring remains a nebulous concept. However, it has been defined in generic terms. The Oxford Dictionary of English (Soanes & Stevenson, 2003) refers to caring as showing kindness and concern for others, and points to the work and practice of looking after others. However, when used professionally, caring cannot be oversimplified. It is a complex, multidimensional concept, that "has been postulated to be a philosophy and science, an ethic, an interactive set of client expectations and nursing behaviours, expert nursing practice, the hidden work of nursing and a synonym for nursing itself" (Rawnsley, 1990, p. 42).

DEFINING NURSE CARING

According to Sullivan and Deane (1994), nurse caring prizes human relationships, and is informed by principles of sharing, sincerity, concern, and moderation. Wolf, Giardino, Osborne, and Ambrose (1994) propose that nurse caring has several tangible dimensions, including "respectful deference to others, assurance of human presence, positive connectedness, professional knowledge and skill, and attentiveness to the other's experience" (p. 107). Pepin (1992) suggests caring may be considered to have two dimensions—love and labour. Love is said to consist of affective (that is, pertaining to feelings) concepts such as altruism, compassion, emotion, presence, connectedness, nurturance, and comfort. It is this aspect of caring that has dominated the nursing literature. Labour, which has received much less attention in the nursing literature, refers to the element of care related to toil and service. It encompasses roles, functions, knowledge, and tasks.

Several theories of nursing have been developed from the standpoint of defining and describing caring practices. Watson (1985) writes of a science (and practice) of caring, and draws upon phenomenological, existential, and spiritual concepts to ground these theories. Along with Astrom, Norberg, and Hallberg (1995), Watson sees caring as the ethical and moral ideal of nursing that has humanistic and interpersonal qualities, and believes nursing as art is "lived, expressed and co-created in the caring moment" (p. xvii). Walters (1994) also linked caring with art.[1] He saw caring as an "aesthetic activity," an activity associated with the artistic aspects of nursing (and its creative expression), something that is not easily captured in words.

Wolf, Giardino, Osborne, and Ambrose (1994) propose caring as an aspect of nursing work that is invisible and may not be recognized

---

[1]Past tense used in this instance because Dr. Walters is deceased.

except when the actions and attitudes that compose caring are not in evidence. Johns (2001) takes this idea of caring's invisibility and elusiveness a step further, and asks the question, "If we do not know caring, how can we practise it and how can we teach it?" (p. 244). He proposes a "framework for revealing the nature of caring" (p. 237) through storied reflection. Johns reveals the essential complexities of nurse caring and challenges the idea that caring can only be known epistemologically. Instead, he posits eleven perspectives which he constructs as "threads," that together reveal the essential nature of caring. These eleven threads he names as the ontological thread, the philosophical pattern, the personal knowing thread, the epistemological thread, the practical thread, the expertise thread, the ethical thread, the existential thread, the relational thread, the systems thread,and the transforming thread.

Feminist and nurse, Falk Rafael (1996), suggests that caring may be considered either "ordered caring, assimilated caring, or empowered caring" (p. 4). She proposes that ordered caring is problematic for nurses, being merely about following orders and allowing "only a severely limited scope of caring, one that is devoid of knowledge, power or ethics" (p. 11). To illustrate this point, Falk Rafael points out the kindness and gentleness shown by nurses toward psychiatric patients as they were led towards the Nazi gas chambers. Assimilated caring is described as a form of caring in which the feminine construct of caring is grounded in (male) scientific discourses. This appropriation of a male construct is proposed as giving legitimacy to the essentially female activity of caring.[2] Falk Rafael positions empowered caring as the most desirable and effective form of caring. This form of caring is grounded within a feminist perspective, and involves the use of power, knowledge, and ethics. Falk Rafael (1996) proposes the acronym of CARE (credentials, association, research, expertise) to encapsulate the elements of this empowered caring.

Holistic caring, another form of nurse caring, has been proposed by Williams (1997) as a global concept with four dimensions, which she calls physical caring, interpretive caring, spiritual caring, and sensitive caring. Holism is viewed as a concept crucial to the effective practice of nursing. It is the term used to describe the belief that a patient is a person with social, physical, mental, and spiritual components (Williams, 1997). Holism is positioned as central to notions of professional

---

[2]For more about the gendered nature of caring, see Chapter 11.

caring, and is so intrinsic that it is often taken for granted or viewed as a given. Therefore, it often is not described or examined in discussions on professional caring. The use of a holistic perspective is said to facilitate an ethos that recognizes the uniqueness and value inherent in individuals, and allows for the provision of individualized nursing care.

DIFFERENTIATING PROFESSIONAL AND INFORMAL CARING

The importance placed on the concept of caring in nursing has seen many attempts by nurses to construct the notion of "professional caring." What is essentially a subjective, intimate, and personal construct has been turned into one that is professional, objective, and able to be readily achieved between strangers. No matter how desirable it may be to position caring as the essence of nursing, there is inherent difficulty with reconstructing caring so as to make it a professional characteristic unique to nursing and nurses. Caring is an attribute intrinsic to human existence. It is not unique to, or especially connected with, nursing (Morse, Solberg, Neander, Bottorf, & Johnson, 1990; Webb, 1996).

In order to support the assertion that caring is the essence of nursing, one needs to be able to reconstruct caring as a professional characteristic that is different and superior to unpaid family-based or "informal caring."[3] In an exploration of women's caring in personal and family situations, Wuest (1997) interviewed twenty-one women from diverse social backgrounds who were involved in informal caring. The caring behavior of these women was found to consist of "connectedness, availability and responsibility." These "caring connections were maintained through acts of nurturance, attending and being with" (p. 51). These findings have similarities to the constructions of professional caring held by nurses (Swanson, 1993), suggesting that caring in and of itself is not unique to nurses. As suggested by Falk Raphael (1996), the knowledge and particular skills held by nurses permit a particular type of caring that complements and supports the informal caring given by carers in the community who have a personal relationship with the recipients of their care.

---

[3]*Informal caring* is a term used to describe the nature of caring available to people through their own social or family networks; for example, care provided by mothers, fathers, spouses, siblings, and other loved ones.

EXPERIENCING NURSE CARING

Defining caring as a concept central to nursing is not only important for the discipline itself, but is highly relevant to the recipients of our care, that is, our patients and potential patients. However, patients and members of the wider community are often not included in these discussions. Nevertheless, if nurses claim to be caring professionals who have the desire to provide care that is effective and meaningful to patients, we really need to find out what nurse caring means to patients and communities of people. Thus, we may develop better understandings about patients' care needs and expectations.

Kralik, Koch, and Wootton's (1997) study of patients' experiences of being nursed revealed that nurses deliver care in a manner that can be described as "detachment" or "engagement." Engagement captured psychosocial qualities, including compassion, kindness, cheerfulness, availability, gentleness, and friendliness, while detachment reflected negative characteristics, such as feeling depersonalized and being treated roughly by nurses. Though nursing was examined from the perspective of patients, the study revealed some consistencies between patients' views and ideas about nurse caring, and those held by nurses.

In a pilot study, Dyson (1996) aimed to elicit constructions of behaviors and attitudes that embody caring from the perspective of registered nurses. Findings revealed that nurses in the study conceptualized caring as essentially an interpersonal construct and considered attributes such as kindness, friendliness, sensitivity, consideration, giving of self, honesty, sincerity, and expertise as evidence of caring attitudes and behaviors. Similarly, Wolf (1986) described nurse-identified caring behaviours such as attentive listening, comforting, and honesty. Twelve years later, a study of patients and nurses aimed at exploring their perceptions of the importance of caring behaviors revealed significant differences between the views of patients and nurses, with nurses placing a higher value on the emotional affective aspects of caring than patients (Larssen, Peterson, Lampic, von Essen, & Sjoden, 1998). Webb (1996) also found that nurses judged the interpersonal aspects of their work as more caring, while patients were found to value technical know-how and clinical competence above interpersonal dimensions of caring. By contrast, the nurses perceived clinical competence as a given and do not regard it as an indicator of nurse caring (Webb, 1996).

The differences in perceptions of caring between nurses and patients is worthy of consideration. In Western industrialized societies, technological skills and expertise are viewed as high-status and the domain of "professionals." In times of vulnerability, such as when people are ill, they like to be assured they are in the care of competent health professionals, and perhaps view technological proficiency as evidence of such competence and expertise. The interpersonal aspects of caring so highly idealized by nurses may be viewed by patients as nonprofessional caring, or the type of caring available to them within their own social worlds (informal caring). As Pepin (1992) states, caring that occurs at home differs from caring that occurs in institutions (such as hospitals), since it is mainly affective in nature.

META-ANALYSES OF CARING SCIENCE IN NURSING

Sherwood (1997) conducted a meta-analysis of 16 qualitative studies of caring in nursing literature. Her work attempted to develop an outcome-based operational model of caring through a meta-synthesis that aggregated findings from all 16 studies. Four essential patterns of outcomes emerged and these four patterns related to:

- Caring interactions
- Caring knowledge
- Intentional response
- Therapeutic outcomes

From the 16 qualitative studies on caring, it was found that caring cannot be split into formal parts such as being versus doing, instrumental versus expressive, what the nurse does and how, how much the nurse does, or technology versus human touch. Caring knowledge is about a way of being that encompasses diverse ways of knowing, being, and doing into one integrated whole. It cannot be isolated and fragmented.

Swanson (1999) conducted a meta-analysis of data-based investigations of the concept of caring, including interpretive and empiric-analytic investigations. Her work reviewed 130 publications between 1980 and 1996; these publications included data from 2,314 participants. She categorized these empirically based, nursing research findings into five levels:

- **Capacities**—found empirically to include compassionate, empathic, knowledgeable, positive and reflective capacities

- **Commitments/concerns**—found empirically to include recognition of dignity and worth of each person, focus on the other's experience, connection with other, doing the right thing, and being present to the self
- **Conditions**—found empirically to include: *patient-related conditions,* i.e., communication, personality, health problems, care needs, nurse-patient relationship, patient attractiveness, and status; *nurse-related conditions,* including personal and professional resources, constraints, and demands; and *organization-related conditions,* i.e., personnel or role related, technology, administration, work or practice conditions
- **Caring Actions**—which were categorized under Swanson's original middle range theory of caring and placed within her organizing framework: *maintaining belief; knowing; being with; doing for; enabling*
- **Consequences**—which were about outcomes or consequences of caring or noncaring. These findings parallel the work of Halladorts-dottir (1999) whose work on caring and noncaring reaffirmed the vivid imagery of "caring as a bridge," which implies reaching out to others to address their care needs. By contrast, a noncaring stance or behaviour is perceived as "a wall," which implies closing off the human connectedness that is associated with nursing caring.

These meta-analyses of caring data in the nursing literature confirm tangible aspects of caring and its nature and consequences (both positive and negative). These studies, when considered together, validate the moral/ethical aspects of caring, as well as the tangible outcomes of patient care and the effects on the nurse. In addition, the results of these meta-analyses offer both a celebration of empirical knowledge, as well as areas for further knowledge development.

CARE AND CURE

Rapid developments in medical science, nursing knowledge, and related health technologies have acted to dramatically improve patient outcomes. In most parts of the world, these same technologies have radically and permanently changed the face of nursing (Sandelowski, 1997). They have been the catalyst for a discussion in nursing and health, known as the "care/cure" debate. Johnston and Cooper (1997) have suggested that the health care system in the United States was initially designed to cure illness and disease, rather than care for people and their health. This is an important distinction that remains in many Western health care systems. This provides additional challenge for those whose main imperative is to care rather than cure.

Notions of care and cure have been constructed as dualistic and oppositional. However, it is the contention of several scholars that these two concepts are not truly antagonistic (see, for example, King & Norsen, 1994; Leftwich, 1993). The difference between the roles of nurse and physician are often centered around ideas of the nurse as caring and the physician as curing. Sullivan and Deane (1994) and similarly, Caffrey and Caffrey (1994) position caring (the domain of nursing) as a traditionally feminine activity that has not been conferred the power and status of more masculine defined activities, to which the physician/curer may more easily lay claim.

In 1990, Morse, Solberg, Neander, Bottorf, and Johnson posed the question, "Can a cure be realised without caring?" More than a decade later, this question remains worthy of consideration and discussion. Clearly, caring alone will not meet all the health needs patients have, but as Webb (1996) points out, curing strategies may be insufficient unless accompanied by a caring dimension. Williams (1997), too, suggests caring is, in itself, important to cure. She proposes that caring nurse behaviors have been demonstrated to have positive effects in terms of patients' wellness and, conversely, noncaring behaviors by nurses have been shown to negatively affect patient well-being and recovery.

Florence Nightingale (1859/1946) may well have rejected the idea that nurses have an essential curing role. In her book, *Notes on Nursing*, she states "nature alone cures" (p. 74), but goes on to say "what nursing has to do is to put the patient in the best position for nature to act upon him (sic)" (p. 75). More recently, in defining professional caring, nurses identify elements of both caring and curing, with certain science-based skills and knowledge identified as essential to caring (Beare & Meyers, 1994; Wolf, Giardino, Osborne, & Ambrose, 1994). We know that patients themselves expect nurses to have a high level of proficiency and technical skills, which are readily associated with "cure." However, and as previously discussed, technical proficiency and skill are key aspects of, and embedded within, notions of professional caring (Borbasi, 1996).

King and Norsen (1994) contend that notions of "care/cure" as solely the domain of either nurse (care) or physician (cure) are not helpful or acceptable. Nurses and physicians have both curing and caring dimensions to their practice areas. Webb (1996) urges nurses to overcome the care/cure dichotomy between medicine and nursing and argues it is no longer important to distinguish the care given by specific professional groups, but to focus instead on establishing clear goals of care. Rather than regarding notions of care and cure as being polarized, it is more accurate to say the notions of care/cure are compatible and complementary. Both are acknowledged and accepted as key aspects of nursing's agenda, and both are reflected in the theories of professional caring constructed by nurses.

CONTROVERSIES AND CONUNDRA

Far from being a simple concept, caring is revealed as complex and multidimensional. It remains controversial among members of the profession with the debate continuing about the centrality of caring to nursing (Dyson, 1996). There are conflicting trains of thought that challenge the relevance of caring as a foundational aspect of nursing. In a classic paper, Dunlop (1986) raised questions about whether a science of caring is possible, and resolved that, if it is, it will have to take a hermeneutical form—i.e., a "form that in many ways does violence to our traditional ideas of science," but one that "challenges the male hegemony of science" (p. 669). Nearly a decade later, Walker (1995) also highlighted problems with nurses' attempts to simultaneously represent nursing as both a discourse of science and a discourse of caring. Lea, Watson, and Dreary (1998) suggest that the difficulty in defining the relationship between caring and nursing arises (in part) because "caring and nursing [both] defy precise description" (p. 663) (see also, Kitson, 2003).

Concepts of caring, as they now stand, may be unrealistic and even unattainable, as nurses find it difficult to maintain the level and range of caring behaviors determined by some theories of nurse caring. There are many reasons for this, and again, they are issues that are confronting nurses globally. These issues include a diminishing workforce, patients that are sicker with increasingly complex needs, cultural issues, economic factors, and issues related to social and health policy. All these factors influence the amount of time that nurses can spend with patients, and the level of care we can provide.

The question of whether caring actually is consistent with the issue/s of power and/or professionalization in nursing is increasingly being addressed. Jenner (2002) cautions that "valorizing care" (p. 249) as the principal way that nurses contribute to healing, can mean that nurses become trapped and constrained, and has ramifications for nursing's ability to progress because, although caring is universally acknowledged as necessary and beneficial, it is in conflict with notions of autonomy. Furthermore, because caring is considered central to their practice, and is perceived as inconsistent with notions of power, nurses (who are mostly women) have been reluctant to acknowledge that power is productive. Though attempts have been made to combine the concepts of power and caring, there continues to be some natural friction between the two (Falk Rafael, 1996). Tensions between the concepts of caring and empowerment in relationships between patients and nurses are especially salient. Malin and Teasdale posed a question in 1991 that remains relevant to nurses today, that is, how does the caring professional avoid the cries of paternalism which come with clinical decisions about what is "best" for patients?. This question continues to confound.

Altruism is associated with caring (Pepin, 1992), but it is also problematic because it implies self-sacrifice. Searching for a way to forge a link between altruism and autonomy, Reverby (1987) contends that nurses seek to be allowed to have "caring with autonomy." Kitson (1987) argues that if nurses choose to align themselves with care rather than cure, with the nurturing processes rather than with technology and treatment, then they will need to identify how to organize and put into operation those skills they possess. Successful execution of the caring role is, she believes, "intimately bound up with having the necessary space to practise, sufficient room to manoeuvre and to be able to explore new areas of knowledge and expertise" (p. 324).

The emergence of differing perspectives about the nature of nursing has not been without debate. Some believe that an emphasis on, and alliance to, concepts such as caring and holism, with their attendant rejection of the natural sciences, will do more harm than good to nursing's attempts to become a credible academic discipline and to the process of professionalization. Meeting the demands of the caring imperative that is concerned with cure requires that nurses have considerable knowledge of a range of scientific disciplines such as pharmacology, anatomy, physiology, biochemistry, immunology, microbiology, and physics. Given the need for continued development of the discipline and the need to meet the demands of increasingly technological societies, a sound scientific knowledge base is undeniably essential for nursing. A sound working knowledge of, and competency in, a number of the scientific disciplines is an essential aspect of nursing knowledge and is integral to the caring imperative claimed by nursing.

THREATS TO CARING

The concept of caring is inherently incompatible with the underlying objectives of many of the organizational structures in which nurses find themselves. In many parts of the (Western) world, health care is not intrinsically altruistic; nor is it based on any real system of equity (Duffield & Lumby, 1994). Rather, health care tends to be resourced on a fee for service basis, and access to health care services is, therefore, linked very strongly with an individual's ability to pay for such services. In many instances, health care is looked at with entrepreneurial rather than philanthropic eyes. To investors, provision of health care services may represent an opportunity for profit, and even "whilst appropriating the language and images of nursing for business purposes, many entrepreneurs treat professional nursing care as a commodity to be whittled away until it becomes impotent" (Jackson & Raftos, 1997, p. 38).

This positioning of the wealth of an individual as a major indicator for allocation of (increasingly scarce) health resources is, by its very nature, incompatible with nursing's caring imperative (Williams, 1997). Though low socioeconomic status is not the only factor that influences health and health care disparities, it is increasingly evident "that persons of marginalized cultures and ethnicities are over-represented among the poor all over the world" (Jackson, 2003, p. 347). Because nurses view nursing and health care as resources to be allocated on the basis of need rather than ability to pay, tensions in relation to social inequity and health arise. These tensions are inherent to the working life of many nurses, and compromise the ability of nurses to provide care in the way idealized by the profession.

Although nurses comprise the largest occupational/professional group within the health care system, the system itself is based on a set of values that directly challenge and compromise the very essence of nursing. The health care system is shaped by economic influences such as cost containment and profit margins. This economic impetus has been the catalyst for reexamining the whole concept of "patient care." Attempts have been made to reconceptualize traditional care delivery by coming up with ways of doing more with fewer resources (Johnston &

Cooper, 1997). These new approaches in provision of care are sometimes presented as strategies to improve the quality of patient care but, as Williams (1997) suggests, more frequently they are concerned with institutional and governmental cost-saving.

This key philosophical difference between nursing's caring imperative and the underlying ethos of many (Western) health care systems throws nurses and health administrators into a permanent state of conflict, and has the potential to become a source of professional tension for nurses (Jackson & Raftos, 1997; Johnston & Cooper, 1997; Kralik, Koch, & Wootton, 1997). Large, impersonal institutions may, by their very nature, devalue caring by providing little incentive or opportunity for nurses to demonstrate behaviors associated with caring, or failing to provide an environment where caring can be expressed (Morse, Solberg, Neander, Bottorf, & Johnson, 1990).

Ray (1989) attempted to reconcile the seemingly irreconcilable by proposing a theory of caring compatible with the bureaucratic cultures existing within large organizations. She suggests that it is essential for the discipline of nursing to come to terms with the corporatization of health care, and goes on to indicate that a failure to do so would be disastrous for nursing:

> The transformation of American and other western healthcare systems to corporate enterprises emphasizing competitive management and economic gain seriously challenges nursing's humanistic philosophies and theories and nursing's administrative and clinical practices. The recent refocusing of nursing as a human science and the art and science of human caring places nursing in a vulnerable position. When pitted against the new goal of corporate advancement in healthcare delivery, nursing faces a loss of self-identity and an increased risk of alienation and confusion in this competitive arena. (p. 31)

Using a grounded theory approach, Ray (1989) generated a "theory of the dynamic structure of caring in a complex organization" (p. 31), and proposes this as a means by which nurses can practice within bureaucratic health structures without compromising nursing's caring imperative. This theory proposes several "structural caring categories," which she names as political, economic, legal, technological/physiological, educational, social, spiritual/religious, and ethical. However, Caffrey and Caffrey (1994) suggest that caring will never be accommodated as a core value while profit remains a primary motive of health care systems.

The truth of this statement is evident in a paper exploring the experience of whistleblowers, registered nurses who attempted to challenge managerial practices which severely compromised the standard of care provided to residents of a long-term care institution (Jackson & Raftos, 1997). These nurses described the struggle to maintain their professional integrity by ensuring adequate levels of care, and how they were thwarted in these attempts by management. The nurses were prevented from providing adequate care by forces external to nursing—forces driven by an economic (rather than a caring) agenda. This suggests that, certainly in some settings, nurses have not yet achieved the level of autonomy necessary for the provision of acceptable professional care based on approved standards.

CONCLUSION

Caring is proclaimed and understood as the basis of modern nursing, and nurses have produced vast amounts of literature on aspects of care and caring, and how they may be applied in a nursing context. However, while the concept of professional caring remains difficult to articulate, it is recognized as a complex concept involving the development of a range of knowledge, skills, and expertise. Professional caring has similarities with nonprofessional or informal caring and applies knowledge derived from various disciplines to promote the health and well-being of people.

The major perspectives of caring recognize the importance of various types of knowledge and, with few exceptions, all allude to the expressive, artistic, and scientific perspectives said to construct nursing. Other common themes that characterize the constructions of caring adopted by nurses are holism, compassion, empathy, and communication. Evidence suggests that patients, too, view caring as a perceptible concept and value it highly as an essential and healing aspect of their professional encounters with nurses. However, in contrast to the ways nurses view caring, reflection on what is known about patients' attitudes to nurse caring suggests that, above all, patients want a nurse who demonstrates caring through clinical and technical competence, as well as through interpersonal skills.

Accepting caring as the basis of nursing practice and scholarship is not without problems. Issues of autonomy and power do not fit easily with the concept of caring. Servitude and altruism are intrinsically linked to caring, and these do not enhance nursing's move to professionalism. Many nurses work within organizational structures whose primary motivation lies with in cost containment or the accumulation of wealth rather than a mandate to heal. These economic factors may compromise or even be antithetical to nursing's imperative to care. The caring imperative therefore represents a potential source of stress and occupational conflict for nurses. While it is argued that the need for nursing to place caring as a central concept has never been greater, there are nevertheless concerns that the caring components of nursing are deemed unsophisticated and hence inferior to the therapeutic interventions of medicine and other allied health service providers.

Despite the many creative theories of nurse caring, the tasks of establishing coherent and clear connections between caring and notions such as professionalism, scholarship, and autonomy remain incomplete. Nurses are left with many issues to consider and debate. The conundrum of caring as the basis of nursing practice and scholarship will no doubt continue to captivate and confound nurses for many years to come.

REFLECTIVE QUESTIONS

1. Think for a moment about why you chose nursing as a career. Did the desire to care for people have any role in your decision?
2. Take some time to reflect on your experiences of caring for and being cared for. How would you define caring based on your experiences to date?
3. Consider the differences in the ways nurses and patients perceive nurse caring. What are some of the ways in which these varying perspectives may be more closely linked?
4. In nursing, how could the concept of caring be reconciled with professional concepts such as power and autonomy?
5. Will "caring science" emerge in the future as a stronger force nursing? Why? Why not?

RECOMMENDED READINGS

Greenhalgh, J., Vanhanen, L., & Kyngas, H. (1998). Nurse caring behaviours. *Journal of Advanced Nursing, 27*(5), 927–932.

Hallodorsdottir, S. (1991). Five basic modes of being with another. In D. A. Gaut & M. Leininger (Eds.), *Caring: The compassionate healer.* New York: National League for Nursing.

Swanson, K. (1999).What is known about caring in nursing science. In A. S. Hinshaw, S. Fleetham, & J. Shavere (Eds.), *Handbook of clinical nursing research.* Thousand Oaks, CA: Sage.

Watson, J., & Smith, M. (2002). Caring science and the science of unitary human beings: A transtheoretical discourse for nursing knowledge development. *Journal of Advanced Nursing, 37*(5), 452.

Wuest, J. (1997). Illuminating environmental influences on women's caring, *Journal of Advanced Nursing, 26,* 49–58.

REFERENCES

Astrom, G., Norberg, A., & Hallberg, I.R. (1995). 'Skilled nurses' experience of caring. *Journal of Professional Nursing, 11*(2), 110–118.

Beare, P., & Myers, J. (1994). *Principles and practice of adult health nursing.* St Louis: Mosby.

Benner, P. (1984). *From novice to expert: Excellence and power in clinical nursing.* California: Addison-Wesley.

Benner, P., Hooper-Kyriakidis, P., & Stannard, D. (1999). *Clinical wisdom and interventions in critical care: A thinking-in-action approach.* Philadelphia: W. B. Saunders.

Borbasi, S-A. (1996). Living the experience of being nursed: A phenomenological text. *International Journal of Nursing Practice, 2*(4), 222–228.

Caffrey, R., & Caffrey, P. (1994). Nursing: Caring or codependent? *Nursing Forum, 29*(1), 12–17.

Dunlop, M. (1986). Is a science of caring possible? *Journal of Advanced Nursing, 11*(3), 661–670.

Duffield, C., & Lumby, J. (1994). Caring nurses: The dilemma of balancing costs and quality. *Australian Health Review, 17*(2), 72–83.

Dyson, J. (1996). Nurses' conceptualizations of caring attitudes and behaviours. *Journal of Advanced Nursing, 23,* 1263–1269.

Falk Rafael, A. (1996). Power and caring: A dialectic in nursing. *Advances in Nursing Science, 19*(1), 3–17.

Hallodorsdottir, S. (1999). The effects of uncaring. *Reflections Magazine, International Sigma Theta Tau, Fourth quarter,* 28–30.

Jenner, E. A. (2002). *The paradox of care in the 21st Century: An analysis of the stereopticon of gender, popular media, and nursing.* Unpublished doctoral thesis, University of Illinois at Urbana-Champaign.

Jackson, D., & Raftos, M. (1997). In uncharted waters: Confronting the culture of silence in a residential care institution. *International Journal of Nursing Practice, 3*(1), 34–39.

Jackson, D. (2003). Culture, health and social justice. *Contemporary Nurse, 15*(3), 347–348.

Johns, C. (2001). Reflective practice: Revealing the [he]art of caring. *International Journal of Nursing Practice, 7*, 237–245.

Johnston, C., & Cooper, P. (1997). Patient-focused care: What is it? *Holistic Nursing Practice, 11*(3), 1–7.

King, K., & Norsen, L. (1994). The care/cure, nurse/physician dichotomy doesn't do it anymore. *IMAGE: Journal of Nursing Scholarship, 26*(2), 89.

Kitson, A. L. (1987). Raising standards of clinical practice:The fundamental issue of effective nursing practice. *Journal of Advanced Nursing, 12*(3), 321–329.

Kitson, A. (2003). A comparative analysis of lay caring and professional (nursing) caring relationships. *International Journal of Nursing Studies, 40*(5), 503–510.

Kralik, D., Koch, T., & Wootton, K. (1997). Engagement and detachment: Understanding patients experiences with nursing. *Journal of Advanced Nursing, 26*(2), 399–407.

Larsson, G., Peterson, V., Lampic, C., von Essen, L., & Sjoden, P. (1998). Cancer patients and staff ratings of the importance of caring behaviours and their relations to patient anxiety and depression. *Journal of Advanced Nursing, 27*(4), 855–864.

Lea, A., Watson, R., & Dreary, I. (1998). Caring in nursing: A multivariate analysis. *Journal of Advanced Nursing, 28*(3), 662–671.

Leininger, M. (1984). *Care: The essence of nursing and health.* Detroit, MI: Wayne State University Press.

Leftwich, R. (1993). Care and cure as healing processes in nursing. *Nursing Forum, 28*(3), 13–17.

Malin, N., & Teasdale, K. (1991). Caring versus empowerment: Considerations for nursing practice. *Journal of Advanced Nursing, 16*, 657–662.

Morse, J., Solberg, S., Neander, W., Bottorf, J., & Johnson, J. (1990). Concepts of caring and caring as a concept. *Advances in Nursing Science, 13*(1), 1–14.

Nightingale, F. (1859/1946). *Notes on nursing.* London: Harrison Book Company.

Pepin, J. (1992). Family caring and caring in nursing. *IMAGE: Journal of Nursing Scholarship, 24*(2), 127–131.

Rawnsley, M. (1990). Of human bonding: The context of nursing as caring. *Advances in Nursing Science, 13*(1), 41–48.

Ray, M. (1989). The theory of bureaucratic caring for nursing practice in the organizational structure. *Nursing Science Quarterly, 13*(2), 31–42.

Reverby, S. (1987). A caring dilemma: Womanhood and nursing in historical perspective. *Nursing Research, 36*(1), 5–11.

Sandelowski, M. (1997). (Ir)reconcilable differences?: The debate concerning nursing and technology. *IMAGE: Journal of Nursing Scholarship, 29*(2), 169–174.

Sherwood, G. D. (1997). Metasynthesis of qualitative analyses of caring: Defining a therapeutic model of nursing. *Advances in Nursing Science, 3*(1), 32–42.

Soanes, C., & Stevenson, A. (2003). *Oxford Dictionary of English.* Oxford: Oxford University Press.

Sullivan, J., & Deane, D. (1994). Caring: Reappropriating our tradition. *Nursing Forum, 29*(2), 5–9.

Swanson, K. (1993). Nursing as informed caring for the well-being of others. *IMAGE: Journal of Nursing Scholarship, 25*(4), 352–357.

Swanson, K. (1999). What is known about caring in nursing science. In A. S. Hinshaw, S. Fleetham, & J. Shavere (Eds.), *Handbook of Clinical Nursing Research.* Thousand Oaks, CA: Sage.

Walker, K. (1995). Courting competency: Nursing and the politics of performance in practice. *Nursing Inquiry, 2*(2), 90–99.

Walters, A. J. (1994). *Caring as a theoretical construct.* Armidale: University of New England Press.

Watson, J. (1985). *Nursing: The philosophy and science of caring.* Boulder: Colorado Associated University Press.

Watson, J. (1988). *Nursing: Human science and human care: A theory of nursing.* New York: National League for Nursing.

Webb, C. (1996). Caring, curing, coping: Towards an integrated model. *Journal of Advanced Nursing, 23,* 960–968.

Williams, S. (1997). Caring in patient-focused care: The relationship of patients' perceptions of holistic nurse care to their levels of anxiety. *Holistic Nursing Practice, 11*(3), 61–68.

Wolf, Z. R. (1986). The caring concept and nurse identified caring behaviours. *Topics in Clinical Nursing, 8*(2), 84–93.

Wolf, Z., Giardino, E., Osborne, P., & Ambrose, M. (1994). Dimensions of nurse caring. *IMAGE: Journal of Nursing Scholarship, 26*(2), 107–111.

Wuest, J. (1997). Illuminating environmental influences on women's caring. *Journal of Advanced Nursing, 26,* 49–58.
Woodward, W. (2003). Preparing a new workforce. *Nursing Administration Quarterly, 27*(3), 215–222.

7

Nursing Theory

F. Beryl Pilkington and Debra A. Bournes

LEARNING OBJECTIVES

Upon completion of this chapter, readers will be able to:

- Discuss the difference between the discipline and the profession of nursing
- Appreciate the history of nursing theory
- Identify different paradigmatic perspectives in nursing
- Articulate the importance of nursing theory
- Demonstrate an understanding of how nursing theory can guide practice
- Begin the process of choosing a nursing theory to guide practice

KEY WORDS

Theory, concept, model, philosophy, paradigm

INTRODUCTION

Over the past half century, nursing has evolved as a field of study that requires formal education to master. As a field of study, nursing has a body of knowledge that is unique to nursing. This theoretical knowledge was developed to guide nursing practice, education, and research, such that members of the nursing profession can be equipped to provide the kind of service that is needed and valued by society. And yet, for various reasons that are beyond the scope of this chapter, nursing theory often does not get the attention it deserves in nursing education. Suffice it to say, that it is our premise that a basic understanding of nursing theory is essential to prepare nurses to provide nursing service that is meaningful and responsive to societal needs.

The chapter begins with a discussion of why nursing theory matters, which we felt was a logical starting point. We then briefly explain what a theory is, before proceeding to a discussion of the phenomena of concern to nursing. As we point out, delineating the phenomena of concern to nursing is important because that is what determines the focus of nursing theories. Next, we provide a brief synopsis of the history of nursing theory development, so that the reader can appreciate the progress that has been made to date. We then turn our attention to a discussion of nursing paradigms. Here, we show how the various nursing theories can be organized into groups according to similarities and differences in their world views. Next, we talk about how to choose a nursing theory. Finally, to illustrate how one's choice of theory makes a difference in practice, we offer a brief case study followed by an illustration of how a nurse would be guided using two alternative theories, Parse's theory of human becoming and the Roy adaptation model.

This chapter does not provide in-depth information about any particular nursing theory; however, we hope that it will inspire you to further investigate different theories so that you can find one that you would like to use to guide your practice. To that end, as you read this chapter, think about the kind of nurse you want to be, and the kind of nurse you would want for yourself or your family member if you required nursing care. We begin by inviting you to consider why nursing theory matters.

WHY NURSING THEORY MATTERS

For over a century, a formal education has been required in order to become a nurse, a fact that begs the following questions: What is it that nurses learn in school? What is the knowledge that guides nursing practice? and What is the nature of nursing knowledge? To answer such questions, it is necessary to differentiate between nursing as a discipline and nursing as a profession (for example, see Nunnery, 1997; Parker,

2001; Parse, 1999). According to Parse (1999), the discipline of nursing is the knowledge base (nursing theories), and the profession consists of those who are guided in their practice by the knowledge base. The profession is "persons educated in the discipline according to nationally regulated, defined, and monitored standards . . . set up to preserve health care safety for members of society" (Parse, 1999, p. 275). Members of the profession are responsible for regulation and standards of practice and education based on disciplinary knowledge (Parse, 1999). In the case of nursing, the knowledge required by members of the profession is very broad in scope, encompassing knowledge from the natural sciences, medicine, the social sciences, ethics, and law, as well as nursing theoretical knowledge. For instance, nurses must know about acute and chronic health conditions and they must have expertise in administering medications, performing diagnostic tests and procedures, and operating various machines. In other words, nurses must, without a doubt, be able to provide safe, competent, medical care. But, as Mitchell and Cody (1999) point out, the delivery of health care services is facilitated and improved when medical science is complemented by unique nursing knowledge, and this resides in nursing theory. Unique nursing knowledge is essential for establishing nursing's distinct contribution to health care.

Unfortunately, what nurses learn in school continues to focus heavily on knowledge from other disciplines and hardly on nursing theory. Practicing nurses often say that they do not use any particular theory; and yet, all knowledge is inherently theoretical. And so, although many nurses may not recognize the source of their theoretical views, close examination of their practice would show that their knowledge is drawn primarily from medical science, with a smattering of psychology and social science theory. What this means is that nurses often find it difficult to articulate to others what nursing is and, thus, feel invisible and undervalued, even though they may know on a personal level that they make a significant difference to the health and wellbeing of those in their care (Krejci, 1995).

Being able to articulate our unique contribution is crucially important if we expect nursing to be regarded as a discipline and a profession. Nursing theoretical knowledge can guide nurses in talking about their contribution to the health care team. When nurses are unable to articulate what nursing is, they are in danger of being viewed merely as substitute labor, as the sociologist Lindsay (cited in Lindsay, Twohig, & McGillis-Hall, 2003) called nurses at a recent national symposium. In her presentation of a study about the ways health professionals work together, or fail to work together, Lindsay cited examples of nurse practitioner and nurse anaesthetist participants who described things like "being given patients while the doctor goes golfing." It is no wonder, then, that she used the term *substitute labor* when referring to nurses who take on the medical and technical tasks that others, mostly the physicians, do not want to do.

What does this mean for nursing as a discipline and as a profession? What is our unique nursing focus? What makes our presence essential? What is going to stop any health professional from taking on our role? The fact that nursing is often invisible in its work underscores the importance of nurses knowing about, understanding, and committing to nursing theory as a guide to practice.

WHAT IS A THEORY?

Theories represent the formal knowledge of a discipline—that is, the knowledge that can be shared with others. Dictionary definitions of the word theory include the following: "the analysis of a set of facts in their relation to one another . . . abstract thought . . . the general or abstract principles of a body of fact, a science, or an art . . . a plausible or scientifically acceptable general principle or body of principles offered to explain phenomena" (Mish, 1999, p. 1223). These definitions indicate that theories are abstract representations consisting of a set of interrelated concepts and principles that describe, explain, or predict some phenomenon or phenomena.

Concepts provide the building blocks of theories. A concept is "an abstract or generic idea generalized from particular instances" (Mish, 1999, p. 238). Concepts can be more or less abstract. For instance, the concepts, *John Smith, person,* and *human being,* range from very specific to very abstract, but they all refer to the same kind of entity. This example shows how that the more abstract a concept is, the more encompassing it is of particular instances. A theory defines the concepts that are important to understanding some phenomenon of interest and specifies how these concepts are interrelated. The statements that specify the interrelationship of concepts are called *principles* or *propositions.*

Just like concepts, theories can also be more or less abstract and at the same time, they vary in scope. On that basis, Fawcett (2002) has classified the works generated by American theorists (in descending order of abstraction) as either philosophies, conceptual models, grand theories, or mid-range theories. According to her, conceptual models are very abstract or general, while grand theories are "broad in scope and substantively nonspecific; their concepts and propositions are relatively abstract. Middle-range theories, in contrast, are more circumscribed and substantively specific; their concepts and propositions are relatively concrete" (p. 501). However, there is no consensus in the nursing theory literature on how extant theoretical works should be classified with regard to level of abstraction and scope. For instance, Marriner, Tomey, and Alligood (2002) categorize Jean Watson's theory of human caring as a philosophy, while Fawcett (2000) calls it a middle-range theory. For the sake of simplicity, in this chapter, we will refer to all theoretical formulations in nursing as theories. Now that we have established what a theory is, we will turn our attention to the phenomena of concern in nursing theories.

PHENOMENA OF CONCERN TO NURSING

The term *phenomenon* indicates an object or event that is perceptible through the senses (Mish, 1999). Every discipline generates theories in order to describe, explain, or predict the *phenomena* that are of central concern to it. A number of nurse scholars have undertaken to delineate the central phenomena and, hence, the boundaries, of the discipline of nursing. This is an important project, because it shows nurses and others what nursing knowledge is about and the nature of nursing's contribution to human health and health care. For example, Kim's (2000) typology of theoretical thinking in nursing includes the domains of *client, client-nurse, practice,* and *environment.* Taking a more synthesized approach, Newman, Sime, and Corcoran-Perry (1991) described the focus of the discipline as "caring in the human health experience" (p. 3). Another formulation, offered by Parse (1997) is "the core focus of nursing . . . is the human-universe-health process" (p. 74). (The hyphens between the concepts are meant to indicate that they are a "unitary construct" (p. 74); that is, they are inseparably interrelated.)

Perhaps the most widely recognized representation of the phenomena of concern to nursing is that of the *metaparadigm* comprising the concepts of *person, environment, health,* and *nursing* (Fawcett, 1984, 2000). A metaparadigm is a broad, organizing framework for a discipline.

Fawcett (2000) proposed that a metaparadigm for nursing ought to a) identify a domain that is distinctive from the domains of other disciplines; b) encompass all phenomena of interest to the discipline in a parsimonious manner; c) be perspective-neutral; and d) be international in scope and substance. She went on to argue that her metaparadigm schema meets all of the above criteria, whereas other classifications of nursing phenomena do not. However, close examination of her propositions, which state how the four metaparadigm concepts are interrelated, reveals that they are not perspective-neutral (Bunkers, 2002). Indeed, all existing representations of a metaparadigm for nursing appear to reflect the world view of their proponents. That this is so attests to the reality that, as humans, our efforts to know and understand things are shaped by what we already know and believe (Mezirow, 1991).

We have been looking at the phenomena of concern to nursing because that seems a logical starting point for exploring nursing theories. We will now briefly overview the historical evolution of nursing theories.

HISTORY OF NURSING THEORY

Florence Nightingale is often called the first nurse theorist. She envisioned nursing as a human service based on knowledge that was different from that of medicine and which required education to learn (Dunphy, 2001). Although Nightingale (1859/1992) did not set forth a theory per se, her *Notes on Nursing* certainly laid the groundwork for theoretical development in the discipline. There, she wrote:

> The very elements of what constitutes good nursing are as little understood for the well as for the sick. The same laws of health or of nursing, for they are in reality the same, obtain among the well as among the sick. (p. 6)

Nightingale was the first to suggest the metaparadigm of nursing by pointing out the interconnection between persons, their environment, and health (Dunphy, 2001). For her, nursing "ought to signify the proper use of fresh air, light, warmth, cleanliness, quiet, and the proper selection and administration of diet—all at the least expense of vital power to the patient" (Nightingale, 1859/1992, p. 6). In her view, the goal of nursing was to enable persons to maintain or restore health by managing the environment and putting persons in the best condition for nature to act upon them (Nightingale, 1859/1992).

Since Nightingale's day, American nurse scholars have led the way in developing theoretical knowledge in nursing. That is perhaps because as early as the 1930s, some American nurses were obtaining higher education. At the time, graduate education was only available in other disciplines. However, nurses who obtained higher education became interested in developing and specifying nursing knowledge, in order to advance nursing education and nursing practice. One of the pioneers who sought to establish the uniqueness of nursing is Virginia Henderson. Her definition of nursing, first published in 1955, is still quoted around the world (Gordon, 2001). Sometimes called the twentieth century Florence Nightingale, Henderson identified the components of basic nursing care according to needs for healthful living. She is also known for advocating that nurses evaluate the quality of nursing care from the perspective of patients (Gordon, 2001). Another pioneer, Hildegard Peplau (1952/1991), emphasized the centrality of the nurse-person relationship in nursing practice, regardless of the setting.

Following the establishment of graduate education in nursing, there was a wave of theoretical developments in the 1970s and 1980s. Perhaps the most innovative thinker of her time was Martha E. Rogers, whose *Introduction to the Theoretical Basis of Nursing* (1970) described humans as irreducible energy fields that are coextensive with the environmental field. Rogers' world view of nursing, known as the *Science of Unitary Human Beings* (Malinski & Barrett, 1994), was radically different from that of her contemporaries, who were heavily influenced by the dominant model of medical science. Rogers' influence shows up in the works of contemporary theorists Rosemarie Rizzo Parse (1981, 1998), Margaret Newman (2000), and, to some extent, Jean Watson (1985, 1999), although the work of each theorist is quite distinct. Other theorists (King, 1981; Neuman, 1995; Roy, 1976) borrowed concepts from the natural and social sciences to synthesize theories unique to nursing.

Despite the burgeoning of theory development in nursing in the 70s and 80s, nurse scholars often encountered resistance when trying to publish in clinical and research journals, a reality that led Rosemarie Rizzo Parse to establish *Nursing Science Quarterly* in 1988. At that time it was the only journal devoted exclusively to advancing nursing theory in research, practice, and education. However, works related to nursing theories can be found today in a variety of nursing journals. An excellent Internet resource to access information about nurse theorists and their works is *The Nursing Theory Page* maintained by the Hahn School of Nursing, at the University of San Diego. The URL is http://www.san diego.edu/nursing/theory.

If you visit the Web site and browse through the information about the many nursing theories in existence, you will find that there are similarities and differences among them, which have led nurse scholars to attempt to classify nursing theories into various paradigmatic perspectives.

NURSING PARADIGMS

When examining the history of theory development in nursing, it is readily apparent that very different perspectives of nursing have emerged. These different perspectives are known as world views, or *paradigms. Merriam-Webster's Dictionary* (Mish, 1999) defines a paradigm as "a philosophical or theoretical framework of a scientific school or discipline within which theories, laws, and generalizations and the experiments [or research] performed in support of them are formulated" (p. 842). A paradigm, then, is a way of thinking about, and approaching the study of, the phenomenon/phenomena of concern to a discipline. It is the mark of a mature discipline that there is more than one paradigm, and indeed, such diversity leads to innovations in knowledge development that advance the discipline.

In *A Simpler Way,* a book about a new paradigm for understanding the organization of human endeavors, Wheatley and Kellner-Rogers (1996/1999) point out that "no one knows what information an individual will choose to notice" (p. 82). This idea also applies to nursing, because no one knows what theoretical perspective an individual (practitioner, researcher, administrator, or educator) might choose to notice, to be inspired by, or to use. And yet, each individual's choices will significantly shape how s/he will engage in practice, research, administration, or education. That is why it is important to have different paradigmatic perspectives—*different perspectives lead to different ways of being, when lived out in practice, research, education, or administration.*

All disciplines have at least two paradigms. Psychology, for example, has psychoanalytic, behavioral, existential-phenomenological, and other paradigms that have given rise to distinctly different approaches to research and practice. Similarly, the discipline of nursing has at least two paradigms, and possibly three (as you will see below, it depends on the author), which specify different approaches to inquiry and practice.

There has been vigorous debate in the nursing literature about paradigms and how to delineate them (Cody, 1995, 2000; Mitchell & Cody, 1992; Thorne et al., 1998; Watson, 1985). This paradigm discourse originated with nurse scholars' attempts to identify and clarify the similarities and differences in the way that different theorists have represented nursing. Perhaps the first to attempt to classify nursing theories according to distinct paradigms was Parse (1987), who identified two paradigms: *simultaneity* and *totality*. Subsequently, Newman (1992) proposed three paradigms (*particulate-deterministic, integrative-interactive*, and *unitary-transformative*), and Fawcett (1993) proposed yet another three paradigms (*reaction, reciprocal interaction*, and *simultaneous action*). Each of these authors used somewhat different criteria to delineate paradigms, but with the same aim—to differentiate theoretical works on the basis of "philosophic claims about the nature of human beings and the human-environment relationship" (Fawcett, 1993, p. 56). Such philosophic claims reflect underlying beliefs and values, and therefore they are *ontological* claims, that is, they are concerned with the nature of reality or existence (Audi, 1995/1998).

To better understand how paradigms reflect philosophical assumptions, let's briefly examine the totality and simultancity paradigms (the theoretical schema for organizing nursing knowledge proposed by Parse in 1987). The assumptions about human beings and health that underpin these paradigms have evolved from different philosophical traditions (Parse, 1987) and thus, they provide distinct knowledge bases from which to conduct research and guide practice (Parse, 2000). The totality paradigm is grounded in contemporary empiricism (postpositivism), wherein it is assumed that "reality exists independent of any knower, and this reality is composed of separate, possibly related, building blocks that can be combined in myriad ways to form entities" (Bunkers, Petardi, Pilkington, & Walls, 1996, p. 34). Human beings are viewed as the sum of biological, psychological, sociological, and spiritual elements (or variables), and health is variously defined, for example, on a continuum from illness to wellness, as adaptation to stimuli, or as self-care ability. Nurses in the totality paradigm make judgments about health in comparison with predefined norms. Research focuses on discovering, predicting, and verifying causal relationships, so that predictability and control are viewed as both possible and desirable (Bunkers, Petardi, Pilkington, & Walls, 1996; Parse, 1981, 1987, 1998). Practice focuses on, for example, goal attainment (King, 2001), adaptation (Roy & Andrews, 1999), universal self-care requisites and demands (Orem, 1995), and conservation of energy (Levine, 1990).

In contrast, the assumptions about humans, universe, and health that underpin simultaneity paradigm theories are that humans are unitary (that is, indivisible, unpredictable, and ever changing) and in mutual process with the universe (Parse, 1987, 1998). The simultaneity paradigm is philosophically consistent with human science, as opposed to natural science. Dilthey was the first philosopher to use, and to define, the term *human science* (Polkinghorne, 1983). Dilthey believed that methods of inquiry used for knowledge development in the empirical science tradition wrongly ignore life as it is lived and experienced by human beings (Mitchell & Cody, 1992). He said that human sciences would fulfill their potential only if they were theoretically grounded in human experience (Mitchell & Cody, 1992). The assumptions underlying this definition of human science specify humans as intentional, free-willed, unitary wholes who continuously participate in life events and who interrelate with all aspects of their environments. Human experience is believed to be shaped by dynamic, temporal, historical, and cultural influences (Mitchell & Cody, 1992; Parse, 1981, 1998; Polkinghorne, 1983; Watson, 1985, 1999).

Human science focuses on the meanings, values, patterns, and relationships of humans as they experience them (Parse, 1981; Watson, 1985). For instance, in nursing, research with a human science perspective focuses on understanding life patterns (Newman, 2000), human-environment pattern manifestations (Butcher, 1996; Carboni, 1995; Cowling, 1998), and universal human lived experiences as they are described by individuals, families, or communities (Parse, 1998). No attempt is made to compare an individual's description with predefined norms or objective data. Whatever is disclosed by the person, family, or community is respected and accepted as their lived reality. As a human being, the researcher affects, and is affected by, the research process (Mitchell & Cody, 1992). Practice focuses on pattern appreciation (Cowling, 1990), health patterning (Barrett, 1998), pattern recognition (Newman, 2000), and quality of life from the person's, family's, and community's perspectives (Parse, 1981, 1998, 2003).

Regardless of how you classify nursing paradigms, it is irrefutable that the unique knowledge of the discipline of nursing is embedded in the diverse theories and frameworks set forth by nurses. Some examples of these theories and frameworks are the self-care deficit theory (Orem, 1995), the science of unitary human beings (Rogers, 1990), the theory of human caring (Watson, 1985, 1999), the theory of nursing as caring (Boykin & Schoenhofer, 2001), the Roy adaptation model

(Roy & Andrews, 1999), the theory of health as expanding consciousness (Newman, 2000), the human-becoming theory (Parse, 1981, 1998), the theory of goal attainment (King, 1981, 2001), humanistic nursing theory (Paterson & Zderad, 1976), the Neuman systems model (Neuman, 1995), the theory of culture care diversity (Leininger, 2001), and others. The depth and breadth of theoretical thinking in nursing is vast, but what all theories of nursing have in common is that, in some way, they explicate the nature of the human-universe-health interrelationship. As such, they provide unique knowledge bases from which to conduct research and practice—theories that, if known, understood, and embraced, can be *lived day by day* in practice situations, research projects, education opportunities, and administrative decisions.

The task of all nurses is to uncover their own beliefs in light of the assumptions about the human-universe-health process (or humans, health, environment, and nursing) embedded in existing nursing theories. Nurses must then choose the theoretical perspective that "represents [their] most profound beliefs about human beings and health" (Cody, 1999, p. 5). It is not that one theory is better than the other, but rather, they are different, and consequently lead to different modes of inquiry and different methods of practice (Parse, 2000).

Take, for instance, two concepts connected with nursing practice that come from different theories: *true presence* (Parse, 1981, 1998) and *caring* (Leininger, 2001; Watson, 1985, 1999). True presence is the term given to the mode of practice that emerges from the human-becoming school of thought (Parse, 1981, 1998). According to Parse (1981, 1998), true presence emerges in the nurse-person process as "a special way of 'being with' in which the nurse is attentive to moment-to-moment changes in meaning as she or he bears witness to the person's or group's own living of value priorities" (Parse, 1998, p. 71). Living true presence incarnates the nurse's beliefs that humans are unitary (that is unpredictable, indivisible, and ever changing), open, and free to choose meaning in any situation. It means embracing the belief that humans coexist and cocreate with others, ideas, objects, and situations at multidimensional realms of the universe (Parse, 1981, 1998); and, the belief that health is the way humans live daybyday a personal commitment to what is important for them (Parse, 1994).

Different from true presence, caring, as a mode of being in practice, emerges from multiple nursing perspectives (see, for example, Leininger, 2001; Watson, 1985, 1999) that guide practice and research in very distinct ways. For example, Leininger's ethnonursing focuses on *culture care patterns and values*, whereas Watson's view of caring focuses on *ontological caring competencies* and advanced caring-healing modalities (for example, therapeutic touch, meditation, and others) with the goal of promoting wholeness and health (defined as the harmony of body-mind-spirit). The challenge for all seasoned and novice nurses is to plumb the depths of their own values and beliefs about phenomena of concern to the discipline, and to carefully consider which of the theories has the potential to guide them in ways congruent with how they want to be known in nursing.

CHOOSING A THEORY

As already indicated, choosing a theory involves careful reflection upon one's values, beliefs, and assumptions in relation to those that underpin the various nursing theories, in order to discover which theory best reflects the way one wants to be known as a nurse. This reflective process exemplifies critical thinking, which is "carefully choosing a direction in light of personal tacit and explicit knowing" (Parse, 1996, p. 139); that is, it involves both rational and intuitive processes. With respect to choosing a theory, the rational aspect of choosing involves an examination of the logic of conceptual elements of different theories. Such examination requires reading some of the primary works written by a theorist of interest. In addition, textbooks that provide an analysis and evaluation of nursing theories (for example, Fawcett, 2000) can be helpful. The intuitive aspect of choosing entails sensing a *good fit* between one's own world view and that represented by a particular theory. Reading articles that show how particular theories guide practice or research can be especially helpful to the process of choosing a theory that reflects who one is and how one wants to be known as a nurse.

To give readers a flavor of how different theories guide practice differently, we present below the story of a young woman with cancer. Following the story, we describe how Parse's (1981, 1998) human-becoming theory and the Roy adaptation model (Roy & Andrews, 1999), respectively, can be used to focus nursing practice.

NURSING THEORIES IN PRACTICE

Margo Pronk's story (Pedwell, 1999) can be used to illustrate the way two different nursing theories could guide nurses' thinking and action.

Margo is a young woman with metastatic breast cancer. In March 1998, she was admitted to an intensive care unit when the tumors in her lungs made it difficult for her to breathe on her own. The doctors experimented with several medications but they came to the point that they did not know what else to do for her. "Here was this person hanging on to life because she loved it so much but she had so much wrong with her that she shouldn't have been living" (Pedwell, 1999, p. 88). Margo made it clear that she wanted to live. She was adamant that her "life [was] worth living" (Pedwell, 1999, p. 88). Margo's goal was to go home to the farm where she lived with her husband. In order to do so, and in spite of being told she was being unrealistic, she learned to use a home ventilator. Margo did not die that summer as everyone had thought she would. In fact, she had what she called her best summer ever. Margo said, "I always envisioned myself as healthy. I visualized being with my husband and doing the fun things we liked to do, like skiing and skating and dancing. . . . At first it was terrifying to be home . . . but soon we were pushing the barriers . . . the risks were important for me to take . . . we took the ventilator along on a canoeing and camping trip, and we even went sailing" (Pedwell, 1999, p. 88).

Practice Guided by the Human Becoming Theory

Parse's (1990, 1994, 1998) work guides nurses to view quality of life as what individuals say life is like for them, to view health as the way individuals live a commitment to what is important for them daytoday, and to make the goal of nursing quality of life from the person's, family's, and community's perspectives. Nurses guided by the human-becoming theory focus on practicing in ways that honor individuals' perspectives of health and quality of life. In this example, Margo was living her personal commitment to be at home and to spend time with the people, places, and activities she valued. She defined her own health and made it clear that her life was worth living. Guided by the human becoming theory, nurses practicing with Margo would not have focused on her medical prognosis (though they would certainly have been there to provide whatever medical-related care was necessary). Rather, nurses practicing with Margo would have focused on honoring her priorities and respecting her freedom to make choices about what was best for her and her family. In true presence (Parse, 1998), the nurses would be available to learn about Margo's hopes, wishes, and goals by listening intently and going with Margo as she talked about the meaning of her situation (illuminating meaning) and lived paradoxical experiences (for example, when Margo described being afraid but at the same time unafraid of what was happening, and feeling certain, yet at the same time uncertain, about what she wanted to do). And nurses would bear witness as Margo connected with patterns of relating with the people and ideas and objects and events in her life (synchronizing rhythms), and set in motion plans to go on with her life in the ways she considered most important (mobilizing transcendence) (Parse, 1998).

Practice Guided by the Roy Adaptation Model

The Roy adaptation model (RAM) (Roy, 1976; Roy & Andrews, 1999) guides nurses to view human beings as holistic, adaptive systems, and health as a state and process of being and becoming whole through adaptation. Humans are believed to respond to internal and external environmental stimuli through four adaptive modes (e.g., physiological, self-concept, role function, and interdependence). The goal of nursing is to promote and support the client's adaptive responses. In this example, the nurse would begin by doing a thorough assessment of Margo in relation to the four adaptive modes. Next, nursing diagnoses would be formulated that identified priority problems to be addressed by nurses. For example, in the physiological mode, one nursing diagnosis might consider the potential for inadequate respiration related to Margo's degree of mobility while using a home ventilator. In the self-concept mode, diagnoses might identify the potential for maladaptive coping and grieving related to Margo's apparently unrealistic expectations about her activity level and her possible denial of her approaching death. Guided by the RAM, nurses practicing with Margo would have created a nursing care plan that focused on supporting and promoting Margo's adaptive responses to the focal, contextual, and residual stimuli that were threatening her ability to adapt to her situation. For instance, with regard to the potential for inadequate respiration, a nursing intervention might be to design an education session for Margo and her spouse on how to perform emergency ventilation should the machine malfunction while they were away from home. And, in regard to the diagnoses concerning potential for maladaptive coping and grieving, nursing interventions could include encouraging Margo and her spouse to share their thoughts and feelings about her death and dying, and assisting them to identify the supports that they needed to help them cope. In addition, the nurse could refer them to counseling with a social worker or chaplain, if they agreed. Finally, the nurse would evaluate outcomes by comparing the progress that Margo had made toward meeting the expected outcomes as specified in the nursing care plan.

CONCLUSION

In this chapter, we have discussed how nursing is a discipline with a body of knowledge that is unique to nursing and that serves as a guide to nursing practice, research, education, and administration. (Although space did not permit us to explore the use of nursing theories except in practice, there is ample nursing literature on their application in these other areas.) Our intent was to provide readers with a basic understanding about the existing range of theories and some insight into how they can be used to guide practice and inquiry. We hope that this chapter is just a starting point and that you continue to investigate different theories. We are reasonably confident that there is a nursing theory awaiting your discovery that can help you on your journey to becoming the kind of nurse you want to be.

REFLECTIVE QUESTIONS

1. What will be the most important aspect of your work as a nurse?
2. What does health mean to you?
3. When you hear the word "patient," what ideas come to mind?
4. How might nursing theory help you set your priorities in nursing practice?

RECOMMENDED READINGS

Fawcett, J. (2002). *Analysis and evaluation of contemporary nursing knowledge: Nursing models and theories.* Philadelphia: F. A. Davis.

Mitchell, G. J., & Cody, W. K. (1992). Nursing knowledge and human science: Ontological and epistemological considerations. *Nursing Science Quarterly, 5,* 54–61.

Parker, M. (2001). *Nursing theories and nursing practice.* Philadelphia: F. A. Davis.

Parse, R. R. (1998). *The human becoming school of thought: A perspective for nurses and other health professionals.* Thousand Oaks, CA: Sage.

Watson, J. (1999). *Postmodern nursing and beyond.* New York: Churchill Livingston.

REFERENCES

Audi, R. (Ed.) (1998). *The Cambridge dictionary of philosophy.* New York: Cambridge University Press. (Original work published 1995)

Barrett, E. A. M. (1998). A Rogerian practice methodology for health patterning. *Nursing Science Quarterly, 11,* 136–138.

Boykin, A., & Schoenhofer, S. O. (2001). Nursing as caring. In M. Parker (Ed.), *Nursing theories and nursing practice.* Philadelphia: F. A. Davis.

Bunkers, S. S. (2002). Analysis and evaluation of contemporary nursing knowledge: Nursing models and theories. *Nursing Science Quarterly, 15,* 172–173.

Bunkers, S. S., Petardi, L. A., Pilkington, F. B., & Walls, P. A. (1996). Challenging the myths surrounding qualitative research in nursing. *Nursing Science Quarterly, 9,* 33–37.

Butcher, H. K. (1996). A unitary field pattern portrait of dispiritedness in later life. *Visions: The Journal of Rogerian Nursing Science, 4*(1), 41–58.

Carboni, J. T. (1995). The Rogerian process of inquiry. *Nursing Science Quarterly, 8,* 22–37.

Cody, W. K. (1995). About all those paradigms: Many in the universe, two in nursing. *Nursing Science Quarterly, 8,* 144–147.

Cody, W. K. (1999). Affirming reflection. *Nursing Science Quarterly, 12,* 4–6.

Cody, W. K. (2000). Paradigm shift or paradigm drift?: A meditation on commitment and transcendence. *Nursing Science Quarterly, 13,* 93–102.

Cowling, W. R. (1990). A template for unitary pattern-based nursing practice. In E. A. M. Barrett (Ed.), *Visions of Rogers' science-based nursing.* New York: National League for Nursing.

Cowling, W. R. (1998). Unitary case inquiry. *Nursing Science Quarterly, 11,* 139–141.

Dunphy, L. H. (2001). Florence Nightingale: Caring actualized: A legacy for nursing. In M. Parker (Ed.), *Nursing theories and nursing practice.* Philadelphia: F. A. Davis.

Fawcett, J. (1984). *Analysis and evaluation of conceptual models of nursing.* Philadelphia: F. A. Davis.

Fawcett, J. (1993). From a plethora of paradigms to parsimony in worldviews. *Nursing Science Quarterly, 6,* 56–58.

Fawcett, J. (2000). *Analysis and evaluation of contemporary nursing knowledge: Nursing models and theories.* Philadelphia: F. A. Davis.

Fawcett, J. (2002). *Analysis and evaluation of contemporary nursing knowledge: Nursing models and theories.* Philadelphia: F. A. Davis.

Gordon, S. C. (2001). Virginia Avenel Henderson: Definition of nursing. In M. Parker (Ed.), *Nursing theories and nursing practice.* Philadelphia: F. A. Davis.

Kim, H. S. (2000). *The nature of theoretical thinking in nursing* (2nd ed.). New York: Springer Publishing.

King, I. M. (1981). *A theory for nursing. Systems, concepts, process.* Albany, NY: Delmar.

King, I. M. (2001). Imogene M. King: Theory of goal attainment. In M. Parker (Ed.), *Nursing theories and nursing practice.* Philadelphia: F. A. Davis.

Krejci, J. W. (1995). Synchronous connections: Nursing's little secret. *Journal of Nursing Care Quality, 9*(4), 24–30.

Leininger, M. M. (2001). Theory of culture care diversity and universality. In M. Parker (Ed.), *Nursing theories and nursing practice.* Philadelphia: F. A. Davis.

Levine, M. E. (1990). Conservation and integrity. In M. Parker (Ed.), *Nursing theories in practice.* New York: National League for Nursing.

Lindsay, S., Twohig, P., & McGillis-Hall, L. (2003, November). Health human resources. Symposium conducted at the inaugural national symposium, Strengthening the Foundations: Health Services and Policy Research, of the Canadian Institutes of Health Research, Institute of Health Services and Policy Research, Montreal, Canada.

Malinski, V. M., & Barrett, E. A. (Eds.) (1994). *Martha E. Rogers: Her life and work.* Philadelphia: F. A. Davis.

Marriner Tomey, A., & Alligood, M. R. (2002). *Nursing theorists and their work* (5th ed.). St. Louis: Mosby.

Mezirow, J. (1991). *Transformative dimensions of adult learning.* San Francisco: Jossey-Bass.

Mish, F. C. (Ed.) (1999). *Merriam-Webster's collegiate dictionary* (10th ed.). Springfield, MA: Merriam-Webster.

Mitchell, G. J., & Cody, W. K. (1992). Nursing knowledge and human science: Ontological and epistemological considerations. *Nursing Science Quarterly, 5,* 54–61.

Mitchell, G. J., & Cody, W. K. (1999). Human becoming theory: A complement to medical science. *Nursing Science Quarterly, 12,* 304–310.

Neuman, B. (1995). *The Neuman systems model* (3rd ed.). Stamford, CT: Appleton & Lange.

Newman, M. A. (1992). Prevailing paradigms in nursing. *Nursing Outlook, 40,* 10–13, 32.

Newman, M. A. (2000). *Health as expanding consciousness* (2nd ed.). Sudbury, MA: Jones and Bartlett.

Newman, M. A., Sime, A. M., & Corcoran-Perry, S. A. (1991). The focus of the discipline of nursing. *Advances in Nursing Science, 14*(1), 1–6.

Nightingale, F. (1992). *Notes on nursing: What it is, and what it is not.* Philadelphia: Lippincott. (Original work published 1859)

Nunnery, R. K. (1997). *Advancing your career: Concepts of professional nursing.* Philadelphia: F. A. Davis.

Orem, D. E. (1995). *Nursing: Concepts of practice.* St. Louis, MO: Mosby-Year Book.

Parker, M. (2001). *Nursing theories and nursing practice.* Philadelphia: F. A. Davis.

Parse, R. R. (1981). *Man-living-health: A theory of nursing.* New York: Wiley.

Parse, R. R. (1987). *Nursing science: Major paradigms, theories, and critiques.* Philadelphia: Saunders.

Parse, R. R. (1990). Health: A personal commitment. *Nursing Science Quarterly, 3,* 136–140.

Parse, R. R. (1994). Quality of life: Sciencing and living the art of human becoming. *Nursing Science Quarterly, 7,* 16–21.

Parse, R. R. (1996). Critical thinking: What is it? *Nursing Science Quarterly, 9,* 139.

Parse, R. R. (1997). The language of nursing knowledge: Saying what we mean. In I. M. King & J. Fawcett (Eds.), *The language of nursing theory and metatheory.* Indianapolis, IN: Sigma Theta Tau International Center Nursing Press.

Parse, R. R. (1998). *The human becoming school of thought: A perspective for nurses and other health professionals.* Thousand Oaks, CA: Sage.

Parse, R. R. (1999). Nursing: The discipline and the profession. *Nursing Science Quarterly, 12,* 275–276.

Parse, R. R. (2000). Paradigms: A reprise. *Nursing Science Quarterly, 13,* 275–276.

Parse, R. R. (2003). *Community: A human becoming perspective.* Sudbury, MA: Jones and Bartlett.

Paterson, J. G., & Zderad, L. T. (1976). *Humanistic nursing.* New York: Wiley.

Pedwell, S. (1999). Personal prescription. *Canadian Living, 24*(3), 87–88.

Peplau, H. E. (1991). *Interpersonal relations in nursing.* New York: Springer Publishing. (Original work published 1952)

Polkinghorne, D. (1983). *Methodology for the human sciences.* Albany, NY: State University of New York Press.

Rogers, M. E. (1970). *An introduction to the theoretical basis of nursing.* Philadelphia: F. A. Davis.

Rogers, M. E. (1990). Nursing: Science of unitary, irreducible human beings: Update 1990. In E. A. M. Barrett (Ed.), *Visions of Rogers' science-based nursing.* New York: National League for Nursing.

Roy, C. (1976). *Introduction to nursing: An adaptation model.* Englewood Cliffs, NJ: Prentice-Hall.

Roy, C., & Andrews, H. A. (1999). *The Roy adaptation model* (2nd ed.). Stamford, CT: Appleton & Lange.

Thorne, S., Canam, C., Dahinten, S., Hall, W., Henderson, A., & Kirkham, S. (1998). Nursing's metaparadigm concepts: Disimpacting the debates. *Journal of Advanced Nursing, 27,* 1257–1268.

Watson, J. (1985). *Nursing: Human science and human care.* Norwalk, CT: Appleton-Century-Crofts.

Watson, J. (1999). *Postmodern nursing and beyond.* New York: Churchill Livingston.

Wheatley, M. J., & Kellner-Rogers, M. (1999). *A simpler way.* San Francisco: Berrett-Koehler Publishers. (Original work published 1996)

8

Research in Nursing

Robert Anders, John Daly, David Thompson, Doug Elliott, and Esther Chang

LEARNING OBJECTIVES

Upon completion of this chapter, readers should have gained:

- An understanding of the role of research in the development of contemporary nursing
- An appreciation of the need for a range of approaches to research in nursing
- Basic knowledge and understanding of research processes in nursing
- An appreciation of the contribution of research to the development of knowledge and clinical practice standards in nursing
- An understanding of research critique and research dissemination processes in nursing

KEY WORDS

Processes, research traditions, quantitative, qualitative, dissemination, critique, evidence

INTRODUCTION

This chapter introduces the reader to the basic concepts and processes of research. Within the United States, nursing research in rapidly maturing into a significant contributor to new knowledge. The first federal funding for nursing research began in 1946 when a Division of Nursing was established within the Office of the Surgeon General, Public Health Services. The current National Institute of Nursing Research was established as a Center for Nursing Research in June 1986 after a national task force found that nursing research was appropriate to the National Institutes of Health (NIH) research mission. In 1993 the Center became one of the 25 Institutes and Centers with the NIH. The initial funding was $16 million and by the turn of the century had increased to over $90 million dollars. (See http://www.nih.gov/ninr/research/diversity/mission/html)

The mission of NINR is to foster basic and clinical research to provide a scientific basis for the care provided across the life span. The funding supports interdisciplinary research on health promotion and risk reduction, clinical topics, as well as quality of life projects. NINR provides funding through a variety of mechanisms that are designed to strengthen the ability of nurses to conduct interdisciplinary research as well as to provide funds for established nurse researchers. Post-doctoral and pre-doctoral nursing students can also apply to NINR to support their research.

There are many private sources of funds for nursing researchers. However, the funds are more limited and in many cases are designated only for pilot studies. These funds are provided by organizations such as the American Nurses Foundation and the International Honor Society, Sigma Theta Tau. In most states and communities, there are also a number of private foundations that have limited funds to support nursing research.

A current NINR priority is to fund research aimed at improving health disparities, particularly among specific population groups. Groups targeted for special focus include Hispanics, African-Americans, Asians, Asian Pacific Islanders, Native Americans, and Native Alaskans. NINR also recognizes that health disparities are interlinked with social, economic, gender, and age factors. In addition, gays and lesbians may have specific health needs that NINR identified as potentially not being met.

The American Association of Colleges of Nursing (AACN) indicates, among other competencies, that the baccalaureate degree nurse uses theory and research-based knowledge in the direct and indirect delivery of care to patients (ACCN, 1998). AACN suggests that key competencies of a baccalaureate registered nurse include, among other things, the ability to:

- Formulate a plan of care that also includes using research findings related to nursing care and collaborative discharge planning
- Participate in the research process and use interpreted research findings to plan, implement, and evaluate discharge plans
- Use research findings of factors that contribute to the maintenance or restoration of health
- Use the research processes and logical reasoning
- Use research findings to facilitate the development of client coping mechanisms during alterations in health status
- Use research findings to assist in the development of clinical practice guidelines

Without an understanding of research, the baccalaureate nurse will not be able to meet these outcome competencies. Thus, the graduate must have a basic understanding of the key concepts in nursing research.

WHAT IS RESEARCH?

Research is a rigorous process of inquiry designed to provide answers to questions about phenomena of concern in an academic discipline or profession. In the Merriam Webster Dictionary (http://www.m-w.com/cgi-bin/dictionary) research is defined as "(a) careful search or inquiry after or for or into; endeavor to discover new or collate old facts etc. by scientific study of a subject, course of critical investigation." In this definition, scientific study implies systematic inquiry according to an established tradition.

Research is a complex subject and field comprising a number of well established but diverse traditions. In a chapter such as this, it is possible to present only broad brushstrokes to familiarize the reader with key ideas underpinning research processes in nursing. To develop in-depth knowledge and understanding of any one or a range of research traditions, processes, and methods, further study and reading from a variety of sources will be necessary.

Research traditions can be investigated in relation to their philosophical underpinnings, and in the course of your reading about research, you will encounter a number of essentially different paradigms. A research paradigm is an overarching framework that is based on values, beliefs, and assumptions. This framework contains theory about the nature of reality and guidelines for the methods to be used in carrying out research using (or within) the paradigm. In addition, the ideas within the paradigm have implications for the type of knowledge being sought in a research study, the way in which the study will be carried out, and the way in which outcomes from the work will be used.

Since nursing is a complex field, researchers use positivist, feminist, and interpretive research paradigms, among others. Quality research is labor, skill, and resource intensive; therefore a number of important decisions must be made before embarking upon a research project. For example, all research must be ethical, and this means adhering to strict guidelines (National Health and Medical Research Council, 1992) and obtaining the necessary approval from institutional ethics committees.

Research has the potential to serve a number of purposes in a practice-based discipline such as nursing. Research in nursing is necessary to:

- test commonly held assumptions
- widen understanding of a subject
- stimulate self-action/study
- develop best practice (i.e., research-based practice)
- explain behaviors
- make predictions
- assist in the formation of a body of nursing knowledge

The four As of Research (Crookes & Davies, 1998, p. xi) are:

1. Awareness (including access)
2. Appreciation
3. Application
4. Ability

The aim of the first three As of research is not to produce research workers but to cultivate and nurture nurses to:

- accept research as a normal and integral aspect of nursing practice
- read and understand research reports
- apply research findings to clinical practice (i.e., evidence-based practice)
- influence colleagues on the use of research data
- accept responsibility for their own professional development

TYPES OF NURSING RESEARCH

Nursing research has traditionally been described as using either *quantitative* or *qualitative* approaches. Oakley (2000, p. 42) notes that the "quantitative-qualitative" dichotomy functions chiefly as a gendered way of knowing. The qualitative is the soft, the unreliable, the feminine, the private—the world of the subjective experience. The quantitative and the experimental are hard, reliable, masculine, public; they are about objectivity. As Oakley points out, the two terms are relative: much quantitative research measures quality, and numbers frequently occur in qualitative research.

Quantitative Research

The term *quantitative research* refers to studies that seek to measure some concept or phenomenon of interest, for example blood pressure, pain, or student attitudes to learning about research. The quantitative research paradigm is also called positivist, reductionist, or empirical. Quantitative reasoning is termed deductive, which means the thinking leads from a known principle to an unknown and is used to test a particular research hypothesis.

Quantitative research encompasses a range of research designs and associated methods; the most common designs used in health care research are listed in Table 8.1. Selection of an appropriate design relates to the research question being posed (Sackett & Wennberg, 1997). The topic of interest may be framed as a question, objective, or research hypothesis. Each design incorporates a number of variations; readers are directed to any number of nursing research texts for amplification of the designs (e.g., Beanland, Schneider, LoBiondo-Wood, & Haber, 1999; Burns & Grove, 2001; Crookes & Davies, 1998).

Quantitative studies rely on sampling a smaller group of individuals who have similar characteristics to the overall population of interest. Inclusion and/or exclusion criteria (defined in Table 8.2) are developed to guide the selection of subjects. In experimental studies, the independent variable (an intervention) is manipulated by randomly assigning subjects to a treatment or control group while the (dependent) variable of interest is measured and other related variables are controlled, for example Randomized Controlled Trial (RCT).

TABLE 8.1   Common Quantitative Research Designs

Design	Purpose
Descriptive	Examines characteristics of a single sample; clarifies concepts; generates questions about potential relationships between variables (e.g., case study, cross-sectional analysis)
Correlation	Examines (describes, predicts or tests) relationships between two or more variables, but does not infer a cause-and-effect relationship
Quasi-experiment	Tests a cause-and-effect relationship, but without control or randomization (e.g., case control, cohort)
Experiment	Tests a cause-and-effect relationship using randomization, manipulation of an intervention, and control of other variables (e.g., randomized controlled trial [RCT], laboratory experiment)

Measurement of the concepts of interest are conducted using single or multiple measuring instruments (also called tools); these can be physiological (e.g., heart rate monitor, blood glucometer) or psychological/psychometric (e.g., anxiety scales, functional status, quality of life). Ideally, an instrument should exhibit characteristics that are valid, reliable, and responsive. Well-developed instruments generally have had the above characteristics rigorously tested over time, and have been accepted as a useful research tool. Development of new instruments is time consuming and resource intensive since the validity, reliability, and responsiveness must be tested, and modification of items (questions) may be required to improve the performance of the instrument.

Instrument validity refers to whether the instrument actually measures what it is intended to measure. There are numerous subforms of validity that have been used to describe increasing rigor for testing an instrument's performance, for example:

- face (on the face of it, appears to measure the concept)
- content (appears to include all major elements of the concept; often assessed by an expert panel of relevant professionals)
- criterion-related (examines the instrument against another or the 'gold-standard' criteria)
- construct

The aim is for an instrument to have appropriate construct validity, which is the extent that an instrument accurately measures a theoretical

TABLE 8.2 Glossary of Common Quantitative Research Terms

Term	Meaning
Descriptive statistics	Description of characteristics (e.g., frequency, percentages) but no inferring of relationships between variables
Exclusion criteria	A list of characteristics that exclude an individual from being recruited into a study (e.g., less than 24 hours admission in hospital; presence of other illnesses that may influence patient outcomes)
Explanatory variable	Independent variable; the intervention being manipulated to exhibit a change in the outcome variable
Inclusion criteria	A list of the characteristics required for a subject to be included in a study (e.g., patients admitted for cardiac surgery: 16 years of age or older; English language skills [reading and writing] sufficient to complete the study questionnaires)
Inferential statistics	Statistical procedures used to test an hypothesis about the relationships between two or more variables (e.g., t-tests, analysis of variance, regression modeling) and the application of study findings to the population being studied (generalizability)
Measuring instrument	The tool used to measure the concept of interest (e.g., questionnaire; biochemical test)
Normal distribution	Distribution of scores for a particular variable follow a bell-shaped pattern around the mean score for the sample
Outcome variable	Dependent variable; measurement of the concept being studied
Primary research	Original research conducted on subjects
Sample	A selected group of subjects which have similar characteristics to the population from which they were drawn (i.e., representative); allows for generalization of results from the study sample to the wider population
Secondary research	A study where data from previous primary research studies are re-investigated (e.g., systematic review; clinical practice guidelines)

construct or trait that is established over time, following repeated use and testing of the instrument in various studies. With any instrument, there is the possibility of measurement error. The aim of a good study or instrument is to minimize the chance of that error.

Reliability relates to the accuracy with which the instrument measures the concept being investigated, and which can be tested in terms of stability (test-retest: similar scores on repeated testing for a stable trait), homogeneity (internal consistency: all parts of the instrument measure the same characteristics), and equivalence (inter-rater reliability: consistency between observers using the same instrument with the same subjects). There are a number of statistical tests for reliability that is commonly expressed as a correlation coefficient, ranging from 0.0 to 1.0. A reliability of 0.80 is considered the minimal acceptable coefficient for a developed instrument.

Responsiveness is the ability of an instrument to detect clinically important changes in the variable of interest with a patient (study subject) (Harris & Warren, 1995). This is the opposite characteristic to stability, and relates to the precision of measurement for the instrument. Unfortunately, assessment of this performance characteristic has been minimal when compared with reliability and validity testing (Deyo & Carter, 1992).

In addition to the glossary at the end of this book, Table 8.2 explains some common quantitative research terms used in this chapter. More detailed glossaries are available in specific nursing research texts (e.g., Crookes & Davies, 1998; Martin & Thompson, 2000).

Quantitative studies collect numerical data to answer the questions or objectives posed. Therefore, all variable information is transformed to numbers prior to data management and analysis. Data analysis procedures can be descriptive or inferential, depending on the design and the levels of measurement for each variable, that is, nominal, ordinal, interval, or ratio. The categories must be mutually exclusive and collectively exhaustive:

- *Nominal:* Assigns values to classify characteristics into nonordered categories, for example sex, religion, diagnosis. The assigned numbers do not convey any relative order or weight between the values, for example 1 = male, 2 = female; in this instance there is no implication that '1' is ordered higher than '2' or that '2' is twice the score of '1';
- *Ordinal:* Values are ordered in a logical way in providing a relative ranking; for example pain, levels of mobility, self-care; use of Likert Scales—'Strongly Agree', 'Agree', 'Undecided', 'Disagree', 'Strongly Disagree';
- *Interval:* Values exhibit a rank ordering with equal distance between values, for example temperature; scores on a linear analogue scale (from 1 to 10);
- *Ratio:* Values have the above characteristics plus a meaningful baseline (absolute zero), for example weight, height, heart rate.

Data management and analysis are commonly undertaken using software packages (e.g., MS Excel spreadsheet software can handle certain statistical analysis procedures; Statistical Package for the Social Sciences [SPSS] is a comprehensive analysis package). Study designs and methods that provide findings using inferential statistics allow the researcher to infer that the results from this sample of subjects (e.g., patients) can be applied to the wider population being investigated. Inferential statistics are further categorized into parametric or nonparametric procedures. Parametric tests are used when the following assumptions are met: the sample was drawn from a normal distribution; random sampling was used; and data were measured at least at interval level.

As beginning research consumers, students must consider the objectives of the study and the related purposes for the statistical tests performed. Table 8.3 can be used to critique papers for consistency between the purpose, the level of measurement, and the actual tests that are appropriate to answer those questions. More in-depth information regarding the actual statistical tests is beyond the scope of this chapter, but can be found in comprehensive research texts.

Qualitative Research

Qualitative research includes a range of research designs and methods. This field of research has its roots in philosophy, anthropology, history, and sociology (Denzin & Lincoln, 1994). Qualitative research refers to research that is focused on human experience, including accounts of subjective realities; it is conducted in naturalistic settings involving close, often sustained, contact between the researcher and research participants (Oiler Boyd, 1993). Naturalistic research is often referred to as field research (Polit & Hungler, 1995) because it is conducted in the field. This label may be applied to a range of contexts, for example a community health center or an intensive care unit.

The qualitative researcher approaches the research project with a different set of values and beliefs from the purely quantitative researcher. These differences relate to the world view (ontology) of the researcher, notions about epistemology (ways of knowing) and research methodology. For example, in the positivist paradigm concepts such as control, precision, objectivity, testing, one truth, prediction, and cause-effect are valued, and individual perceptions are not considered. In the qualitative or interpretive paradigm, the opposite applies and value is placed on subjectivity, multiple truths may be accommodated, and

TABLE 8.3   Statistical Purposes and Related Parametric and Nonpara-metric Tests

Statistical Purpose	Parametric	Nonparametric
Compares *mean scores* for two independent samples	Two sample (unpaired) t-test *[interval/ratio data]*	Mann-Whitney U test *[ordinal data]*
Compares *mean scores* for two sets of observations from the same sample	Paired t-test *[interval/ratio data]*	Wilcoxon matched pairs test *[ordinal data]*
Compares *mean scores* for three or more sets of observations	One-way Analysis of Variance (ANOVA)	Kruskall-Wallis ANOVA by ranks
Compares proportions from two samples	Chi-square (c^2) test	Fisher's exact test
Compares *proportions* from a paired sample	McNemar's test	No equivalent
Assesses strength of straight line *association* between two variables	Product moment correlation coefficient (Pearson's r)	Spearman's rank correlation coefficient (r^s)
Describes *relationship* between two variables, allowing one to be *predicted* from the other	Simple linear regression	Nonparametric regression
Describes *relationship* between a dependent variable and several predictor variables	Multiple regression	Nonparametric regression

Adapted from Beanland et al., 1999; Burns & Grove, 2001; Greenhalgh, 1997.

individuals who participate in this type of research are regarded as research participants, not research subjects as with the positivist approaches. Variables, hypotheses, cause-effect relationships, and randomization are not considered in qualitative approaches. This type of research takes the *emic* perspective, i.e., the insider's point of view (Holloway & Wheeler, 1996). Consequently, sampling approaches in qualitative research often deliberately seek people who have lived the experience under investigation. Reasoning in qualitative research is inductive, but may involve a process of induction-deduction.

Qualitative research methods are mostly descriptive in nature (Sarantakos 1993) and allow exploration of a range of human experiences that are of interest in a discipline such as nursing. For example, the experience of suffering for people living with terminal cancer, the characteristics of cultural groups, including their health beliefs, or the question "What is comfort for recipients of nursing?" might be described. It may be possible to study these phenomena using a quantitative approach, but this could be very limiting. The advantage of using a qualitative approach is that the phenomena may be studied more holistically taking account of shared human reality (Oiler Boyd, 1993), there is a focus on human experience, research participants are valued and treated as equals by the researcher, and it is possible to develop a rich description of the experience under investigation with implications for nursing knowledge and often nursing practice. Qualitative research, then, involves broadly stated questions about human experiences and realities, studied through sustained contact with persons in their natural environments, and producing rich, descriptive data that help us to understand those persons' experiences. The emphasis is on achieving understanding that will, in turn, "open up new options for action and new perspectives that can change people's worlds" (Oiler Boyd, 1993, pp. 69–70).

Qualitative studies are commonly carried out on small numbers of research participants and involve in-depth inquiry into the phenomenon of concern. The data in qualitative research are presented in the form of words rather than numbers as in quantitative research (Miles & Huberman, 1994, p. 1). For example, in many approaches to qualitative research work, the researcher may interview the research participants and audiotape the conversation, which is later transcribed for data analysis. In this way, narrative text is often assembled by the researcher while working with the research participants. This text can be analyzed and broken down into themes to reflect core ideas or recurring features in the data (Miles & Huberman, 1994). This process involves intensive reflection on the part of the researcher. The qualitative paradigm is often referred to as the interpretive paradigm because it centers on interpretation and creation of meaning by human beings, and their subjective reality.

Researchers must understand the socially constructed nature of the world and realize that values and interests become part of the research process (Holloway & Wheeler, 1996).

The qualitative researcher can choose from a range of research approaches and this selection will be linked to the aims or purposes of the study. Each approach incorporates a way of structuring the study, selecting the research participants, and collecting and analyzing the data. Some examples are provided below. Readers are directed to any number of nursing research texts for amplification of the approaches to qualitative research described below (Denzin & Lincoln, 1994; Munhall & Oiler Boyd, 1993; Holloway & Wheeler, 1996).

Phenomenology is a philosophy and a descriptive research method designed to uncover the essence and meaning of lived experiences, for example suffering or grieving. "The focus of phenomenological inquiry . . . is what people experience regarding some phenomena and how they interpret those experiences" (Polit & Hungler, 1995, p. 197).

Ethnography is a qualitative research approach that is applied to study of the culture of a group. Culture may "be broadly defined as the learned social behavior or the way of life of a particular group of people. Ethnography provides knowledge (theory) that can be used to help us understand our own culture(s) and those of others" (Germain, 1993, p. 237). The ethnographer sets out to uncover insiders' (emic) view of the culture under study as opposed to the outsiders' (etic) view (Polit & Hungler, 1995).

Grounded theory is a research process designed to lead to generation of theory through study of a particular human context. This involves a "search for social processes present in human interaction" (Hutchinson, 1993, p. 181).

In the course of your reading and learning about research processes in nursing, you will discover that in some instances, researchers mix quantitative and qualitative research processes in research design; qualitative research processes may be considered soft and less rigorous by proponents of positivist research; and evaluative criteria for establishing the scientific validity of qualitative research are the subject of ongoing debate. Sicne the content of this chapter is introductory, you can also expect to learn of other research traditions, paradigms, and methods during your undergraduate education.

DEVELOPING RESEARCH QUESTIONS

Research ideas come from many sources. Some ideas are derived from theoretical considerations, while others arise from the need to solve practical problems or to improve the quality of care. Having a good idea is often not enough—you need to translate that idea into research questions. This section discusses how to develop research questions based on the amount of knowledge and/or theory about the topic, and describes the importance of a thorough review of the literature to identify relevant theory and research.

A research question needs to be clearly stated as an "explicit query about a problem or issue that can be challenged, examined, and analyzed and that will yield useful new information" (Brink & Wood, 1993, p. 2). Although there are no specific rules and procedures for asking research questions, the way research questions are worded can have an effect on the research design and methods that follow.

Research questions can be classified into levels based on the amount of knowledge and/or theory about the topic.

Level I research studies are known as exploratory, with little or no literature on either the topic or the population to be researched. Questions at Level I are designed to explore the topic or a single population, since the area under study has not been adequately researched. Hence, the question is always *What is?* or *What are?* The question is asked in a way that leads to an exploratory research design.

Level II research studies build on the results of studies at the first level. There is existing knowledge and theory about the topic and population. Questions at Level II examine relationships between variables. A variable is a characteristic being measured that can vary or be manipulated among the subjects under study. Level II questions ask *What is the relationship?* and the topic often contains two or more variables. Statistical analysis is used to determine the significance of the relationship between the variables. All Level II questions lead to correlation designs.

Questions at *Level III* require considerable knowledge of the topic. Research at this level begins at knowing the relationships between variables; therefore, questions at Level III are designed to examine why this relationship exists, with a rationale and with an explanation. "All Level III questions lead to experimental designs" (Brink & Wood, 1993, p. 16).

When formulating a research question, it is important that you discuss your topic and question with your colleagues or experts in the field, since this will assist you with the development and refinement of the research question. Often, the initial research question is formulated too broadly for the time frame that is available or to make the appropriate observations. Consider the following example: Do undergraduate students taught in a supportive environment increase their learning capabilities as graduates? Before this can be answered, a number of issues have to be clarified. What exactly is a supportive environment? What does it mean to increase their learning capabilities? How do we measure learning capabilities? How do we determine learning capabilities in graduates? Until you can define the terms and determine how to measure the variables they represent, you cannot answer the original question. Frequently, researchers have to narrow the topic area or, in some cases, the types and number of settings or the number of participants they include in the study. Ultimately, this process of narrowing the topic must also be consistent with the research design and methods of the study.

REVIEWING THE LITERATURE

Whether you begin with a vague idea of a research study or a well-developed research plan, every research study needs to be considered an extension of previous knowledge and thereby stimulate research. There are many reasons for reviewing the literature before beginning a research endeavor. First, your research question may have been addressed and answered, or a review can be the initial source of ideas for a research question. By being familiar with and understanding what has already been done with existing research and theory, you can devise your research study to explore any newly identified questions (Bordens & Abbott, 1996). The review will also assist you to establish a theoretical context and rationale for your study. From a practical (methodological) perspective, the review can reveal research strategies, measuring instruments, experimental techniques and analysis. It allows you to learn from the strengths and limitations of other researchers' work in regard to successful outcomes and assumptions. A further advantage is that a review of the literature also keeps you up to date with current research work that has been undertaken in the area of interest.

WHERE DO WE FIND THE RESEARCH?

Literally hundreds of research journals, dissertations, reports, and books are published each year. One of the most important steps in the research process is conducting a thorough literature review. Students are often faced with the dilemma of how extensive a review is necessary. There is no formula to determine whether a specific number of articles will provide the necessary background for the study. The number of references will depend on how familiar you are with the area under investigation, and the scope of the review will depend on how much research is available in that area. Checking the reference list at the end of recent articles can often assist in the process. Experienced researchers know that maintaining an up-to-date review of the literature is an ongoing process throughout the research project.

To begin with, it is important to differentiate between primary and secondary sources. A primary source is written by the study author/s themselves. A primary source includes information on the rationale of the study, its participants, design, methods of collecting data, procedure, results, outcomes, limitations, recommendations, and references. Most research articles published in professional journals are primary sources. A secondary source is one that summarizes information from primary sources presented by other authors. When an author cites a previous study in the review of literature section, that is a secondary source. Both primary and secondary sources are important; however, secondary sources should not be substitutes for primary sources. Avoid over-reliance on secondary sources, and make every effort to obtain the primary sources that are important to you.

Many libraries also provide reference sources in computer databases to assist students in locating references on a specific topic and to undertake their own computer searches. A computer search will generate complete bibliographic citations, often including abstracts of many articles published in a particular area of interest. A variety of indexes and databases are available, providing bibliographic listings of articles, abstracts, conference proceedings, and books. The reader is advised to consult a handy research guide to nursing and health literature (Guyatt & Rennie, 2002).

INDEXES, ABSTRACTS, AND DATABASES

Some cumulative indexes provide abstracts, while others do not publish abstracts. Abstracts are short summaries of the article. Abstracts give more information about the article, as titles can be misleading in their description of the content. All indexes provide bibliographic citations, giving the authors' names, article title, journal volume and issue number, date, and pages. Each academic discipline has an index to its collection of journals. Most indexes and databases in the medical field use medical subject headings. When a topic is not found in the subject headings, you need to find some related terms that have been adopted by most of the journal publishers. Many journals also publish key words with an article that refers to these headings. A valuable index and database for research in the health science literature is the Cumulative Index to Nursing and Allied Health Literature (CINAHL), which has all nursing journals and several allied health disciplines listed. Another important index and database is Indexis Medicus (Medline), which provides a bibliography of medical reviews (Guyatt & Rennie, 2002). The Cochrane Collaboration publishes the Cochrane Library, which focuses primarily on systematic reviews of controlled trials of therapeutic interventions. Updated quarterly, the Cochrane Library is available in CD-ROM format or over the Internet. Other important abstract indexes that may be of relevance to your topic are the Education Resources Information Centre (ERIC), Psychology Abstracts, Sociological Abstracts, cancer therapy abstracts (CANCERLIT), and Dissertation Abstracts International. Excerpta Medica publishes abstracts related to specialized topics in the field of medicine, including rehabilitation and physical medicine, gerontology, and many others (Portney & Watkins, 1993).

THE ROLE OF PEER-REVIEWED JOURNALS IN DISSEMINATING RESEARCH

Peer-reviewed journals serve many important functions, including facilitation of expert review of manuscripts, reporting the findings of research studies or theoretical papers, dissemination of papers which have been approved for publication following peer review, and serving as a resource for scholars and researchers involved in compiling and/or developing knowledge in an area of nursing research or practice. Criteria which must be met before a paper is approved for publication in a refereed journal vary from one to another, but all editors will be concerned with a standard of excellence which must be met (particularly in regard to scientific merit), relevance of the paper in terms of its potential to contribute to incremental development of knowledge in the area, as well as the literary standard of the work. There are many international peer-reviewed journals in nursing. Each has its own aims, purposes, and requirements that must be followed by nurses wishing to submit their work for peer review with a view to being published in the journal. Most university libraries hold extensive collections of refereed journals in hard copy across a range of disciplines, and lately some journals such as *Nursing Research* are available online, negating the need for hard copies stored on library shelves. The Nursing Collection is a CD-ROM comprising a number of journals, and which allows for downloading of full-text articles.

HOW NURSES CAN USE RESEARCH

In recent times, nursing and other health professionals have been interested in the quality of patient care and establishing standards for best clinical practice, by examining the evidence base. Findings from research studies are commonly disseminated at conferences and in professional journals. Some studies are designed to inform clinical practice. For example, studies may describe a clinical practice, or compare two (or more) different ways of performing a practice. Other types of studies may shed light on patients' experiences of phenomena that are poorly understood, for example hope or suffering.

As noted earlier, not all nurses need the ability to conduct research, but all clinical nurses need research utilization skills in order to practice in a professional manner and in accordance with the best available evidence. Research utilization skills involve the Four As mentioned earlier in this chapter and include abilities in *accessing* the literature, an *awareness* of important and recent studies applicable to their area of practice, an *appreciation* of the study findings, and *application* of the findings in relation to their own practice setting. These skills are important, but clearly different from the *ability* to undertake primary research. The ability to critique studies is therefore a fundamental skill for undergraduate nurses to master in preparation for professional practice as registered nurses. Current registered nurses also need these skills in terms of continuing professional development. However, the skill is not easily attained, and does not magically appear at the end of a single university research course. Rather, the ability is additive in that it is related to experience, practice, and reflection over time. In fact, it is an ability that relates to lifelong learning since it is an area where we can always learn and improve our skills.

EVIDENCE-BASED PRACTICE

The critique of an individual research paper can be extended to multiple papers on the same topic, resulting in a literature review. This is a common assessment item for nursing students. An adaptation of this narrative literature review is a systematic review (SR), which addresses a well-defined question, provides specific information on the process undertaken to minimize bias in the review process, and uses a systematic approach to assess the quality of each study reviewed (Droogan & Cullum, 1998). The question for an SR has a specific clinical focus with four components:

1. a specific patient population and setting
2. a clinical condition of interest
3. exposure to a clinical intervention
4. measurement of a specific outcome (Cook, Mulrow, & Haynes, 1997, p. 368)

The search strategy describes the databases (e.g., CINAHL; Medline) and/or journals searched by hand. Selection of articles occurs by keywords in the article title or abstract, followed by a preliminary review prior to final selection of the papers for inclusion in the SR. Included studies are then assessed according to stated criteria. A systematic review may also include the pooling and analysis of data from the studies investigated; this process is called a meta-analysis.

A number of organizations are now developing repositories of systematic reviews to appropriately guide clinical practice (Cochrane, 1972). The Cochrane Collaboration is an international network of individuals from different disciplines committed to the preparation, maintenance, and dissemination of SRs of research evidence about the effects of health care (http://www.general@cochrane.co.uk). The Cochrane Library contains three main sections: the Cochrane Database of Systematic Reviews (CDSR) that includes the complete reports of all the SRs that have been produced by members of the Cochrane Collaboration and the protocols for the Cochrane SRs that have been published outside the collaboration, and the Cochrane Controlled Trials Registry (CCTR) that contains the references to clinical trials that Cochrane investigations have found by searching a wide range of sources (Guyatt & Rennie, 2002). A critique and examples of systematic reviews in nursing was published by Droogan and Cullum (1998).

The majority of the current systematic reviews are related to medicine. This is not surprising, given the number of studies and journals devoted to topics in the various medical subspecialties. As noted previously, the gold standard for examining cause-and-effect questions in clinical practice is the randomized controlled trial (RCT). Thus, a hierarchy of study designs for studies of effectiveness have been developed (NHS Centre for Reviews and Dissemination, 2001):

Level 1:	Experimental studies (e.g., RCT with concealed allocation)
Level 2:	Quasi-experimental studies (e.g., experimental study without randomization)
Level 3:	Controlled observational studies
Level 3a:	Cohort studies
Level 3b:	Case control studies
Level 4:	Observational studies without control groups
Level 5:	Expert opinion based on pathophysiology, bench research or consensus

It is important to remember that RCTs should rank high in the hierarchy only when they are well conducted. If there are no good RCTs, then well-conducted quasi-experimental and observational studies should be considered. Quality criteria for the assessment of all of these study designs have been produced (NHS Center for Reviews and Dissemination, 2001), though it is important to remember that quality is a construct about which there are differing views. The Centre for Evidence-Based Nursing (Droogan & Cullum, 1998) is currently involved in systematic reviews of specific clinical practices that are of importance to nurses (see their Web site for current projects: http//www.york.ac.uk/depts/hstd/centres/evidence/cebn.htm).

It should be borne in mind, however, that nursing uses a variety of research paradigms and methods to answer questions that cannot be appropriately investigated by RCTs. We therefore need to consider how to evaluate non-RCT observational studies of nursing practice so that these findings can also guide nursing care. Further, how do we incorporate findings from qualitative studies which have no generalizability to the patient group in question, but which may provide valuable insights of patient experiences in guiding quality nursing practice? The development of the necessary frameworks to address these issues is not yet formed or developed to an adequate level nationally or internationally. The aim, therefore, is to foster systematic reviews of relevant studies on clinical nursing so that the best available evidence, regardless of the research design, will provide for quality nursing practice.

CONCLUSION

An understanding of basic concepts and processes in research is central to professional nursing practice. Ideally, quality nursing care is based on the outcomes of quality research processes. It is envisioned that, in time, one of the hallmarks of the nursing profession will be the widespread utilization of research evidence to provide the best, safest, and most appropriate care. All nurses engaged in nursing practice require research utilization skills in order to make judgments about how relevant and applicable research findings are to practice. Nursing is a complex, practice-based discipline in which a range of researchable questions will always require answers in order to extend knowledge. This in turn requires use of a range of research paradigms and methods.

REFLECTIVE QUESTIONS

1. What processes could be followed in formulating a research problem in nursing?
2. What advantages, if any, might qualitative research designs have over quantitative research designs in clinical nursing research?
3. What are the critical features of a comprehensive review of the literature?

RECOMMENDED READINGS

Burns, N., & Grove, S. K. (2001). *The practice of nursing research: Conduct, critique, and utilization*, 4th edition. Philadelphia: Saunders.

Crookes, P. A., & Davies, S. (Eds.) (1998). *Research into practice: Essential skills for reading and applying research in nursing and healthcare.* Edinburgh: Ballière Tindall.

Guyatt, G., & Rennie, D. (Eds.) (2002). *Users' guides to the medical literature: A manual for evidenced-based clinical practice.* Chicago: AMA Press.

Holloway, I., & Wheeler, S. (1996). *Qualitative Research for Nurses.* Oxford: Blackwell Science.

Martin, C. R., & Thompson, D. K. (2000). *Designs and Analysis of Clinical Nursing Research Studies.* London: Routledge.

Oakley, A. (2000). *Experiment in Knowing: Gender and Methods in the Social Sciences.* Cambridge: Polity Press.

REFERENCES

American Association of Colleges of Nursing (1998). *The essentials of baccalaureate education for professional nursing practice.* Washington, DC: AACN.

Beanland, C., Schneider, Z., LoBiondo-Wood, G., & Haber, J. (1999). *Nursing research: Methods, critical appraisal and utilisation.* Sydney: Mosby.

Bordens, K. S., & Abbott, B. B. (1996). *Research design and methods: A process approach* (3rd ed.). Mountain View, CA: Mayfield.

Brink, P. J., & Wood, M. J. (1993). *Basic steps in planning nursing research.* Boston: Jones and Bartlett.

Burns, N., & Grove, S. K. (2001). *The practice of nursing research: Conduct, critique, and utilization* (4th ed.). Philadelphia: Saunders.

Cochrane, A. L. (1972). *Effectiveness and efficiency: Random reflections on health services.* London: Nuffield Provincial Hospitals Trust.

Cook, D. J., Mulrow, C. D., & Haynes, R. B. (1997). Systematic reviews: Synthesis of best evidence for clinical decisions. *Annals of Internal Medicine, 126,* 364–371.

Crookes, P. A., & Davis, S. (Eds.) (1998). *Research into practice: Essential skills for reading and applying research in nursing and healthcare.* Edinburgh: Baillicrc Tindall.

Denzin, N. K., & Lincoln, Y. S. (1994). Introduction: Entering the field of qualitative research. In N. K. Denzin & Y. S. Lincoln (Eds.), *Handbook of qualitative research.* Thousand Oaks, CA: Sage.

Deyo, R. A., & Carter, W. B. (1992). Strategies for improving and expanding the application of health status measures in clinical settings: A researcher-developer viewpoint. *Medical Care, 30* (5 suppl.), 176–186.

Droogan, J. E., & Cullum, N. (1998). Systematic reviews in nursing. *International Journal of Nursing Studies, 35,* 13–22.

Germain, C. P. (1993). Ethnography: The method. In P. L. Munhall & C. Oiler Boyd (Eds.), *Nursing research: A qualitative perspective,* 2nd ed. New York: National League for Nursing.

Greenhalgh, P. (1997). *How to Read a Paper.* London: BMJ Publishing.

Guyatt, G., & Rennic, D. (Eds.) (2002). *Users' guides to the medical literature: A manual for evidence-based clinical practice.* Chicago: AMA Press.

Harris, M. R., & Warren, J. J. (1995). Patient outcomes: Assessment for the CNS. *Clinical Nurse Specialist, 9*(2), 82–86.

Holloway, I., & Wheeler, S. (1996). *Qualitative research for nurses.* Oxford: Blackwell Science.

Hutchinson, S. A. (1993). Grounded theory: The method. In P. L. Munhall & C. Oiler Boyd (Eds.), *Nursing research: A qualitative perspective* (2nd ed.). New York: National League for Nursing.

Martin, C. R., & Thompson. D. R. (2000). *Design and analysis of clinical nursing research studies.* London: Routledge.

Miles, M. B., & Huberman, A. M. (1994). *Qualitative data analysis* (2nd ed.). Thousand Oaks, CA: Sage.

Munhall, P. L., & Oiler Boyd, C. (1993). *Nursing research: A qualitative perspective.* New York: National League For Nursing Press.

National Health and Medical Research Council (1992). *Notes on human experimentation.* Canberra: Australian Government Printing Service.

NHS Centre for Reviews and Dissemination (2001). *Undertaking Systematic Reviews of Research On Effectiveness.* CRD's guidance for those carrying out or commissioning reviews. CRD Report No. 4, 2nd ed. York: NHS Centre for Reviews and Dissemination.

Oakly, A. (2000). *Experiments in knowing: Gender and method in the social sciences.* Cambridge: Polity Press.

Oiler Boyd, C. (1993). Philosophical foundations of qualitative research. In P. L. Munhall & C. Oiler Boyd (Eds.), *Nursing research: A qualitative perspective* (2nd ed.). New York: National League for Nursing.

Polit, D. F., & Hungler, B. P. (1995). *Nursing research: Principals and methods* (5th ed.). Philadelphia: Lippincott.

Portney, L. G., & Watkins, M. P. (1993). *Foundations of clinical research: Applications to practice.* Norwalk, CT: Appleton & Lange.

Sackett, D. L., & Wennberg, J. E. (1997). Choosing the best research design for each question: It's time to stop squabbling over the 'best' methods. *British Medical Journal, 315*(7123), 1636.

Sarantakos, S. (1993). *Social research.* Melbourne: MacMillan.

9

Ethics: A Patient-Centered Approach

Gladys L. Husted and James H. Husted

LEARNING OBJECTIVES

After reading this chapter you will be able to:

- Discuss the ethical nature of nursing practice
- Compare the contemporary nonpractice-based ethical systems and a practice-based system and their appropriateness to bioethical decision making in the health care arena
- Explore the relevance of context to a justifiable bioethical decision
- Differentiate between ethics and bioethics

KEY WORDS

Agreement, context, ethics, nursing ethics, bioethics, ethical decision making

INTRODUCTION

Ethics arose from the necessity of making decisions in the face of adversity. Ethics is the branch of philosophy that is concerned with right and wrong—the determination of what actions ought to be taken, and what changes ought to be brought about in common—and uncommon—situations.

For bioethics, that which produces and protects the well-being of patients and professionals is considered "ethical." That which fails to do this when it could be achieved, or which harms patients and professionals when this could be avoided is considered "unethical."

This chapter will examine some commonly applied theories of ethics in nursing and health care, along with the authors' own practice-based "symphonological" theory, which is based on the individuality of each patient and nurse, and the implied "agreement" they share. An essential issue raised by this discussion is: Should ethics be based on "norms and rules" that apply to all, or should it allow for adaptation to the individual situation? The authors' theory is based on the latter, and will be discussed in more detail later in the chapter.

NURSING AND BIOETHICAL PRACTICE

Nurses are becoming more and more aware of the ethical responsibilities of their practice. "Unless nurses are able to engage in the process of ethical reasoning and apply . . . expertise to a given bioethical dilemma, there is no chance to exercise the ability to judge" (Clark & Taxis, 2003, p. 237).

If a nurse regards her[1] patient as a carbon copy of herself, she will never be able to apply "expertise to a given bioethical dilemma." Every patient is unique—and *real*. To accept her patient's right to be different from herself is the first ethical decision a nurse ought to make.

The second decision is the mirror image of the first. It is the decision that, while no patient will have motivations or a personality structure identical to her own, no patient is entirely different. *All* humans share in common with all other humans the fact that they can be benefited or harmed. And, this fact makes a difference to them.

Ethical reasoning and clinical judgment share a common process, and each serves to inform the other. "As the nursing profession continues to confront and manage health care problems in a changing world, many gray areas exist. Although uncertainty will always exist, it is wise to seek clarity of process and purposes, particularly for nurses who are new to the profession" (Scotto, 2003, p. 289).

---

[1]For simplicity of expression, we have used the female pronoun for the nurse, and the male pronoun for the patient.

AGENCY

For bioethics, one disability sets apart and defines every patient regardless of the specific nature of his affliction. This is the *loss of agency*—the power to act on his purposes. Specific afflictions: appendicitis, a broken leg, pneumonia, high blood pressure, psychosis, etc., are the objectives of nursing and medicine's technical attention. The loss of agency is the object of a health care system's ethical attention. Every patient suffers an impaired ability to take the actions that further his life and allow him to flourish. Recovery of this ability is the overall objective of the health care sciences. The science of health care is a human science.

All of bioethics, properly so called, is directed to this end. There cannot be a separate set of ethics for every sort of disability. The onset of sickness or disability—the loss of well-being and agency—sets the standards and purposes of the health care setting and of ethical awareness in relation to the disabled.

Research and technology consistently increase the potentials and the complexities of the health care sciences. "Nurses and nursing are at the center of issues of tremendous and long-lasting impact . . . nurses cannot afford to limit their actions" (Milstead, 2004, p. 22). This includes their ethical actions. The most efficient way to limit ethical actions—or to keep them limited—is to make them irrelevant to the profession.

THE FOCUS OF BIOETHICS

"He who would be everything will be nothing."
—Rabbi Akiba, c. 40 BC–40 AD

Bioethics—ethics as it relates to the practice of the health care professionals—came into existence as an independent discipline around 1970. At its best, bioethics gives health care professionals a tremendous professional advantage. It limits and focuses the sphere of their ethical attention.

The fundamental elements of bioethics, which form its essential nature, are:

- The nature and needs of humans as living, thinking beings
- The purpose and function of the health care system in society
- The awareness, at least implicit, of a human individual's essential moral status

Bioethics, in limiting its sphere of attention to interactions in the health care setting, can exquisitely refine actions and interactions according to their appropriateness to the health care setting. Bioethics can also vastly increase one's ability to analyze ethical puzzles outside the health care setting. While a broader, less focused, ethical study will produce little skill in a nurse's professional actions.

Professional ethics must be purposeful. "Bioethics is a system of standards to motivate, determine, and justify the choice of actions directed to the pursuit of vital and fundamental goals" (Husted & Husted, 2001, p. 49).

Where there are no vital and fundamental goals—no long-term goals—ethical awareness is both irrelevant and inconceivable. But we all have basic and life serving purposes. These sometimes come into apparent conflict. Or the best choice among alternative courses of action may not be obvious. Then our ability to call upon ethical awareness and to exercise ethical analysis becomes first in importance.

THE SPECIFIC AND THE 'IN GENERAL'

Constantine Stanislavski was, easily, the most famous acting coach of all time. One of his most fertile observations to actors was "That which is 'in general' is the enemy of art" (1964, p. 107). By "in general" he meant that which is usually the case in situations of a certain sort, but not necessarily true in a given concrete situation. The "in general" is the opposite of the "in context." It replaces that which is relevant and beneficent with that which is quite possibly irrelevant and harmful.

Stanislavski advised that an actor should study the person he is portraying and achieve an understanding of *that individual.* This observation is true of nursing as well. It is the purpose of the assessment skills that nurses must learn.

CONTEMPORARY NONPRACTICE-BASED ETHICAL SYSTEMS

Skillful ethical comportment will deteriorate to a merely competent level if we apply norms and principles to complex practical situations where we have the potential for skillful recognition of patterns and intuitive responses. Strategies of adjudication and the search for certitude through the application of norms and principles, though comforting, do not produce expert skillful ethical comportment. (Benner, Tanner, & Chesla, 1996, pp. 276–277)

Ethical decisions are the most important decisions we make. It is strange, but true, that while contemporary nonpractice-based ethical systems lead us to begin with the experience of an "ethical" dilemma, they provide no guidance to experience, analysis, and understanding. They skip over the steps of discourse, discovery, and the search for insight—steps necessary to a thought process—to a ready-made decision and a purpose that may have no relation to the context a nurse and patient face. The patient is no longer the center of professional concern. Actions are not determined by contextual awareness. Below we will examine these systems as they relate to nursing.

Deontology—A Duty Ethic

Deontology is "the theory that action, in conformance with formal rules of ethical conduct, are obligatory regardless of their result" (Angeles, 1992, p. 60). A deontological theory of ethics is "one which holds that at least some acts are morally obligatory regardless of their consequences for human weal or woe" (Edwards, 1972, p. 343). Deontology views ethics as "doing one's duty."

Deontology is not a theory that is designed to promote happiness or well-being. There is no purpose to the duties that deontology proposes beyond the duties themselves. It is not an orientation toward human values. It is essentially indifferent to human values. It is not an expression of benevolence. The sense of duty is inherently self-righteous. The consequences of actions prompted by duty are ethically irrelevant. Nothing is good except good (duty-driven) intentions. But intentions are not sufficient to the ethical practice of a nurse. And duties, as such, are entirely irrelevant. At their best, they are designed to provide a patient with what is appropriate "in general."

Take this case: An 18-year-old boy is in the intensive care unit of the hospital. He is critically ill and is very frightened. The policy of this hospital only allows visits every two hours for ten minutes in the ICU. The boy is pleading with his nurse to allow his mother or father to stay with him. If the nurse follows deontology, she will not permit this, because it is against a rule—a norm or principle.

Utilitarianism—An Ethic of Utility

Utilitarianism is the theory that "one should act so as to promote the greatest good (pleasure) of the greatest number of people. An act is morally right if it brings about a greater balance of good over evil than any other action that could have been taken" (Angeles, 1992, p. 307). It is a theory in which the end justifies the means (Gibson, 1993).

Thus, utilitarianism is concerned with benefiting the majority, rather than the needs and desires of individuals. Nursing, since nurses deal with individual patients, is particularly unsuited to a utilitarian standard. People who enter nursing "to serve the greatest possible number" suffer a confusion that will have a very negative impact on their career satisfaction. All the time they spend with individual patients is time taken away from the pursuit of their chosen ethical standard. Ethically, a utilitarian could devote attention to an individual patient only when she had nothing "better" to do. In the practice of their profession nurses never have anything better to do than giving attention and care to their patients. "The greatest number" exemplifies the "in general."

Take this case: A 9-year-old boy is dying of leukemia. He comes into the hospital at least once a week for a blood transfusion. On a particular day he tells his nurse that he does not want the blood transfusions anymore. She asks him if he understands what will happen if they are stopped. He says that he knows that he will die. The family and physician are consulted. They are adamant that the transfusions continue to keep him alive as long as possible since he is so young. They refuse to discuss it with him.

From a utilitarian perspective, this might provide the greatest good for the greatest number. The child becomes unimportant in the decision making process. Unfortunately, decisions are often made in the health care setting simply because they follow the wishes of the greater number. It is especially common with children and elderly patients. Many nurses find that this is the most common ethical dilemma they face.

Relativism—An Ethic of Customs

Relativism means that "what is ethical or unethical is determined by the customs, beliefs, and practices of a society, culture, or religion" (Angeles, 1992, p. 244). Relativism implies that ethical values are not essentially connected to human well-being. There is no beneficiary to receive the benefits provided by relativism. Relativism leaves no way to determine when a culture is mistaken. But, a culture, according to relativism, cannot be mistaken. The thoughts and values of individuals are unimportant—or even meaningless. The standard is whatever a society deems best "in general."

Take this case: A man is a member of a religious group that forbids its members from receiving blood. He desperately needs to have a number of blood transfusions and he wants to receive them. All other available means have failed. But he is fearful that his family will find out about it, so he has refused the transfusions. A nurse who accepts relativism will accept his refusal as final. A nurse who is concerned about her patient receiving the care that he actually needs and wants, will discuss with him the possibility, for instance, of having the transfusions during the night when his family will not be present.

"If a patient wishes to go against a custom of his culture he has a right to do so. . . . When families bring pressures to bear on the individual to comply with cultural customs, so much so that the person does not stand up for his own personal wishes, the health care professional must support the patient and encourage him to take the course that supports his well-being" (Zoucha & Husted, 2000, p. 339). While cultural values are important, they can only be as important as the importance placed on them by the individual person. To do otherwise, would be to treat the patient as if he were a mere extension of his culture.

Emotivism—An Ethic of the Subconscious

"Emotivism promotes ethical actions in accordance with the emotions of those involved. Rational thought has no place in choices made by an emotivist, making this type of decision making inappropriate in the health care arena" (Scotto, 2004, in press).

An unsophisticated form of emotivism, even if unrecognized, is far and away the most influential ethical system and is characterized by the following thought process: If I feel that something is right, then it is right. If I feel that something is wrong, then it is wrong. "Emotivism is an outgrowth of ethical noncognitivism. It is an implicit kind of knowledge recognized in the form of emotional attitudes. . . . Ethical noncognitivism is the position that statements containing implicit or explicit references to moral values do not contain descriptive knowledge, are not informative in that sense, and hence are neither true nor false" (Angeles, 1992, p. 84).

This system displaces reason-based relationships with emotional responses, and logical guidance with urges arising from the subconscious. There is no objective guidance in one's feelings. There is no nurse-patient relationship possible between those who are guided by their emotional urges.

The emotivist's primary object of attention is her feelings. Her emotional responses to facts displace the facts. An emotivist will allow her feelings about a patient to shape the quality of the care she gives him, and to determine whether she, the nurse, will be caring and nurturing or callous and indifferent. Her feelings, she assumes, will guide her to what is best "in general."

Take this case: A woman is admitted to the hospital because of dehydration. She is two months pregnant. During a routine exam a lump is discovered in her neck. Tests reveal that it is cancer of the thyroid. She decides to have the treatment for cancer even though she knows that it will, in all probability, harm her child. The nurse caring for her feels that she has no right to do this and that she should wait until she gives birth to the baby. Her care of this woman ceases to be "caring," since she only attends to her patient's physical needs.

Many nurses, some without realizing it, feel a certain way about a person because of the disease, the treatment decision, or some personal characteristic, which then change the way in which they give care. This is done without any assessment, analysis, or communication with the person. A nurse who acts on her feelings will not get into the context of her patient, let alone the context of her practice. She does not evaluate why she "feels" a certain way or she rejects the professional irrelevance of her feelings.

A circumstance cannot be objectively evaluated by reference to an emotion. An emotion must be objectively evaluated by reference to the circumstance.

Nurses would have great difficulty remaining competent in their practice if they failed to consider consequences, did not relate to patients as individuals, made decisions based on some relativist standard, or acted on emotions without reference to the patient's situation. Most nurses do not do this. Nurses are concerned about their individual patients and have a caring attitude toward them. They want to give the best care that they can, given what is possible in the situation. This is very fortunate for patients. The following is an approach that helps nurses to continue to give the best care that they can.

A PRACTICE-BASED APPROACH TO BIOETHICAL DECISION MAKING

A practice based ethic is derived from, and intended to be, appropriate to the self-determination of individual patients, the human purposes that guide individuals in a health care setting, and the role of individual health care professionals acting in harmony with the intrinsic purposes of the health care system. A practice-based ethic is an approach to ethical interaction derived from professional responsibility and from a nurse's determination to be a good nurse. Its purpose is to establish intelligible interactions between health care professionals and their patients.

There are different ways to approach ethical decision making in health care. The *symphonology* approach is a practice-based theory for bioethical decision making that we have developed for professionals in the health care arena, with an emphasis on nurses and their agreement with their individual patients (Husted & Husted, 2001). It is described here to give readers a sense of how ethical decision making can be approached in a systematic way with the patient as the central focus. The symphonological theory of bioethical decision making is based on the principle that the nurse-patient relationship is grounded in a mutual agreement—which includes agreement on context, the role of the nurse, and the individuality of the patient. ("Symphonia" is the Greek equivalent of "agreement.") It is derived from, and is therefore intended to be appropriate to, the situation of the patient, the purpose of the health care setting, and the role of the nurse. It is based on a shared state of awareness, the foundation on which ethical interactions between nurse and patient occur. Figure 9.1 illustrates the basic elements of this theory.

The practice-based symphonological approach to the ethical aspects of professional practice begins with the agreement that unites nurse and patient in their interactions. This agreement is reached under many different conditions and in many different ways, but the simple, commonplace process is as follows: A health care professional walks into a patient's room where the patient is lying in a bed. Right there the agreement is set up: "You are my patient, I will be your nurse" and "You are my nurse, I will be your patient."

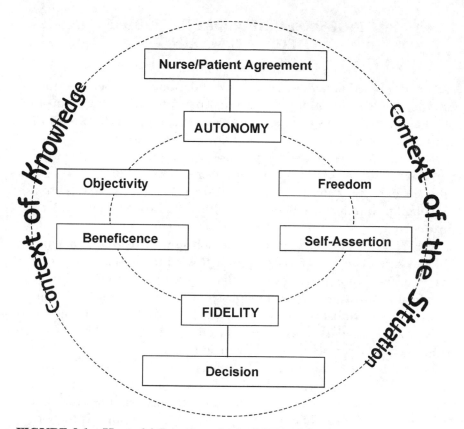

FIGURE 9.1   Husteds' Symphonological Ethical Decision Making Guide
©Husted & Husted, 2001.

Professional and Patient Roles

The following definitions and standards underlie this guide to bioethical decision making (Husted & Husted, 2001).

Definition of "Patient"

A patient is one who, through illness or disability, has lost the power to take certain actions. Being forced into a state of passivity, he requires help in order to regain the ability to take the actions his survival or self-fulfillment requires. This establishes the purpose of the health care setting. The health care setting functions in order to return a patient to a state of agency—to make it possible for him to act on his own behalf. His disability, whatever else it may entail, makes him unable to take the actions his flourishing, or even his survival, requires.

Definition of "Nurse"

A nurse is the agent of a patient, doing for a patient what he would do for himself if he were able. It is her patient who provides the nurse's reason for being a nurse. It is her patient who enables the nurse to discover what it is to be a nurse. The nurse provides much of what the patient lacks. She has the ability to take well-informed actions. Without the actions that a nurse provides, in many cases, the patient could not survive. In many more cases, he could not live successfully. In nearly every case, he could not flourish on his own as well as he does under the care of an ethically competent nurse.

Centrality of the Patient

In the roles established for them in the health care setting, the patient is the natural center of the nurse's attention. Patients are the reason-for-being of the nursing profession. What a nurse is, in being a nurse, *is defined in terms of a patient.* A professional nursing ethic, therefore, if it is relevant to practice, will be patient-centered.

Patients are individuals whose circumstances have brought them into a relationship with health care professionals. A professional ethic relates a nurse and patient internally. This ethic centers a nurse's attention on the context of her patient. Patients are unique individuals. A nursing ethic, to the extent that it is practice-based, focuses a nurse's attention on the circumstances and the motivations of individuals whom a nurse must recognize as similar to her, but also different from her.

The Nurse-Patient Agreement

This agreement is a shared state of awareness on the basis of which interaction occurs. Agreement is the "jumping off point" of *every* interaction. The role of the nurse and the context of the patient determine the terms of their agreement. Even if a patient is not able to actively participate in this interaction, the agreement (through the bioethical standards) is in place.

Bioethical Standards

Bioethical standards act as guides to bioethical decision making within a given context. They are the virtues that explain an individual's purposes, actions, and values. These standards function best—or perhaps only—when interactions are guided by the objective commitments and expectations implied in the nurse-patient agreement:

- *Autonomy* refers to the uniqueness of every individual. In order to interact with a patient, a nurse must recognize his uniqueness.
- *Freedom* refers to an individual's self-directedness. A nurse has an obligation to help a patient exercise his freedom of choice.
- *Objectivity* refers to the desire to know something apart from emotion or personal prejudice. A nurse has to help herself and her patient achieve and sustain the exercise of objective awareness.
- *Self-Assertion* refers to the power and right of an individual to control his or her time and effort. It implies a person's self-ownership. It also implies the right of a patient to make his own decisions and initiate his own actions. A dedicated nurse is his ally in this effort.
- *Beneficence* refers to the act of assisting a patient's effort to attain that which is beneficial and to avoid that which is harmful. This is the life-centered motivation of the nurse-patient agreement and interaction. The illustrious Chinese philosopher, Confucius, describes it magnificently: "The man of beneficence is one who, desiring to sustain himself, sustains others, and desiring to develop himself, develops others" (Fung, 1948, p. 43). This is a nurse's ideal attitude.
- *Fidelity* refers to adherence to the terms of an agreement. It also refers to an individual's faithfulness to his or her autonomy. For a nurse, it is a commitment to the obligation she has accepted as part of her professional role, and the rights she possesses by virtue of her human nature. A patient places his life, health, and well-being in the care of a nurse. At a minimum, he is entitled to expect fidelity from her.

Health Care Context

The nurse functions both as a professional and as a human being within a variety of contexts. These contexts influence directly or indirectly the way in which the nurse performs caring tasks (Gastmans, 1998, p. 126).

A decision made out of context, based on external assumptions or derived from "in general" practices cannot be an appropriate decision for a particular patient in a particular context. A context is the interweaving of the relevant facts of a situation—the facts it is necessary to act upon to bring about a desired result—and the knowledge one has of how to deal most effectively with these facts. A context consists of two distinct but dynamically interrelated elements:

- *The context of the situation*—The interweaving of the relevant facts of a situation that are fundamental to understanding the situation and to acting effectively in it.
- *The context of knowledge*—An individual's awareness of the relevant aspects of a situation that are necessary to understanding the situation and to acting effectively in it.

Ethical Dilemma: An Example

The following is a sample ethical dilemma which is analyzed via the symphonological bioethical decision-making model:

Edgar has been in the hospital for almost 12 weeks. His prognosis is very poor, but the family remains insistent on the patient's remaining a full code, despite the physician's opinions on the poor prognosis and his present and future quality of life. Edgar has multiple medical problems, including metastatic cancer. He has been heard to say on a number of occasions, "I do not want to live." He is now semicomatose and cannot make his wishes known. The family remains unrealistically optimistic.

Using he criteria we have outlined above reveals the following:

Autonomy: If the desires of Edgar's family are given priority, his autonomy is violated since his wishes and theirs contradict each other.
Freedom: Not to honor Edgar's wishes is a violation of his freedom. It is the more so since there is no possibility of his achieving freedom in the future.
Objectivity: The family's optimism is a subjective feeling in conflict with the objective facts.
Self-assertion: Assertion of one's values for another person is not an ethical standard. It is not justifiable to take over a patient's right to self-assertion in order to satisfy the family's unrealistic expectations.

Beneficence: The benefit that Edgar has to lose and the harm he faces are much greater than the benefit that his family has to lose, or the harm they face. Forcing him to act against his will is a maleficent action.

Fidelity: The nurses and other health care professionals working with Edgar have an agreement with him, not with his family. His family's emotions are not a justification for breaking that agreement. The family should be told directly, but with sensitivity, of Edgar's prognosis.

Analysis using the bioethical standards produces a well-rounded justification for a nurse's decisions. Further, it provides a rational framework for those decisions and the greatest possible certainty that they are objectively justifiable.

The experience that is gained with each decision can be and ought to be retained. But, no "in general" decisions can ever be taken whole and placed onto another situation. As in all resolutions, *the unique person within a context* is of central importance.

CONCLUSION

Nursing is engaged in an exciting discovery of its meaning as an ethical practice. This calls for a set of nursing ethics that direct its efforts toward the role of the nurse and the meaning of a professional practice that are grounded in an ethical approach that is relevant to the internal nature and purposes of the health care system. Early efforts to develop nursing ethics focused on the nurse as primarily duty-driven. Reasoning and critical thinking were not considered important components of nursing practice. Today, they are—and this attitude is gaining momentum.

The American Nurses Association (ANA) has long been involved in analyzing the ethical practice of nursing and in setting standards as a guide for practice. The latest ANA Code of Ethics recognizes the critical skills and independent thinking of nurses. This code provides ethical standards for both students and practitioners of nursing. Its nine provisions are included in Table 9.1.

Nursing is an intricate part of the health care system. Nurses have more intimate and continuous contact with patients than any other

TABLE 9.1   ANA Code of Ethics for Nurses

1. The nurse, in all professional relationships, practices with compassion and respect for the inherent dignity, worth, and uniqueness of every individual, unrestricted by considerations of social or economic status, personal attributes, or the nature of health problems.
2. The nurse's primary commitment is to the patient, whether an individual, family, group, or community.
3. The nurse promotes, advocates for, and strives to protect the health, safety, and rights of the patient.
4. The nurse is responsible and accountable for individual nursing practice and determines the appropriate delegation of tasks consistent with the nurse's obligation to provide optimum patient care.
5. The nurse owes the same duties to self as to others, including the responsibility to preserve integrity and safety, to maintain competence, and to continue personal and professional growth.
6. The nurse participates in establishing, maintaining, and improving health care environments and conditions of employment conducive to the provision of quality health care and consistent with the values of the profession through individual and collective action.
7. The nurse participates in the advancement of the profession through contributions to practice, education, administration, and knowledge development.
8. The nurse collaborates with other health professionals and the public in promoting community, national, and international efforts to meet health needs.
9. The profession of nursing, as represented by associations and their members, is responsible for articulating nursing values, for maintaining the integrity of the profession and its practice, and for shaping social policy.

Source: American Nurses Association (2001). *Code of Ethics for Nurses with Interpretive Statements.* Washington, DC: American Nurses Publishing. Available with interpretive statements at www.ana.org.

health care professionals. Because of this, nurses have a very specific role to fulfill in regard to bioethics.

Acquiring skill in bioethical decision making is similar to acquiring any other skill. A person must be active in the experience and learn the skill from an immediate vantage point. One does not learn insightful bioethical decision making from passive contemplation or hearsay.

By mastering bioethical decision making a nurse becomes active in promoting a patient's benefit and her own. By interacting with what is important in a patient's life, a nurse increases her patient's well-being, strengthens the profession of nursing, and establishes the conditions of pride in herself as a professional.

REFLECTIVE QUESTIONS

1. How might the study of nursing ethics assist nurses to practice nursing in an ethically justifiable and responsible manner?
2. How could a nurse assess the ethical aspects of the patient's context?
3. Using the symphonological model for ethical decision making, how would you counsel a patient who must decide whether to gamble on a "long-shot" treatment?

SUGGESTED READINGS

Johnstone, J. (2000). Informed consent and the betrayal of patient's rights. *Australian Nursing Journal, 8*(2), 40–41.

Husted, G. L., & Husted, J. H. (2004, in press). The Ethical Experience of Caring for Vulnerable Populations: The Symphonological Approach. In M. DeChesnay (Ed.), *Caring for vulnerable patients.* Sudbery, MA: Jones & Bartlett.

Kikuchi, J. F. (1996). Multicultural ethics in nursing education: A potential threat to responsible practice. *Journal of Professional Nursing, 12,* 159–165.

REFERENCES

Angeles, P. (1992). *Dictionary of philosophy.* New York: Harper Collins.

Benner, P, Tanner, C. A., & Chesla, C. A. (1996). *Expertise in nursing practice.* New York: Springer Publishing.

Clark, A. P., & Taxis, J. C. (2003). Developing ethical competence in nursing personnel. *Clinical Nurse Specialist, 17,* 236–237.

Edwards, P. (Ed.) (1972). *The encyclopedia of philosophy* (vol. 2). New York: Macmillan.

Fung, Y-L. (1948). *A short history of Chinese philosophy* (Edited by D. Bodde). New York: The Free Press.

Gastmans, C. (1998). Challenges to nursing values in a changing nursing environment. *Nursing Ethics, 5,* 236–245.

Gibson, C. H. (1993). Underpinnings of ethical reasoning in nursing. *Journal of Advanced Nursing, 18,* 20–27.

Husted, G. L., & Husted, J. H. (2001). *Ethical decision-making in nursing and health care: The symphonological approach* (3rd ed.). New York: Springer Publishing.

Milstead, J. (2004). *Health policy and politics: A nurse's guide.* Sudbery, MA: Jones & Bartlett.

Scotto, C. (2003). A new view of caring. *Journal of Nursing Education, 47,* 289–291.

Scotto, C. (2004, in press). Symphonological bioethical theory. In A. M. Tomey & M. R. Alligood (Eds.), *Nursing theorists and their work.* St. Louis: Mosby.

Stanislavski, C. (1964). *An actor prepares.* Routledge, NY: Theater Arts Book.

Zoucha, R. D., & Husted, G. L. (2000). The ethical dimensions of delivering culturally congruent nursing and health care. *Issues in Mental Health Nursing, 21,* 325–340.

10

The Legal Context of Nursing

Ellen Murphy

LEARNING OBJECTIVES

Upon completion of this chapter, the reader should be able to:

- List three sources of law and provide a nursing example of each
- Describe the contents of typical state Nurse Practice Acts
- Define the elements of a case in malpractice
- Enumerate legally recognized patient rights
- Identify strategies to influence nursing's legal context

KEY WORDS

Patient rights, legislation, malpractice, negligence, duty, informed consent

INTRODUCTION

One of the most authoritative forces that shape the context of nursing practice is that provided by law and the legal system. Like nursing, law interacts with its social context—it both shapes the society it is part of, and is shaped by that society. In other words, law and nursing are both product and part of society. It logically follows that law and nursing also interact—each influences and is influenced by the other. This chapter will review the sources of law and provide examples of each that directly affect nursing practice. These examples will include statutory law (the Nurse Practice Acts); common law (negligence and malpractice); and administrative law (rules of state boards of nursing). Patient rights which have been recognized in statutory and/or common law and a brief examination of criminal law will complete this section.

Finally, the chapter will return to its original thesis—that law not only shapes nursing, but that nurses also shape the law. This fact demonstrates that nurses and organized nursing can influence its legal context.

SOURCE OF LAW

As nurses will recall from their high school social studies courses, law in America's representative democratic republic is "made" by the legislative, judicial and executive branches of government. These branches generate different sources of law. State legislatures and the federal Congress produce statutes. Decisions of state appellate and federal judges form our common law or case law. Administrative agencies, such as state boards of nursing or federal agencies, have rule making authority and can promulgate administrative law. The governors or the United States president have authority to make executive orders that become executive law. Executive orders have less of a direct influence on nursing practice and will not be discussed, other than to note that executive orders to call up the national guard or reserves, or to declare disasters, can influence the context of nursing. Superseding all other sources of law are our state and federal constitutions which form the framework of our governments and allocation of power among individuals, states, and the federal government.

STATUTORY LAW—NURSE PRACTICE ACTS

Statutes that define and regulate the practice of nursing in each state most immediately come to mind as an example of law passed by legislatures. Nurses frequently refer to these as *nurse practice acts*, although they may have different technical titles in various states. Typically, each state's nurse practice act defines the practice of nursing in broad terms and establishes a mechanism to provide the regulation and licensure of nursing practice in that state. The purpose of nurse practice acts and the licensure of nurses is to protect the public's health and safety from unqualified, incompetent, or unprofessional practice. The regulatory mechanism established in every state is implemented by a state board of nursing that has the authority to make rules addressing the educational preparation, licensing, practice, and discipline of nurses. The precise composition of the board of nursing differs from state to state, but typically includes both nurses and consumers. Members are usually appointed by the governor and/or the legislature. Other components typical to most nurse practice acts include: a definition of nursing (frequently referred to as the legal scope of practice); provisions and criteria for the granting of the license (typically graduation from an accredited school or college of nursing, passage of a licensure exam, and possession of "good moral character"); and provisions and criteria for discipline, revocation, or suspension of the license.

Nurses who consult their nurse practice acts to answer a specific question such as "What am I legally required to do?" are often disappointed. While statutes define the general scope of nursing practice for each state, statutory language cannot be so specific as to anticipate every situation a nurse may encounter. For example, most nurse practice acts include some phrase like "treatment of the sick under the supervision of a physician," but the statute does not further differentiate among types of treatment or even define the parameters of supervision.

Nor would nurses want such specificity. Prescriptive language in statutes would effectively freeze the status quo and require a return to the legislature every time nursing practice evolved. This is neither desirable nor practical.

ADMINISTRATIVE LAW—THE REGULATION OF NURSING PRACTICE

Administrative law is a kind of hybrid between statutory (legislature made) and executive (governor or president made) law, since administrative agencies get their authority from the legislature and are usually headed by appointees of the governor or president. Administrative agencies are granted rule-making authority by the statutes that create them (for example, boards of nursing are established and given authority by the nurse practice act statutes). The rules that result and the implementation of those rules are known as administrative law.

All state boards of nursing have rule-making authority. These rules provide nurses more specific guidance for their practice than do nurse practice acts. But board of nursing rules are still not as specific as some nurses may wish. Nurses will find the rules of their state board of nursing in their state's administrative code, which can be assessed via their state government Web site.

Rules of the boards of nursing typically include criteria to be a recognized school or college of nursing; faculty qualifications; more specifics about qualification and processes for licensure; standards of practice; criteria and processes for discipline, license suspension, or revocation.

It is imperative that all nurses know the parameters of their practice set by the legislature and board of nursing in the state where they practice (not the state where they live). These can be accessed by a search engine on the Web or by following links to each state by starting at http://www.ncsbn.org, the Web site for the National Council of State Boards of Nursing (NCSBN). There are minor differences among all states in practice at the entry level; there can be significant differences at the advanced practice levels. The NCSBN Web site also lists the states that have adopted the Nurse Licensure Compact. This Compact allows nurses who hold a licensure in one state to practice in another state, provided both states have adopted the Compact.

When reviewing nurse practice acts and state board of nursing administrative rules, nurses should note especially the processes and criteria for discipline. Very few nurses ever face discipline, but prevention of finding oneself in such a situation remains the best approach. Licensure is a privilege; but once granted, it becomes a property right that cannot be taken away without "due process." Due process requires that nurses have notice of what conduct is expected, be told specifics about any charges against them, have an opportunity to be represented by counsel and confront/refute any evidence against them, and have a decision maker who is impartial.

As a result, it is not easy to lose a license, but it does happen. When it does, it is most often due to behaviors most nurses would agree endanger the public health and safety (e.g., use, diversion, or sale of controlled substances). When the issue is one of poor judgment or lack of sufficient competence, state boards tend to rule in favor of suspension and rehabilitation or remedial learning rather than revocation. Still, all nurses must remember licensure to practice is a privilege and should deliver care according to legal and professional standards.

COMMON LAW—NEGLIGENCE AND MALPRACTICE

Common law sometimes is called case law or judge made law. It results from the compilation of reported appellate court decisions. The most obvious example of common law related to nursing is the law of negligence and malpractice.

Negligence is a subset of the common law categorized as tort law. Tort law deals with injury to persons or property. Negligence law applies when the injury to persons or property results from the nonintentional failure to act reasonably. Malpractice is simply negligence by a professional in the performance of a professional act. Nurses have exposure for both negligence and malpractice in the course of their practice. Whether an action is negligence or malpractice is a technicality that is more important to the attorneys involved and how they approach the case than it is a practical difference for nurses. Practically, the same general elements apply. Knowledge of the elements, and of the evidence used to establish those elements, can be used by the nurse to develop strategies to prevent negligence or malpractice claims (Murphy, 1987).

Elements of a Case in Negligence and Malpractice

The elements of a case are those factors that the plaintiff's (injured patient's) attorney must prove in order to be successful in a suit against the defendant (nurse and/or employing facility). The elements of a case in negligence and malpractice are:

1. *Duty*—The nurse or facility has undertaken a professional/patient relationship and thereby agrees to render reasonable and prudent care. Except for a few exceptions provided by statutes (e.g., the federal Emergency Medical Treatment and Active Labor Act, or some states' Good Samaritan statutes), neither nurses nor facilities have a duty to provide care to everyone who might seek or need their care. Health care is a mutually contracted relationship. Both the provider and the recipient must agree to enter into a caregiving relationship. Nurses who agree to work for a facility also agree to care for the patients that the facility accepts. Once a nurse or facility enters a professional relationship with a patient, the nurse has a duty to provide the amount and the type of care that a reasonable and prudent nurse or facility would have provided. This is what is known as the "legal standard

of care." Most often the judgment as to what constitutes the legal standard of care must be informed by nurse-generated evidence. Examples of this evidence are provided below.

2. *Breach*—The defendant did not do what reasonable and prudent defendants would have done. The health care record and the testimony of material witnesses are key pieces of evidence in determining whether the nurse or facility complied with the legal standard of care. Material witnesses are those with first-hand knowledge of what happened at the time and include both the plaintiff and the defendants, as well as all other persons who may have been present.

3. *Causation*—The link between the defendant's breach of the standard of care and the patient's injury must be a causal one. This element usually requires expert testimony from physicians as to what caused the injury.

4. *Damages*—The money value necessary to compensate the injured plaintiff, i.e., the amount of money necessary to put the plaintiff in the position he would have occupied had the defendants' action(s) not caused the plaintiff's injury. This also requires expert testimony by economists, physicians, and an emerging field of "life plan" experts.

The plaintiff has the burden of proof in negligence and malpractice cases. This means the plaintiff must prove each element by a preponderance of the evidence. Unless the plaintiff proves all four elements, the defendant cannot be found liable of negligence or malpractice.

Evidence of the Legal Standard of Care

A major difference between negligence and malpractice cases is in how the standard of care (what a reasonable and prudent nurse would have done) is determined. In a negligence case, the jury may be allowed to use their own common sense (e.g., that reasonable staff members wipe up spilled water from the floor and failure to do so can cause a fall). The jury usually needs evidence to assist them in determining what a reasonable nurse/facility should have done because lay jurors do not always know what is reasonable and prudent nursing practice. This evidence includes:

1. Expert witness testimony, i.e., another nurse testifying as to what should have been done, based on the professional education

and experience of the expert and the expert's review of the facts of the case.

2. Policies and procedures of the facility. These are very persuasive since they are written by the professionals who actually work in the facility and know its realities.

3. Statutes or administrative rules. If there are laws that specifically address the situation at issue, these are seen as authoritative statements of what is expected reasonable behavior. As noted above, such specificity is rare.

4. National professional association of standards or recommended practices. The American Nurses Association and most specialty nursing organizations have published standards, guidelines, or recommended practices. These statements do not have the force of law but they can be used as evidence to assist the jury in determining what the defendant nurse should have done. Likewise, the standards of professional associations that apply to facilities, such as those of the Joint Commission on Accreditation of Healthcare Organizations (JCAHO), can be admitted as evidence as to what reasonable facilities should have done.

5. Professional literature. Textbooks, journal articles and Web sites can be a source of evidence as to what reasonable and prudent nurses and facilities would have done if a qualified expert attests to their authoritative nature.

Each of the four requisite elements must be proved against the nurse and/or the employing facility. The reason injured plaintiffs can sue both parties is grounded in the legal principle of "respondeat superior," from the Latin, "let the master respond." Under the principle of respondeat superior, the employer is legally responsible for the negligence of its employees (both professional and nonprofessional). It is the relationship as employee, not the status of professional or nonprofessional, that determines whether respondeat superior applies. Respondeat superior is a doctrine of vicarious or indirect liability; that is, one person or entity (the employer) is legally liable if another person or entity (the employee) is found negligent.

Employing facilities can also be directly liable to injured patients. The employing facility, not the individual employee nurse, has a direct duty to its patients to provide the patients with a safe environment (e.g., equipment that works, adequate ventilation, sanitary services, safe food preparation, etc.); safe staffing levels (both in terms of numbers and expertise); and having the policies and systems in place to deliver the right care to the right patient at the right time so as not to cause (or fail to prevent) injury.

The frequently quoted case of *Darling versus Charleston Community Memorial Hospital (1965)* illustrates both direct and indirect hospital liability exposure. One of the questions before the court in that case was whether the hospital had failed to have a "sufficient number of trained nurses for bedside care" (Darling, p. 258) so as to have assessed the progressive gangrenous condition of plaintiff's leg and notified the physician in a sufficiently timely manner so the cast could have been loosened and the ischemia relieved.

It is possible for facilities to be liable to patients even when its employee nurses are not found liable. For example, a hospital was found liable for failure to provide adequate nurse assessment competency to its neonate patient when an adult care nurse was floated to the neonatal unit. The adult care nurse failed to assess a neonate's deteriorating condition in a timely fashion and the neonate ultimately died. The nurse was found not liable because the nurse had done what a reasonable adult care nurse would have done under the circumstances. The hospital was found liable because it failed in its direct duty to provide the level of newborn expertise needed to care safely for this neonate (Northern Trust v. Louis Weiss Memorial Hospital, 1986).

Comparative or Contributory Negligence

American common law recognizes that patients also have a duty to be reasonable and prudent. If a patient's unreasonable conduct (e.g., providing false data; noncompliance with discharge instructions) contributes to the injury, the patient's damage award can be reduced or barred, depending on the jury's determination of the percentage of contribution that was due to the patient's negligence. This principle emphasizes the importance of patient teaching, since patients must know what elements of self-care are expected or needed in order to protect themselves from injury.

PATIENT RIGHTS

Legally recognized patient rights can be created and/or enforced by statutory, administrative, and common law. Patients have a right to be free from injury caused by others, which is enforced by the common law of negligence. Patients have a right to competent care, which is enforced by licensure laws applicable to nearly all health care professions and providing facilities. Patients also have specific legal rights to informed consent or informed refusal of consent to treatment, and confidentiality regarding treatment. Interestingly, patients do not have a legally recognized right to health care in the United States. Except in cases of emergency, American health care is a mutually contracted agreement, which can be premised on ability to pay. Once a patient is accepted by a provider of health care, however, a variety of rights is attached.

Informed Consent

All states' statutes and/or case law recognize the patient's legal right to be informed and to consent prior to receiving health care treatment. The right to consent to treatment was recognized in the seminal case of *Schloendorff versus Society of New York,* which stated, "Every human being of adult years has a right to determine what shall be done with his own body" (Schloendorff v. Society of New York, 1914, p. 93).

Over the rest of the twentieth century, this doctrine evolved to require not only that the patient consent, but that the consent be informed (Cobbs v. Grant, 1972). To be "informed," the patient must understand the risks, benefits, and alternatives to the proposed treatment before consenting. Case law in various states differs about what specific information about the risks, benefits, and alternatives must be provided. Some require the patient be told what a reasonable patient would need to know; others require only what this patient's specific circumstances require he/she know in order to knowledgeably consent; and a few states require only what a reasonable provider would have disclosed (e.g., Canterbury v. Spence, 1972; Karp v. Cooley, 1974). These differences can be subtle and complex and have spawned much debate in the literature, courts, and legislatures.

Despite the distinctions in what must be disclosed, case law is consistent among the states that the professional responsible for providing the required information and obtaining the patient's consent is the person performing the procedure, more often than not, the treating physician. Thus, except for some advanced nurse practitioners, nurses have very limited legal exposure for failure to obtain the patient's informed consent.

What exposure nurses have is limited to following whatever procedure is in place in the facility. Many times, nurses participate in the process that documents that the patient's consent has been obtained or to assure that documentation of the patient's consent is on the health care record prior to receiving treatment or submitting to a procedure. But documenting that consent has been obtained (by the physician) is not the same as obtaining the consent (providing necessary information and having the patient indicate his or her consent). Nurses must know and follow whatever the facility's procedure prescribes; their liability exposure is limited to following those procedures.

Furthermore, nurses should not undertake to provide the patient with additional information about the procedure lest they be deemed to have assumed the duty that otherwise is solely that of the treating physician. However, if the nurse or hospital knows or should have known that the informed consent was not obtained, there may be a legal duty to intervene (Robertson v. Menorah, 1979). That intervention is limited to informing a supervisor or physician of the deficit, or following whatever other action is required by facility policy.

Refusal of Treatment

The corollary to the right to consent to treatment is the patient's right to refuse treatment. (The right to consent would be meaningless without the right to refuse). This is another patient right recognized in most states' statutes and case law. In addition, the federal Patient Self Determination Act (PSDA) requires that patients be explicitly informed of their rights under the applicable state law (e.g., Living Wills or Durable Powers of Attorney for HealthCare), although it does not create any additional federal rights.

The right to refuse consent includes the right to withdraw consent even after consent has been given, as long as medically viable alternatives remain (Schreiber v. Physician's Insurance, 1999). Even more complex, however, is the patient's right to refuse treatment even when that refusal is likely to hasten death. Most states recognize living wills and/or durable powers of attorney for health care that provide mechanisms for patients to exercise this right even after incapacity or incompetence.

In no other area of patients' rights, does the right to refuse treatment involve so many intertwined moral, ethical, religious, social, economic, and cultural dimensions. Nurses should not allow themselves to be placed in positions where they must make decisions regarding commencing or discontinuing life-sustaining treatment unilaterally. Such complex decisions with irreversible results require an interdisciplinary approach and may require consultation with a facilities ethics committee. Broad consultation provides evidence that the ultimate decision was reasonable, if it is later challenged in a legal proceeding.

Confidentiality

Nurses also should know and comply with their facility's procedures to protect the patient's legal right to confidentiality. The parameters of this right are found in state statutes and case law, and more recently in the federal statute known as HIPAA, the Health Insurance Portability and Accountability Act of 1996.

The core provision of all patient confidentiality laws requires that patient care information not be disclosed to outside parties without the patient's knowledge and consent, unless the law provides a specific exception. Implementation of these laws is also very complex and best left to those responsible for facility policy. Nurses should follow the facility policy very closely. In addition, nurses should guard against informal (cafeteria, elevator) or even professional (consultation with a nurse or physician in the hallway or nurses station) conversations that could be overheard by nonauthorized third parties. Care must also be taken that any information provided in person, over the telephone, or via e-mail is given only after authorization that the person is the person claimed to be and is approved by the patient or by policy to receive the information requested.

CRIMINAL LAW

Criminal law is another section of the legal system (separate from the law discussed above which is called civil law). Criminal law also is created by state and federal statutes and case law. However, unlike most other areas of the law pertaining to nurses, criminal law carries with it an element of intent to perform the criminal act and a social sanction of bad conduct and bad person if the act is carried out. A nurse who injures a patient negligently or infringes on confidentiality without intending to do so may cause harm to another person, but is not legally considered a bad person or a bad nurse, because these are nonintentional acts. While the negligent nurse may owe the patient money damages, the purpose of that payment is to compensate the patient, not to punish the nurse. On the other hand, the purpose of criminal law is to deter bad behavior and to punish persons found guilty of criminal behavior via fines or restrictions on personal freedom, such as imprisonment. A nurse found guilty of criminal behavior is legally judged to be a bad person, deserving of punishment.

Controlled substance usage, diversion, and sale comprise a major area of criminal exposure for nurses. Willful killing of patients via drug administration provides high-profile, but extremely rare, instances of nurses in violation of criminal law. Occasionally, nurses who did not intend to kill or injure a patient can still be criminally prosecuted under negligent homicide law if the nurse's behavior was so "reckless" as to rise to a level deserving punishment and deterrence of others. Actions while impaired by drugs or alcohol could place the nurse at risk for a negligent homicide charge if those actions cause a death. Just as driving while impaired or intoxicated is reckless in placing others at risk, so too would trying to deliver nursing care while impaired or intoxicated.

THE INTERACTION OF LAW AND NURSING

Obviously, nursing practice is heavily influenced by its legal context. Statutes and administrative rules regulate nursing, what it is nurses may do, and how they may be disciplined. Common law allows injured patients to sue nurses. Likewise, patients can seek redress for infringements of their rights to consent, to refuse consent, or to have their health information held in confidence. Criminal law can punish reckless conduct. These laws all provide extra incentives for nurses' caution when caring for patients. But it is worth noting that these laws are not totally imposed upon nursing from the outside. Nurses can and should influence the laws that are passed in Congress or the state legislatures. They can do this by voting, joining professional associations, and becoming politically active to influence who gets elected. Nurses, as individuals and as members of professional associations, can lobby legislators to influence the content of the statutes passed.

It is also noteworthy that the majority of the members of the state boards of nursing are nurses who are frequently appointed pursuant to nomination and support from organized nursing associations. Thus, nurses are the primary source of laws regulating nurses.

Nurses can also influence case law. Judges, attorneys, and lay jurors cannot speculate as to what reasonable and prudent nurses do. They must base those conclusions on evidence. This evidence includes nurse-generated information in the form of expert nurse witnesses, policies and procedures drafted by nurses, and refereed articles authored by nurses. For continuing discussion of issues related to law and nursing, readers may wish to consult the *Journal of Nursing Law.*

CONCLUSION

Nursing and the law do interact. Each influences the other. Nurses have a duty to know and comply with the laws that form nursing's legal context. Nurses also have a responsibility to influence the parameters and contact of the law as advocates for their patients and for quality nursing practice.

KEY TERMS

Administrative rules—laws passed by administrative agencies led by appointees of the governor or president.

Civil law—area of the law concerned with the rights and duties of private persons or groups.

Criminal law—area of the law concerned with crimes and their punishments.

Direct liability—liability for one's own negligence.

Evidence—authoritative information, sworn to be true, that is admitted at trial to assist the trier of fact (usually a jury, sometimes the judge) making its decision.

Expert witness—person with specialized knowledge about the professional or technical issue involved who testifies under oath to assist the jury in understanding the situation in dispute. If accepted as qualified by the judge, may testify as to opinion.

Indirect or vicarious liability—liability for the negligence of others.

Malpractice—negligence by a professional performing a professional act.

Material witness—person with first-hand information about a disputed fact who testifies under oath at trial.

Negligence—failure to use reasonable care.

Standard of care—what a reasonable and prudent nurse of similar education and experience would have done under similar circumstances.

Statutes—laws passed by state legislatures or Congress.

Tort law—the area of common law dealing with injury to persons or property.

REFLECTIVE QUESTIONS

1. What strategies can you identify that will make successful suit for nursing malpractice less likely? (Hint: review the elements of negligence.)
2. How can nurses as individuals and collectively influence the law in your state?
3. The evidence used to establish the legal standard of care is mostly generated by nurses. Why is this important?
4. Do the laws related to patients' rights reflect the ethics of patient care? Why or why not?
5. The majority of the members of state boards of nursing are nurses. Is this a good practice for a body charged with protecting the public?

RECOMMENDED READINGS

Northrup, C. S., & Kelly, M. (1987). *Legal issues in nursing.* St. Louis: Mosby.

Guido, G. W. (2001). *Legal and ethical issues in nursing* (3rd ed.). Upper Saddle River, NJ: Prentice Hall.

REFERENCES

Canterbury v. Spence, 464 F 2d, 722 (D.C. Cir. 1972), cert. denied 409 U.S. 1064 (1972).

Cobbs v. Grant, 104 Cal. Rptr. 505(Cal. 1972)

Darling v. Charleston Community Memorial Hospital, 33 Ill.2d 326, cert. denied 383 U.S. 946 (1966).

Health Insurance Portability and Accountability Act (HIPAA), Public Law 104–191, August 21, 1996.

Karp v. Cooley, 349 F. Supp. 827 (S.D. Tex. 1972), aff'd at 493 F. 2d 408 (5th Cir 1974).

Murphy, E. K. (1987). Preventing a successful malpractice claim. *AORN Journal, 46*(0), 106–110.

National Council of State Boards of Nursing, accessible on the Web at www.ncsbn.org

Northern Trust v. Louis Weiss Memorial Hospital, 143 Ill. App. 3d 479 (1986).

Patient Self-Determination Act, Public Law 101–508, Sections 4206 and 4751, 1990.

Robertson v. Menorah, 588 S.W. 2d 134 (Mo) (1979).

Schloendorff v. Society of New York, 211 N.Y. 125, 105 N.E. 92 (1914).

Schreiber v. Physician's Insurance, 223 Wis.2d 417, 588 N.W. 2d 26 (Wis. 1999).

11

Gender Issues In Nursing: A Global Perspective

Sandra Speedy

LEARNING OBJECTIVES

On completion of this chapter, readers will:

- Understand and appreciate the historical development of feminist thinking on concepts such as nursing work and science
- Have examined the role that gender plays in defining the world of nursing work
- Develop an enlarged perspective about how the health care system and health professionals are affected by the issue of gender
- Have briefly explored the influence that feminism has had on the discipline of nursing
- Understand how feminist theory has influenced nursing research
- Have considered the debate about the relative advantages and disadvantages that gender provides for nurses

KEY WORDS

Gender, nursing work, feminism, patriarchy, power, organizational culture

INTRODUCTION

In order to consider a range of gender issues—which have become of increasing interest and relevance to nurses all over the world—this chapter will consider the gendered nature of nursing work. This will involve discussion of the nature of women who provide the majority of the nursing workforce. It will also require some analysis of the nature of nursing work as it is performed by women. Inherent in this discussion will be consideration of the role of science in determining the concept of woman, as well as the work they undertake. The chapter will also consider briefly the influence of feminism on nursing, and the influence of nurses and nursing on feminism. Finally, the chapter will also examine the increasing role played by men in nursing, a gender issue of utmost importance for the future of nursing.

THE GENDERED NATURE OF NURSING WORK

A consideration of the gendered nature of nursing work must examine the concept of woman, since the majority of nurses are women. Whatever views are held regarding women will influence perception of women's work, in this case, nursing work. Perspectives on women are influenced by "scientific" views about the nature of women, although it might also be argued that perspectives on women influence beliefs about the nature of science.

There is a burgeoning body of literature that demonstrates a range of approaches and various viewpoints on woman as object and subject. Women can be examined from sociological, psychological, biological, philosophical, or political perspectives—and from other viewpoints as well. Many of these viewpoints feature devaluation of women, as any examination of the concepts of essentialism, biologism, naturalism, or universalism will demonstrate. In an insightful work, Grosz (1990) suggests that all of these terms, which argue the nature of women (and men, incidentally), fix and define the limits, because they "are commonly used in patriarchal discourses to justify women's social subordination and their secondary positions relative to men in patriarchal society" (p. 333). Gherardi (1994) argues that "masculinity and femininity are symbolic universes of meaning socially and historically constructed" (p. 591). She suggests also that the way we "do gender" in our work "helps to diminish or increase the inequality of the sexes: we use ceremonial work to recognize the difference of gender, and remedial work socially to construct the 'fairness' of gender relationships" (p. 592). There is no question that in nursing each gender experiences "cross-over," necessitating the management of dual presence in what are essentially separate symbolic contexts.

There are problems with constructing a "universal feminism" since allowance must be made for difference and diversity between women, just as there is between women and men. What is worthy of exploration are some of the views about women and nurses within a medical and health professions context, because these views are influenced by the concepts mentioned above. The issue of how women are constructed by science is also relevant here (Kane & Thomas, 2000).

Feminist literature argues that the masculinity of science is an image that has been perpetuated for centuries. This image creation is affected by textbook representations, curriculum organization, classroom behavior, and stereotypical beliefs and attitudes. It distorts science, yet scientific method has not been successful in filtering out patriarchal bias in the scientific construction of women. In the early 1990s, Lather wrote with clarity regarding this:

> The claim of positivistic researchers that their method is sufficient protection against ideological incursion is debunked by feminist critiques of the conceptual and methodological orientations that reflect and reinforce sex-based inequality. Hence the construction of women brings into question that which has passed for knowledge in the human sciences. (Lather, 1991, p. 17)

The masculinity of science is only an illusion (albeit a powerful one), not an intrinsic part of its nature. Science is a social construct, and "its development is inextricably linked with social relations, not least the relations between men and women" (Kelly, 1985, p. 76). This leads, of course, to using male as the norm and female as the referent, a strategy that has been exposed and rejected in a wide range of disciplines, including psychology, sociology, psychiatry, medicine, education, and biology. As long ago as the 1970s, it was pointed out that male medicine misunderstood the female body, and these debates have now extended to cover all aspects of women's health, not just those of childbirth and reproduction.

In nursing and medicine, the presence of increasing numbers of women at all levels of authority indicate a modicum of success in producing woman-friendly services and conditions. This has come about only because women have been forced to reclaim their healing role, which was given a boost by the knowledge and insights in the classic treatise written by Ehrenreich and English (1979) documenting the exclusion of womenashealers from professionalized, modern medicine. There has long been "increasing institutional awareness of the deficiencies and sexism of specific institutional practices" (Evans, 1997, p. 42). This has had both positive and negative effects. For the latter, it has resulted in some feminists "beating up" on nurses, thus earning the title "anti-nurse." This behavior is:

> predicated on the belief that nurses willingly capitulate to male (and/ or medical) dominance, thereby making it difficult for 'real feminists' to achieve their goals. This . . . 'complicity hypothesis' . . . sees nurses as compliant with patriarchal demands to remain oppressed. (Buchanan, 1997, p. 82)

Using this argument, nurses may be viewed as either the embodiment of the "ideal" woman, conforming to masculine desires, or as the "bad mother, thwarting women in their endeavors and assisting the medical profession in torturing women patients" (Buchanan, 1997, p. 82). In some ways, this historical debate could be seen as unfortunate; in other ways, it suggests that there can be growth for women and nurses if we critically consider all sides of this argument.

Of course, we do not need feminists to beat up on nurses–nurses do that very well to each other, whether they are feminists or not (Briles, 1994; David, 2000). Horizontal violence has long been recognized by a range of authors, who suggest that nurses' self-hate and dislike of other nurses is demonstrated by the lack of cohesion in nursing groups, as well as the phenomenon of "eating our young" (Bent, 1993). The systematic oppression of women can assist nurses to recognize the oppressive structures in which they practice, which

> includes recognizing that nurses are placed in a culture that does not value their attributes, rather than 'blaming' them for ranking lower in self-esteem and higher in submissiveness in job-trait studies than do people in other occupations. Nurses must no longer assume that they are inherently inferior to the systems that surround them. (Bent, 1993, p. 298)

This brings us to the work of nursing.

NURSING WORK

The role and function of nursing cannot be separated from those who undertake this activity. It is quite clear that there are particular views held about women and nursing that then create the definitions of women's work and nursing work, and by implication, men's work (David, 2000; Meadus, 2000). Cheek and Rudge (1995) point out that

> the low status of nursing and the way in which the work of nurses is devalued, especially when compared to other health professionals, can at least in part be explained by its gendered nature. (Cheek & Rudge, 1995, p. 312)

Labelling nursing as "women's work" creates a deterrent which "inhibits recruitment of men into the profession and aids promotion of the sex imbalance in the nursing workforce" (Meadus, 2000, p. 9). Nursing is thus viewed as a natural extension of the female role, valuing nurturance, caring, support, care, and concern (Bent, 1993; Brykczynska, 1997; Evans, 1997). These characteristics have been described as encompassing a "tyranny of niceness" (Street, 1995). Nevertheless, researchers have found that these characteristics are selectively eliminated during the educational and socialization process (Doering, 1992). For example, Treacy (1989) noted that current nurse training endorses "compliance, passivity, and ladylike behavior, but it negatively sanctions other female traits such as intuition, empathy, and emotional expression" (p. 88). The descriptors "compliance, passivity and ladylike behavior" are words which, it could be argued, are suggestive of "powerlessness" and "intuitiveness, empathy and emotional expression," are often viewed as unscientific and hence unacceptable in the world of science. As David (2000) also points out, "the gender dialectic is still so fundamental to gender politics that it permeates the traditions of nursing, such as the belief that nursing is woman's work" (p. 86). Because of this, it can be argued that women and nurses are on shaky ground, while men are inhibited from entering the nursing profession.

Evans (1997) points out that nineteenth-century science and rationality perceived the "feminine" as an abstraction, which assisted in marginalizing women within institutional practices. Women, as we have seen, were constructed as hysterical and intellectually inferior, while men were expected to conform to the stereotype of masculine behavior. Thus, "the 'soft' feminine and the 'hard' masculine then receive institutional recognition and confirmation in particular practices" (Evans, 1997, p. 39). Feminists have sought to demonstrate the disjunction between supposed institutional objectivity and actual institutional practice. Specifically, the institution of medicine, for example, defines its values as nongendered, while in practice, they are deeply gendered (Evans, 1997). This has been exposed in many areas, one example being the management of childbirth.

Because the values that dominate our health system are so pervasive and reflect the values of society at large, "it is a struggle for nurses to remain aligned to the person rather than the institution" (Huntington, 1996, p. 170). This creates difficulties in nursing work, as the dominant discourses that shape health, illness, and perceptions of what it is to be a woman (and a man, incidentally) can disadvantage the individual. As Huntington (1996) points out, "we have been left with only male language to explain the fundamentally female practice of healing bodies" (p. 170). The only solution to this problem is to develop an alternative discourse to that constructed and dominated by the orthodox scientific discourse characteristics of the medical world.

Clearly, too, feminist thinking has challenged the cultural code of organizations, designed around masculinity and femininity, which suggests that "gender is deeply embedded in the design and functioning of organizations" (Davies, 1995, p. 44). These workplaces are socially constructed, they are not gender-neutral, and operate on masculine values for their legitimization and affirmation (Gherardi, 1994). Nurses therefore find it difficult to function within such gendered organizations, and frequently resort to blaming the victim—other nurses who also struggle with their day-to-day functioning within a hostile environment. Thus

> [W]omen, in a very important sense, cannot be 'at home' in the public world—it is constructed in such a way that assumes home is somewhere else, somewhere far away and different. (Davies, 1995, p. 62)

However, Kane and Thomas (2000) remind us that nursing has historically provided a haven for women who seek to control their lives within a professional context, although there are significant limits to what can be achieved.

There is a range of other historical scholarly work that demonstrates the further weakening of nursing's value. For example, Gamarnikow (1978) linked nursing to domesticity; Treacy (1989) suggested that the invisibility of nurses' contribution to care reflected the invisibility of much of the work contribution of women to society. Other scholars have pointed out that the sexual division of labor in the home disadvantages women in the workplace, which creates enormous stress for working women, in this case, nurses. This taps into the work of feminist scientists who have "identified 'women's work,' the 'caring professions,' 'unpaid domestic labour,' 'the double shift,' and other manifestations of the apparently 'natural' social division of labour" (Evans, 1997, p. 59).

It has been pointed out by many scholars that caring itself is a gendered construct, since notions of professional caring are derived from traditional concepts of caring as a feminine obligation (Caffrey & Caffrey, 1994; Falk Rafael, 1996; Wuest, 1997; Ekstrom, 1999; Tronto, 1999). Caring in nursing has in the past been constructed as an inherently feminine pastime, and traditionally, has received little social or economic recognition; it has been perceived as women's work, as unintellectual, unskilled, and emotional, and thus likely to perpetuate gender exploitation (Bubeck, 1995). It was long believed that the work nurses undertake in order to provide care does not require any particular skill or knowledge; it has been viewed as a quality women possess "naturally" (Falk Rafael, 1998; Henderson, 2001; Zebroski, 2001).

However, this view has been challenged in more recent times. For example, Meadus (2000) cites research that demonstrates that men enter nursing because of their desire to care for others, thus challenging the stereotype that only women nurses care. He also notes that such men run the risk of being perceived as gay because of this role violation. This viewpoint is challenged by Bubeck (1995) as she notes that "part of the practice of care is to focus on the needs of the other, to become attentive, to be selfless" (p. 114). By the construction of masculinity, caring is very difficult for men; they also escape from the care burden through the public/private split in responsibilities of women and men (Tronto, 1999).

Nursing's detractors have long promoted the idea that nurses are doers rather than thinkers; that is, nurses do not need to think to do nursing, as long as they can do certain tasks. This has, in no small measure, led to a significant devaluation of nursing, assisted by the unequal power relations which characterize the position of nursing vis-à-vis medicine (David, 2000). For many years this view was used to justify the low level education provided to nurses prior to their entry into the higher education system. That caring is assumed not to require knowledge is not without practical consequence. The replacement of registered nurses with less skilled personnel is considered less of a reflection of economic rationalism than a reflection of the idea that caring is unskilled activity intrinsic to domesticity and womanhood. To engender nurse caring as feminine, therefore positioning it as innately instinctive to women, is to deny the advanced knowledge and skills that lie within the therapeutic caring acts of nurses. Despite the fact that "emotional labor" is a vital and necessary part of the nursing labor process, it "tends to be marginalized as a skill that a predominantly female nursing workforce would naturally possess" (Bolton, 2000, p. 580).

Emotional labor can be conceived as a "gift in the form of authentic caring behaviour" which truly reflects the state of "being a nurse" (Bolton, 2000, p. 586). The fact that it is undertheorized and not appreciated is of serious concern (Henderson, 2001). Emotional work can be hard labor, and relief measures are sought to cope with this continuous laboring. Relief can be found in "backstage regions" such as the nurses station, where profound irritation with patients or emotional anguish can be expressed, where nurses can drop their public mask and express their true feelings. As Fineman (1993) indicates, "off-stage settings are not emotion free-ports" (p. 21). Here, implicit feeling rules can come into play; colleagues can express emotion to a degree that will be cathartic, but will also maintain organizational order.

Despite the fact that it is now acknowledged that emotional labor occurs in organizations, and that employers have expectations about what sorts of emotions one should feel in particular contexts, emotional work tends to be privatized and moved out of the realm of organizational responsibility (Boyle, 2002a, 2002b). Emotional labor work involves remaining continuously vigilant and sensitive to the environment, constantly noting and responding to others' emotional states, alleviating resultant distress, and assisting those who are "inappropriately emotional" to regain their stability (Lupton, 1998).

Emotional labor work can be emotionally and physically demanding, but requires skill and competencies that are not acknowledged (Myerson, 2000; Nicolson, 1996). This lack of acknowledgment occurs for three reasons. First, emotional work remains largely invisible. Second, it requires the development of awareness and of a vocabulary to describe this work as a competency. Third, this work is done predominantly by women. Women tend to be more involved in the caring and service industries than men (as in nursing), and also perform much of the backstage or behind the scenes work (Goffman, 1959). While this work may be perceived as trivial, it is usually of a supportive nature, enhancing the intellectual capability or productivity of organizations (Lupton, 1998). This is not to say that men do not do emotional labor; some do.

However, management is still predominantly done by men, and their power to demand emotional labor from both men and women is maintained by management, although it is "often constructed as (non)emotions" (Hearn, 1993, p. 161).

It is important not to forget the value of relationships that nurses develop with their patients, with relatives, and with carers, all of which are part of using the self in caring mode, often critical to recovery, and which can be very demanding. Sandelowski (1997) makes the point that those who engender nursing as female

> inadvertently minimize or deny nursing its record of expertise and innovation within technology, the primary roles nurses have played in the deployment of technology and the power and remuneration that come with technological knowledge and skills in a high-technology culture (Sandelowski, 1997, p. 172).

Traditional expectations which surround caring as a feminine, nursing activity involve subjugation of the self and selfless devotion to duty (Caffrey & Caffrey, 1994). In some circumstances, nurses may experience feelings of powerlessness and eventually burnout, as a result of suppression of their own feelings and needs (Demerouti, Bakker, Nachreiner, & Schaufeli, 2000).

For Benner (1984), caring may be experienced as an empowering, enabling process. Power and caring are gendered concepts, power as "male" and caring as "female," and though relatively few studies examining gender-related differences in nurse caring have been undertaken, there is some evidence to suggest that nurse gender has an influence on how nurse caring behaviors are demonstrated (Greenhalgh, Vanhanen, & Kyngas, 1998; Ekstrom, 1999; Jones, 2001). Because of the gendered nature of power and caring, these two concepts may thus appear as oppositional. Benner (1984) associates power with caring by identifying power characteristics related to the caring dimensions of nursing practice, specifically, transformative power, integrative caring, advocacy, healing power, participative/affirmative power, and problem solving.

Transformative power refers to power that patients claim for themselves in order to take control of a situation, but which is only possible because of the particular way nurses choose to care for such patients. Integrative caring refers to the care nurses provide which enables the patient to be integrated into his or her social world, despite the limitations that illness may impose. Participative/affirmative power refers to the power nurses gain from engagement and involvement with the patient by using the meanings and resources that flow from the specific situation.

Davies (1995) argues that femininity itself is what provides the threat in caring. Nursing stands for a set of qualities that are unacceptable, since they are the "vulnerabilities and dependencies that are edited out of masculinity." She adds that

> Femininity—with its stress on dealing with dependency, acknowledging emotions and intimacy and nurturing others—comes to represent qualities that are feared and denied in masculinity, qualities that at best are seen as to be contained and allocated to a different sphere, and at worst are repressed or treated with contempt (Davies, 1995, p. 183).

Jones (2001) points out that claiming caring as nursing's unique essence creates serious vulnerability for nursing, particularly as caring has such widespread currency within the profession (see also Traynor, 1996; Snellgrove & Hughes, 2000).

Peacock and Nolan (2000) have expressed concern that the "spread of outcome-oriented health services has led to care being redefined as the provision of the finest form of treatment that is financially viable" (p. 1066), or as part of a "business model" of health care (Bolton, 2000). This immediately places the concept and practice of care at risk, as it "creates a tension at the heart of modern health care." As Gattuso and Bevan (2000) point out, the caring relationship is hard to measure, but not to do so in the outcomes context may be dangerous for the future of nursing.

THE INFLUENCE OF FEMINISMS
ON THE DISCIPLINE OF NURSING

The feminisms refer to the variety of theoretical approaches to the advocacy of equal rights for women, accompanied by a commitment to improve the position of women in society. They are informed by a range of theoretical propositions, and includes liberal feminism, socialist feminism, postmodern feminism, and others. This chapter has developed the argument that women and nurses are devalued in general, although some gains have been made in recent years. Feminist nurses, and others, have provided feminist analyses of their clinical practice, their educational understandings and their research. It is most notable that the feminisms have been promoted more by nursing scholars than practitioners, which has led to some uneasiness between the two groups. This may have arisen due to the fact that the feminisms have an "image" problem due to negative stereotypical views of what constitutes a feminist.

In reality, the feminisms are political perspectives that seek to balance societal power, and to gain equalities and autonomies for women in all their diversity. These feminisms offer the opportunity for nurses to recognize and analyze the unequal power relations that have been discussed earlier in this chapter, and to develop a raised consciousness about gender issues (Valentine, 2001; Meadus, 2000).

While it is true that the feminisms have not been adopted wholeheartedly by nurses, they certainly have had an impact (Torkelson, 1996). Some feminists have been hypercritical of nursing and nurses because of the latter's inability to embrace feminist theories; they believe that nursing as a women's profession needs "rescuing," that it is a victim of patriarchy and needs help in recognizing this. As previously noted, some feminists place the blame for the continuance of nursing oppression at the feet of nurses who collude with their oppressors to prevent change in the system (David, 2000). In this way, nurses are viewed as weak and compliant with the dominant forces that seek to retain the status quo, or as deceiving themselves.

Nursing has, however, provided fertile ground for the development of feminist theories, as these theories provide useful perspectives for nurses who work with disempowered and marginalized groups in their practice. Nurses are recognizing that they are also disempowered and marginalized within the health care system, and are developing understandings of these processes in order to action change. But while this is an ongoing process, it certainly is no easy task.

One example of the way feminist theory has influenced nursing will now be explored. While feminist theories have focused on nursing and the development of nursing research, there is a significant halo effect that works against the valuing of nursing research. In accepting the premise that women and nurses are devalued in general, by "scientific" researchers in particular, nursing research itself is devalued, because it is done by women and nurses. The qualities that define a good nurse are quite distinct from those defining a good researcher. Hicks (1997; 1999) argues that "research has fundamentally masculine connotations and nursing is quintessentially feminine," which in itself contributes to the relative paucity of nursing research output. Clearly, two cultures are in collision: nursing and research (Valentine, 2001; Neuman, 1999).

There is a long history of males who, in the past, were the academic, intellectual, and political gatekeepers of Western thought. They constructed and reproduced knowledge. But with the deconstruction and reconstruction of knowledge by feminists who have challenged the "received view," nurses can take advantage of the liberalizing approach inherent in the scholarly work published since the 1970s and 1980s in academic feminism and nursing. Since this time, feminist critics of science have exposed the history and assumptions of science and identified its masculinist practices.

Evans (1997) argues that "women then had to fight and argue their way back into science—and a scientific epistemology and community that they had had little or no part in constructing" (p. 54). Not only were they literally absent from science; there was a wider absence of the feminine and an absence also from the findings and conclusions of science. This was not surprising because "the *questions* that science identified as important were determined by the construction of the social world in which men occupied the public, and women the private, space" (Evans, 1997, p. 54). According to Huntington (1996), this created an opportunity for scientific knowledge to maintain control of women (primarily through their bodies) as men have constructed a knowledge base that is able to be extrapolated to women. She continues, "nurses . . . have not addressed the issue of the place of science in nursing nor the impact this has had on nursing generally, and the nursing of women in particular" (Huntington, 1996, p. 168). This of course has implications for nursing work and nursing research, as it suggests that nurses may be instrumental in maintaining a medical ideology for women patients, calculated to be negative and oppressive (Buchanan, 1997).

Part of the rejection of masculinist science was fostered by scholars, intellectuals, and researchers who adopted the "emancipatory science" perspective promulgated by the Frankfurt School of Sociology and Philosophy. The inaugural address given by Habermas in 1965 entitled *Knowledge and Interest* defined emancipatory science as "one which reveals the relationship of knowledge and interests which the objectivist attitude conceals" (Hagell, 1989, p. 227). This included a rejection of logical positivism as the only or most appropriate approach to research; interpretive and other qualitative forms were deemed by many to be superior for the task at hand in a range of disciplines, including nursing.

In the 1960s, the nursing discipline was given opportunities for development of nursing science that was driven by an empiricist or logical positivist philosophy. Edwards (1999) suggests that nursing was driven to claim its science base for reasons of prestige and status, as well as a need to be perceived as a "successful" profession. Nurse researchers and scholars have long acknowledged the inappropriateness for *all* nursing research to be undertaken using the empiricist model, because many of the questions framed were not valid for nursing knowledge development (Whittemore, 1999). However, if we return to the argument that has been developed, given society's attitudes to women, and hence nurses, there may be more value in conforming to the dominant culture, that is, "scientific research" that is acceptable to masculinist science. This is not appropriate, however, because it will not answer many of the questions nursing asks.

In an important work, Hagell (1989) proposed an alternative approach for the development of nursing knowledge that was underpinned by feminist principles that could assist nurses in finding out what it is that they know, and what it is they experience. This involved reclaiming and renaming nursing's experiences and knowledge of the social world lived in and daily constructed. Doering (1992) also argued for supporting other research approaches, but most particularly, feminism and poststructuralism. These she justifies as

> particularly relevant to nursing because they incorporate the concepts of the female experience and of power. These concepts reflect the historical, social, and political dynamics in which the discipline of nursing operates. They encompass a theme central to nursing, that of powerlessness, characterized by oppression, submission and male domination. (p. 25)

It is important to note, however, that feminist research "permits the recognition and exploration of socio-cultural factors that transcend gender" (Jackson, 1997, p. 87), which signals that, while the concept of oppression is central to feminism, it is clearly shared with other groups (Evans, 1997). Jackson proposes further that

> Accepting that experiences around oppression and struggle are not exclusive to women, permits recognition that institutionalized patriarchy and androcentricity are oppressive to all but those of the dominant class, race and gender. (p. 87)

This insight attempted to deal with the charge by Allen, Allman, and Powers (1991) that feminist research actually marginalizes men. These authors raised the question of whether feminist research involving only women simply "supports a conceptual scheme that reinforces the material subjugation of women" and thus "perpetuates problematic social categories" (p. 50). They concluded that "a better strategy is to deconstruct the dichotomy itself and to expand awareness of the diverse contemporary and historical forms of gendered existence" (Allen, Allman, & Powers, 1991, p. 56), which has subsequently occurred.

It may be reasonable to support the view that the value of feminist research is that it "empowers women and addresses issues that can make a difference to the quality of life for all humankind" (Parker & McFarland, 1991, p. 66). There are those who believe that nursing research should be approached from a much broader perspective and incorporate a range of paradigms. The method used is defined by the questions being asked. Unfortunately, though, the method may be driven by other motives, such as economic rationalism, and the need to obtain research funding, regardless of the ethical and moral imperatives that would normally guide research behavior. But it is clear that the research approach must take into account the context in which it is conducted, and for nursing, this has political and power implications. There is no question that gender is a critical and all-encompassing variable to be acknowledged. And it is feminist theory and practice that has largely been responsible for raising nursing's consciousness in this domain.

MEN IN NURSING

It has long been noted that men are a minority in nursing, despite the fact that their numbers have increased over the decades. In 1996 the nursing workforce in the United States consisted of 4.9% men, while in 1998 men comprised 4.4% of the Canadian workforce (Meadus, 2000). This compares to statistics from Britain, where men have constituted less than 10% of the qualified nursing workforce, while in Australia, it is around 9% (Armstrong, 2002). More specifically, analyses of gender breakdown of the U.K. registration authority indicate that in 1990, 8.37% of registrants were male; in 2000 this figure had increased to 9.75% (see http://www.ukcc.org.au). In the United States, males comprised 8.6% in baccalaureate programs, 9.6% in master's programs, and 6.7% in doctoral programs (American Association of Colleges of

Nursing, 2002). The proportion of male nursing undergraduate students in Australia increased from 11.9% in 1987–1990, to 15.9% in 1995 (Brown, 1998).

Nursing school faculty in the United States comprises 96.3% female and 3.7% male (American Association of Colleges of Nursing, 2002). In a national survey, which examined numerical representation, seniority status, and experiences of men compared with women in the university-based nursing education workforce in Australia, men were found to be over-represented at the highest levels. Fifty-two per cent of deans having control of nursing were males, 19% were professors and associate professors, and 26% were at the next level of senior lecturer (Sharman, Short, & Black, 1996, p. 308). The study indicated that women were supporting men in the workforce and the home, often at the expense of their own career advancement. This is a finding that has previously been highlighted in other traditionally female occupations such as teaching, physiotherapy, occupational therapy, librarianship, and social work (Williams, 1992). What it demonstrates is that males are moving into powerful positions over the largest occupational group in the health workforce, an occupational group that has been traditionally "managed, taught, disciplined and organized almost entirely by women" (MacGuire 1980, p. 160, cited in Sharman, Short, & Black, 1996). There is little doubt that "the ideological climate, socialization processes, and women's family and domestic responsibilities underlie a glass ceiling for women and a glass elevator for men in nontraditional occupations" (Sharman, 1998, p. 56).

While men are relative newcomers to nursing, they are increasingly being promoted to higher levels than women in nursing, despite their disproportionate numbers; furthermore, they seem to have less experience and fewer qualifications (Dolan, 1990). Brown's study (1998) found that in Australia men were over-represented in senior nursing administrative positions. Although men comprised only 8% of the registered nurse workforce, they held 22% of senior nursing positions. Poliafico (1998) indicates that the comparative figure is only 6% in United States, and suggests that there is a common misconception that men hold a disproportionate number of administrative positions. Brown (1998) considers a range of explanations for this discrepancy in Australia. One of the most compelling is that women are seen to be invading the workplace, since workplaces are constructed by men. So it is that

even in 'women's' occupations, such as nursing, where it may be expected that men would be perceived as not fitting in, the overriding culture of the workplace turns this disjunction into a benefit for men. (p. 21)

Thus, men who enter nursing are seen to be "lowering themselves, losing status by undertaking 'women's work'" (Brown, 1998, p. 21), yet are expected to be better workers than female nurses. They retain the benefits of their ascribed gender role; they are seen to be the "breadwinner," to have leadership qualities, and to be worth mentoring (since they are more likely to be serious about their career), and they are more likely to be assisted in accessing "power networks" in nursing. Hicks (1999) argues that if men in these top positions behave consistently with the findings of research studies, then they are most likely to reproduce themselves at these top level positions. This will then serve to widen the gender/power divisions in nursing.

Further evidence that men are being promoted to the highest levels of service in nursing, despite their numerical minority, is provided by Boughn (2001), who notes that "men who go into nursing rise like cream in milk" (p. 23) because they expect practical rewards and set up their lives to achieve and attain these, whereas women fail to recognize their economic and emotional power.

A study which examined senior nursing administrative positions in the United Kingdom found that 8.6% of registered nurses were men, but 50.3% held chief nurse/advisor posts, and 57.8% were directors of nursing education (Gaze, 1987). There has been a disproportionate increase of males in senior nursing positions in the U.K., which has also occurred in the U.S. It should be noted however, that there was a concerted effort in the U.K. to defeminize management within nursing, enabling men to be more easily promoted into these positions (Carpenter, 1977).

Jenkins (1989) notes that Florence Nightingale had a vision that nursing would always be under the control of women; she saw no place in nursing for men, just as there was no place for men in controlling nursing. Mackintosh (1997) and Meadus (2000) believe that the contribution of men to nursing has not been recognized and that it is time for affirmative action in favor of men for nursing to survive the twenty-first century. This means "that the Nightingale image must be counterbalanced by the entry and acceptance of larger numbers of men into the profession" (Meadus, 2000, p. 10).

This view is rejected by other researchers who suggest that nursing, rather than increasing male numbers, should introduce feminist strategies to enhance the power of women nurses, since their lower dispropor-tionate voice in academic writing and actual power in practice requires improvement (Ryan & Porter, 1993). Other research that focuses on the experiences of male nurses suggests that attrition is a major issue, due to the treatment given to males (Morin, 1999; Kelly, Shoemaker, & Steele, 1996).

To counteract the inequities experienced by men in nursing, the American Assembly for Men in Nursing was formed in 1971. Its aims were "to recruit more men into the profession, to provide support to those men who already are nurses, and to increase the visibility of men in nursing" (Poliafico, 1998, p. 43). However, to date, this has not had the desired impact because of the gendered attitudes which are "reinforced and perpetuated by patriarchal societal institutions and processes" (Evans, 1997, p. 231). The solution lies in challenging our stereotypes of femininity and masculinity, and of structural relations.

CONCLUSION

The aim of this chapter is to bring into sharp focus the issue of gender in global nursing. Clearly there are inequities in nursing work that can be documented with respect to control, management, and leadership in nursing. Additionally, there are more subtle ways that gender affects nursing. This chapter has argued that nursing work in all its forms (including clinical practice, education, and research), mostly under-taken by women, is affected severely by gender because of its construc-tion and the context in which nursing is carried out (Valentine, 2001). Becoming aware of such systematic oppressions is the first step in chang-ing paternalistic structures and systems that operate to disadvantage nurses, their patients, and the overall health care system. David (2000) suggests that nurses "must reframe the sociopolitical reality and give it back," otherwise they will continue to be "shackled in servitude, [and] denied freedom to acknowledge the full benefit of their health and healing practices" (p. 90). This has been described as "talking back," which requires courage, awareness, and the understanding of the role of language in creating and maintaining oppression. This is what the feminisms seek to contribute to the profession of nursing. David (2000) asks, "If nurses take action and use their willfulness to socially construct their own context, taking ownership and power, they will define what is left of nursing in the next century. So, why not?" (p. 93). This will require nurses to be "leader-rebels" in order to regain their power (Heide, 1977). Again, one can only ask, "Why not?"

REFLECTIVE QUESTIONS

1. What do you think the feminisms have to offer the discipline of nursing?
2. Do you believe that the role and function of nursing cannot be separated from nurses who undertake it? If so, why is this? If you disagree, outline your arguments to support your position.
3. What is your view of the debate that men in nursing, despite their numerical minority, have (or do not have) the majority of leadership positions? If this is true, why do you think it has happened? What implications does this have for nursing as a profession?

RECOMMENDED READINGS

Davies, C. (1995). *Gender and the professional predicament in nursing.* Buckingham: Open University Press.

Evans, J. (1997). Men in nursing: Issues of gender segregation and hidden advantage. *Journal of Advanced Nursing, 26,* 226–231.

Horsfall, J. (2000). Feminism in nursing. In J. Greenwood (Ed.), *Nursing theory in Australia: Development and application.* Sydney: Harper Educational Publishers.

Kane, D., & Thomas, B. (2000). Nursing and the 'f' word. *Nursing Forum, 35*(2), 17–25.

Lumby, J. (1997). The feminised body in illness. In J. Lawler (Ed.), *The body in nursing: A collection of views.* Melbourne: Churchill Livingstone.

Torkelson, D. J. (1996). Feminist research. *Journal of Neuroscience Nursing, 28*(2), 121–125.

REFERENCES

Allen, D. G., Allman, K. K. M., & Powers, P. (1991). Feminist nursing research without gender. *Advances in Nursing Science, 13*(3), 49–58.

American Association of Colleges of Nursing (2002). Annual state of the schools. Retrieved February 14, 2003 from http://www.aacn.nche.edu/media/annualreport02.pdf

Armstrong, F. (2002). Not just women's business: Men in nursing. *Australian Nursing Journal, 9*(11), 24–27.

Benner, P. (1984). *From novice to expert: Excellence and power in clinical nursing.* Menlo Park, CA: Addison Wesley.

Bent, K. N. (1993). Perspectives on critical and feminist theory in developing nursing praxis. *Journal of Professional Nursing, 9*(5), 296–303.

Bolton, S. C. (2000). Who cares? Offering emotion work as a 'gift' in the nursing labor process. *Journal of Advanced Nursing, 32*(3), 580–586.

Boughn, S. (2001). Why women and men choose nursing. *Nursing and Healthcare Perspectives, 22*(1), 14–24.

Boyle, M. V. (2002a). You wait until you get home: Emotional regions, emotional process work and the role of off-stage support. Paper presented at the *Third Emotions in Organisational Life Conference*, Bond University, Gold Coast, Ghana

Boyle, M. V. (2002b). Sailing twixt Scylla and Charybdis. *Women in Management Review, 17*(3/4), 131–141.

Briles, J. (1994). *The Briles report on women in healthcare. Changing conflict to collaboration in a toxic workplace.* San Francisco: Jossey-Bass.

Brown, C. R. (1998). *Gender segmentation in the paid work force: The case of nursing.* Unpublished doctoral thesis. Griffith University, Queensland, Australia.

Brykczynska, G. (Ed.) (1997). *Caring: The compassion and wisdom of nursing.* London: Arnold.

Bubeck, P. E. (1995). *Care, gender and justice.* Oxford: Clarendon Press.

Buchanan, T. (1997). Nursing our narratives: Towards a dynamic understanding of nurses in literary texts. *Nursing Inquiry, 4*(2), 80–87.

Caffrey, R., & Caffrey, P. (1994). Nursing: Caring or codependent? *Nursing Forum, 29*(1), 12–17.

Carpenter, M. (1977). The new managerialism and professionalism in nursing. In M. Stacey, M. Reid, C. Heath, & R. Dingwall (Eds.), *Health and the division of labour.* London: Croon Helm.

Cheek, J., & Rudge, T. (1995). Only connect . . . feminism and nursing. In G. Gray & R. Pratt (Eds.), *Scholarship in the discipline of nursing.* Melbourne: Churchill Livingstone.

David, B. A. (2000). Nursing's gender politics: Reformulating the footnotes. *Advances in Nursing Science, 23*(1), 83–94.

Davies, C. (1995). *Gender and the professional predicament in nursing.* Buckingham: Open University Press.

Demerouti, E., Bakker, A. B., Nachreiner, F., & Schaufeli, W. B. (2000). A model of burnout and life satisfaction amongst nurses. *Journal of Advanced Nursing, 32*(2), 454–464.

Doering, L. (1992). Power and knowledge in nursing: A feminist poststructuralist view. *Advances in Nursing Science, 14*(4), 24–33.

Dolan, B. (1990). Project 2000: The gender mender? *Nursing Standard, 4,* 52–53.

Edwards, S. D. (1999). The idea of nursing science. *Journal of Advanced Nursing, 29*(3), 563–569.

Ehrenreich, B., & English, D. (1979). *For her own good: 150 years of experts' advice to women.* London: Pluto.

Ekstrom, D. N. (1999). Gender and perceived nurse caring in nurse-patient dyads. *Journal of Advanced Nursing, 29*(6), 1393–1401.

Evans, J. (1997). Men in nursing: Issues of gender segregation and hidden advantage. *Journal of Advanced Nursing, 26,* 226–231.

Evans, M. (1997). *Introducing contemporary feminist thought.* Oxford: Blackwell Publishers.

Falk Rafael, A. (1996). Power and caring: A dialectic in nursing. *Advances in Nursing Science, 19*(1), 3–17.

Falk Rafael, (1998). Nurses who run with the wolves: The power and caring dialectic revisited. *Advances in Nursing Science, 21*(1), 29–42.

Fineman, S. (Ed.) (1993). *Emotion in organisations.* London: Sage.

Gamarnikow, E. (1978). Sexual division of labour: The case of nursing. In A. Kuhn & A. M. Wolpe (Eds.), *Feminism and materialism.* London: Routledge & Kegan Paul.

Gattuso, S., & Bevan, C. (2000). Mother, daughter, patient, nurse: Women's emotion work in aged care. *Journal of Advanced Nursing, 31*(4), 892–899.

Gaze, H. (1987). Man appeal. *Nursing Times, 83*(20), 24–27.

Gherardi, S. (1994). The gender we think, the gender we do in our everyday organizational lives. *Human Relations, 47*(6), 591–601.

Goffman, I. (1959). *Presentation of the self in everyday life.* New York: Overlook Press.

Greenhalgh, J., Vanhanen, L., & Kyngas, H. (1998). Nurse caring behaviours. *Journal of Advanced Nursing, 27*(5), 927–932.

Grosz, E. (1990). Conclusion: A note on essentialism and difference. In S. Gunew (Ed.), *Feminist knowledge: Critique and construct.* London: Routledge.

Hagell, E. I. (1989). Nursing knowledge: Women's knowledge. A sociological perspective. *Journal of Advanced Nursing, 14,* 226–233.

Hearn, J. (1993). Emotive subjects: Organizational men, organizational masculinities and the (de)construction of 'emotions'. In S. Fineman (Ed.), *Emotion in organizations.* London: Sage.

Heide, W. S. (1977). Assertiveness: The key to power and politics. Paper presented in October at the New York State Nurses Association Convention, New York, New York.

Henderson, A. (2001). Emotional labour and nursing: An under-appreciated aspect of caring work. *Nursing Inquiry, 8*(2), 130–138.

Hicks, C. (1997). The research-practice gap: Individual responsibility or corporate culture? *Nursing Times, 93*(39), 38–39.

Hicks, C. (1999). Incompatible skills and ideologies: The impediment of gender attributions on nursing research. *Journal of Advanced Nursing, 30*(1), 129–139.

Huntington, A. (1996). Nursing research reframed by the inescapable reality of practice: A personal encounter. *Nursing Inquiry, 3*(3), 167–171.

Jackson, D. (1997). Feminism: A path to clinical knowledge development. *Contemporary Nurse, 6*(2), 85–91.

Jenkins, E. (1989). Nurses' control over nursing. In G. Gray & R. Pratt (Eds.), *Issues in Australian nursing 2.* Melbourne: Churchill Livingstone.

Jones, A. (2001). Time to think: Temporal considerations in nursing practice and research. *Journal of Advanced Nursing, 33*(2), 150–158.

Kane, D., & Thomas, B. (2000). Nursing and the 'f' word. *Nursing Forum, 35*(2), 17–25.

Kelly, A. (1985). The construction of masculine science. *British Journal of Sociology of Education, 6,* 33–154.

Kelly, N. R., Shoemaker, M., & Steele, T. (1996). The experience of being a male student nurse. *Journal of Nursing Education, 35*(4), 170–174.

Lather, P. (1991). *Feminist research in education: Within/against.* Geelong, Victoria: Deakin University Press.

Lupton, D. (1998). *The emotional self.* London: Sage.

Mackintosh, C. (1997). A historical study of men in nursing. *Journal of Advanced Nursing, 26,* 232–236.

Meadus, R. J. (2000). Men in nursing: Barriers to recruitment. *Nursing Forum, 35*(3), 5–10.

Morin, K. H. (1999). Mothers: Responses to care given by male nursing students during and after birth. *Image: Journal of Nursing Scholarship, 31*(1), 83–87.

Myerson, D. E. (2000). If emotions were honoured: A cultural analysis. In S. Fineman (2nd ed.), *Emotion in Organizations.* London: Sage.

Neuman, C. E. (1999). Taking charge: Nursing, suffrage and feminism in America, 1873–1920. *Journal of Women's History, 10*(4), 228–235.

Nicolson, P. (1996). *Gender, power and organisation: A psychological perspective.* London: Routledge.

Parker, B., & McFarland, J. (1991). Feminist theory and nursing: An empowerment model for research. *Advances in Nursing Science, 13*(3), 59–67.

Peacock, J. W., & Nolan, P. W. (2000). Care under threat in the modern world. *Journal of Advanced Nursing, 32*(5), 1066–1070.

Poliafico, J. K. (1998). Nursing's gender gap. *RN, 61*(10), 39–43.

Ryan, S., & Porter, S. (1993). Men in nursing: A cautionary critique. *Nursing Outlook, 41*(6), 262–267.

Sandelowski, M. (1997). (Ir)reconcilable differences? The debate concerning nursing and technology. *Image: Journal of Nursing Scholarship, 29*(2), 169–174.

Sharman, E. (1998). The glass elevator: How men overtake women in the nursing higher education workforce in Australia. Unpublished doctoral thesis, University of New South Wales, Sydney, Australia.

Sharman, E., Short, S., & Black, D. (1996). Why so many? The masculine mystique and men in the nursing higher education workforce in Australia. In Conference Proceedings of the Changing Society for Women's Health Conference, Australian National University, Canberra, Australia.

Snellgrove, S., & Hughes, D. (2000). Interprofessional relations between doctors and nurses: Perspectives from South Wales. *Journal of Advanced Nursing, 31*(3), 661–667.

Street, A. (1995). *Nursing replay: Researching nursing culture together.* Melbourne: Churchill Livingstone.

Traynor, M. (1996). Looking at discourse in a literature review of nursing texts. *Journal of Advanced Nursing, 23*(2), 1155–1161.

Treacy, M. P. (1989). Gender prescription in nurse training: Its effects on health provision. In L. K. Hardy & J. Randell (Eds.), *Recent advances in nursing: Issues in women's health.* Edinburgh: Churchill Livingstone.

Torkelson, D. J. (1996). Feminist research. *Journal of Neuroscience Nursing, 28*(2), 121–125.

Tronto, J. C. (1999). Caring: Gender-sensitive ethics. *Hypatia, 14*(1), 112–120.

Valentine, P. E. B. (2001). A gender perspective on conflict management strategies of nurses. *Journal of Nursing Scholarship, 33*(1), 69–79.

Whittemore, R. (1999). Natural science and nursing science: Where do the horizons fuse? *Journal of Advanced Nursing, 30*(5), 1027–1033.

Williams, C. (1992). The glass escalator: Hidden advantages for men in the 'female' professions. *Social Problems, 39*(3), 253–267.

Wuest, J. (1997). Illuminating environmental influences on women's caring. *Journal of Advanced Nursing, 26*(1), 49–58.

Zebroski, S. A. (2001). The gender lens: Caring and gender. *Journal of Comparative Family Studies, 32*(2), 322–324.

12

Becoming Part of a Multidisciplinary Health Care Team

Kathleen M. Nokes

LEARNING OBJECTIVES

At the completion of this chapter, the reader will be able to:

- Identify contemporary trends mandating the use of effective multidisciplinary teams in health care settings
- Analyze benefits of multidisciplinary teamwork
- Apply a model of team process
- Visualize how the beginning registered nurse would function on multidisciplinary teams
- Identify potential sources of conflict between team members and strategies to resolve those conflicts

KEY WORDS

Communication, teamwork, motivation, multidisciplinary, interdependency, conflict

INTRODUCTION

Although the concept of the health care team, with significant input and participation by nursing staff, is not new, continuous quality initiatives and changes resulting from a renewed focus on performance and process improvement have made a significant impact on the way nurses conduct their everyday work through teams (Hetherington, 1998). Health care delivery settings are multifaceted and diverse. Without a systematic method of interdepartmental communications, patients must act as the primary communication link among departments and coordinate their care. But few patients possess the information, expertise, or energy required to assume this role effectively (Irson & McGillis, 1998). Failures to communicate can result in an adverse impact on patient outcomes such as increased morbidity, prolonged lengths of stay, dissatisfaction with care, and increased mortality. In order to address the complex needs of patients, the beginning registered nurse must be prepared to function on multidisciplinary teams.

A team is a group of people who are committed to achieving common objectives (Umiker, 1998). Teams are not simply another way of assigning work groups or leaders, but rather a fundamental commitment to interdependence to address the complexity in the health care environment (Dienemann, 1998). Teamwork in health care organizations is a coordinated effort among several individuals who place the team's goal and interests above their own. The team's customers—both internal and external, such as accrediting agencies and third-party payers—are at the heart of meaningful team work (Hetherington, 1998). Active participation on these teams is challenging, especially for new graduates, who are novices in the culture of the nursing profession, refining multiple skills, and integrating comprehensive patterns of clinical information. Nonetheless, there are compelling reasons for registered nurses to enhance their skills by participating in multidisciplinary teams. Multidisciplinary teams should be used in the decision making process, especially if the issue, options, or patient outcome involve other disciplines (Welch, 2003).

Professional codes of ethics delimit the nature of activities and relationships between professionals and their clients (Hayward, DeMarco, & Lynch, 2000). The eighth provision of the Code of Ethics, approved by the American Nurses Association, states: "The nurse collaborates with other health professionals and the public in promoting community, national, and international efforts to meet health needs" (ANA, 2001, p. 1). Racial and ethnic minorities in the United States tend to receive a lower quality of health care than nonminorities, even when access-related factors such as source of health insurance and income are controlled (Smedley, Stith, & Nelson, 2003). In response, the Institute of Medicine Committee on Understanding and Eliminating Racial and Ethnic Disparities in Healthcare recommended: "5-11: Implement multidisciplinary treatment and preventive care teams" (p. 18) because these teams can coordinate and streamline care, enhance patient adherence throughout follow-up techniques, and address the multiple behavioral and social risks faced by patients (Smedley, Stith, & Nelson, 2003).

Regulatory agencies, such as the Joint Commission for Accreditation of Healthcare Organizations (JCAHO), are placing increasing emphasis on integrated care delivery (Brunt, et al., 1999). Starting in January, 2004, JCAHO surveyors will be searching for evidence of communication and documentation at every stage of interdisciplinary care, which places the patient as the center of the focus, not the individual discipline. It is expected that this new orientation will enhance patient outcomes, reduce redundancy, and avoid situations where disciplines are working in isolation from each other (Briefings on JCAHO, 2003).

This chapter describes multidisciplinary team membership skills for beginning registered nurses. It focuses on the novice nursing practitioner since team building and maintenance skills are complex and are facilitated by leaders who have broad professional expertise.

WHY TEAMS ARE NECESSARY

In the past, health and social service providers often worked in their own spheres of clinical practice, frequently with little understanding of each other's contributions and some degree of indifference to learning about each other's role (Crowell, 2000). As the nursing profession differentiated itself from medicine, a specialized body of knowledge has grown, leading to increased clarity about nursing's unique contribution to the health of populations. Simultaneously, economic factors changed the health care setting and highlighted an increasing recognition of the need for integrated systems in the continuum of care, including primary, acute, home, and rehabilitation settings, with patients moving through these settings using integrated systems of documentation and coordination. As a result, interactions between health, medical, and social team members focus on patient outcomes through open communication channels. Case management is usually achieved through the work of multidisciplinary teams with the purpose of facilitating a patient's progress through the continuum of care (Brunt et al., 1999). A team approach generally is the most effective means of achieving the goal of optimum patient outcomes.

As a student of nursing preparing to work in a rapidly changing health care system, it is essential to understand the significance and responsibilities of being an active participant on multidisciplinary teams. This requires not only insights about the potential contributions of nurses with different expertise, but also an understanding of the contributions of other team members (Griffiths & Crookes, 2000). There is a connection between the quality of relationships among team members and the success of different teams in achieving their goals (Crowell, 2000). Since optimum patient outcomes will be facilitated through open communication between team members, nurses need to be aware not only of their potential contributions, but also how other health and social service providers and consumers can provide valuable input.

TYPES OF MULTIDISCIPLINARY TEAMS

There are different types of interdisciplinary teams: unit-based teams, composed of direct care providers; clinical teams; and shared governance support teams, composed of nurse managers; and department directors that focus more on administrative issues. Clinical teams are usually composed of providers with clinical expertise in a specific area and may consist of clinical nurse specialists, nutritionists, therapists, and primary care providers, such as physicians, nurse practitioners, and physician assistants. Some examples of clinical teams are wound care, pain/palliative care, ostomy care, or discharge planning. Shared governance support teams may also be referred to as committees and address policy, quality assurance, ethics, or governmental affairs (Blais, Hayes, Kozier, & Erb, 2002). Committee or team members are generally selected in terms of their individual functional roles and employment status rather than because of their personal characteristics.

Unit-based teams often meet weekly and address problems related to impeded quality and/or efficiency of care delivery, along with strategies to improve communication and create a sense of community (Irson & McGillis, 1998). Beginning registered nurses will probably join existing unit-based teams. Hetherington (1998) surveyed nurses working in a medium-sized hospital and a large ambulatory clinic about their team-related experiences. She found that prior experience with teams along with past level of involvement were the best predictors of nurses' belief that their participation on the team was important to improved patient care. Nurses who believed that they learned something in the team process were more likely to want to be on more teams. She also found that serving on perceived "go nowhere" or "dead end" teams was tantamount to slowly killing pride in work and enthusiasm for teamwork.

MODELS OF HOW EFFECTIVE TEAMS WORK

Ecologic models emphasize interdependence among component parts and use available resources in order to foster connectedness among individuals and increase the sense of community and commitment to the organization's goals (Irson & McGillis, 1998). An integrated team-building model is known as the Team Spirit Model (Crowell, 2000). This model will be described more fully as an illustration of how teams function and evolve through different stages.

Components of the Team Spirit Model drawn from the field of organizational development view team development as a series of five stages; the model also integrates concepts from new science which views the stages more as a spiral. Because the stages are interdependent, they are dynamic and there are times when events may be a reflection of more than one stage. There is a continuous ebb and flow or rhythm experienced by the team members as they build on their consonances and work through their dissonances. The team is an expression of human spirit when viewed from a spiritual perspective. The concept of service is at the core of the Team Spirit Model. Consonances of service include contribution, aligned execution, and mutual support. Dissonances of service include depletion, uncoordinated action, and unsupportiveness. This integrated model consists of five interdependent stages: initiating, visioning, claiming, celebrating, and letting go.

Initiating Stage: Getting to Know Each Other

There can be many differences between team members based on gender identity, values, principles, educational preparation, and clinical perspectives. By helping new team members through the phases of orientation, the team leader builds cooperation, communication, and cohesion among all team members (Costello-Nickitas, 1997). The team serves as a bridge between standards set by professional groups and the needs of the operating unit where the members are functioning (Newhouse & Mills, 2002). New team members should be oriented prior to the first team meeting, so that they have a beginning understanding about the composition of the team along with its history. The leader, using a directive style, should tell the new employer what to do, demonstrate how to do it, why the work is important, and relate how the team's work fits into the big picture (Umiker, 1998). During the initial meeting, the new team member should learn about the duration of the team, the different clinical perspectives of the team members, the role/function of the registered nurse that is being replaced, and that person's role on the team. Knowing that the new employee may be frightened, insecure, and stressed, the team leader should be highly supportive (Umiker, 1998).

Membership on the team depends upon the needs of the patient population and the purpose of the team. The patient, along with the support system, is an essential team member. Table 12.1 describes different team members in addition to nurses, but the patient characteristics

TABLE 12.1   Common Members of Multidisciplinary Teams

Type of Provider	Primary Purpose
Physician	Diagnosis and treatment of disease or injury through the use of medications and/or surgery
Nutritionist/Dietitian	Educate and advise individuals and groups on dietary management of disease and health promotion
Occupational Therapist	Perform functional assessments and intervene to optimize client's levels of independence in activities of daily living
Physical Therapist	Assess, treat, and prevent issues associated with movement
Social Worker	Counsel, refer, and assist with obtaining different entitlements
Speech Therapist	Treat communication and swallowing disorders
Clergyman/woman	Provide spiritual counseling, pastoral care, and emotional support
Pharmacist	Review medication orders, prepare medications, evaluate for drug interactions
Respiratory Therapist	Treat breathing and pulmonary conditions

(Griffiths & Crookes, 2000)

will determine the composition of the team membership. Teams should include employees in many central hospital services such as housekeeping and phlebotomy, in addition to more holistic direct-care providers (Lake, Keeling, Weber, & Olade, 1999). For example, if most of the clients on the medical unit are hospitalized with HIV infection acquired through injecting drugs, a harm reduction specialist would be on the team to assist patients to avoid relapse and learn new coping skills. Although the registered nurse may have completed the fewest years of formal professional education as compared with other professional team members, the amount of time that nurses spend with the patients provides a holistic perspective that can enhance the effectiveness of the plans developed by the team. The new member should also plan to meet with the team leader after the first meeting to clarify any misconceptions and answer questions that arose during the meeting. When the orientation phase is over, usually after a minimum of three meetings (Thompson & Roda, 1999), issues that have arisen should be addressed by the group during the team meeting. As employees develop confidence in their ability, the team leader should back off, give more latitude, and encourage the team members to solve their own problems (Umiker, 1998).

Visioning: Sharing Meaning and Mission

The mission and function of the team tend to be described to new members during the orientation meeting. However, integration onto the team shapes how the team achieves its stated mission. Even though each member brings his/her own values and unique expertise to the team processes, it is the team leader's responsibility to ensure that a drift too far from the stated mission does not occur. Periodic evaluations of how a specific meeting agenda is keeping the team on track in accomplishing broad goals should be scheduled at regular intervals. Shared meaning emanates from trust and understanding of different perspectives, and how they can contribute to the mission of the team. In order to enhance understanding of the contributions of the different disciplines represented at the meetings, each member should review the position descriptions of the different team members.

Claiming: Doing the Work

Team members from different disciplines share knowledge, skills, and expertise so that information from their discipline can be collected, evaluated, and discussed by other team members (Stepans, Thompson, & Buchanan, 2002). As a team member, registered nurses contribute particular expertise in discussing health history, interpreting medical records, and offering information about the physical and developmental stage of the patient, explaining medication use, including dose and drug interactions, and delineating implications of diseases/disorders on patient outcomes. During the working stage, the team works on achieving its stated mission by completing specific tasks and projects. Evidence of progress towards goals is represented by data that is clearly portrayed and concise in its message (Newhouse & Mills, 2002).

In a well functioning team, members leave meetings feeling energized. The team leader ensures that the contributions of each group member are valued and rotates assignments, such as keeping meeting notes and arranging room assignments. Establishing tentative time frames for achievement of specific objectives is essential to ensure that the members continue to value the benefits of working on the team (Thompson & Roda, 1999). Attendance at team meetings along with participation by most of the members can signal whether team members believe that their meeting time is being well used. Characteristics of effective teams include shared leadership, joint decisionmaking, consistent implementation of plans, and solid interpersonal relationships and collegiality (Stepans, Thompson, & Buchanan, 2002).

Celebrating: Recognition, Awards, Rewards

Taking time to recognize professional achievements can motivate team members and assist them in learning more about other team members so as to build cohesion. As a strategy for spending more time with team members in a more relaxed setting, newer team members can volunteer to participate in the preparations for the celebration of professional team achievements.

Letting Go: Really Communicating

A difficult, but essential, part of sustaining team spirit is effective communication. The team leader sets the tone and allows for various roles and sides of an issue to emerge in a safe environment. Helpful ground rules include defining a purpose for each meeting, starting and ending meetings on time, using and adhering to a set agenda that is approved by all the members, and setting the time of the next meeting at the end of the current meeting so scheduling conflicts can be addressed and everyone can leave knowing when they will return with completed assignments. The team leader recognizes that different team members will have conflicting opinions, and thus works to create an honest environment in which trust between members can grow. New members will observe how different team members respond to a member who introduces controversial issues, and this response will shape their willingness to contribute to the group. Recognizing that service is the core of the team building model will help the group to stay oriented on its mission: optimal patient outcomes.

It is possible that a representative from a key professional discipline, such as medicine, will not participate in the case management team meetings. Since communication is essential across all the professional disciplines, alternate strategies of communication will be necessary, such as written summary notes on the patient's medical record (Annis, 2002). Interdisciplinary documentation systems will promote the work of multidisciplinary teams. If physicians are to ensure high-quality care for patients, they will need to improve collaboration skills as they work in an environment of increased interdependence where relationships are complex (Newhouse & Mills, 2002).

POTENTIAL CONFLICTS WITHIN THE TEAM

Teams often fail because of unrealistic mandates from upper management, lack of purpose and direction, poor leadership, and breakdowns in communication (Umiker, 1998). Team members will report to their immediate supervisor along with the team leader, which can result in confusion. For example, registered nurses will report to the nursing manager on his/her unit, while the team leader will report to the functional director for the clinical area, such as oncology or women's health (Newhouse & Mills, 2002).

Hospitals can be a natural stage for conflict, since there is a diverse mix of professions and departments and each one views their perspective as being the right one for the patient's needs (Crowell, 2000). It is expected that team members who have been educated differently and who, by nature, gender, or personality, chose their profession, will have diverse thinking patterns and approaches to solving problems. Each discipline and department has long established rules of behavior about how to achieve specific goals and priorities. The tempo of the work also will differ, from extreme urgency to a more reflective process, and team members generally feel most comfortable with familiar rhythms.

Teamwork does not follow a straight line, but rather takes a path requiring time, energy, and skills (Costello-Nickitas, 1997). Professionals must contend with the need to validate professional identity in a competitive work environment and be cognizant of political liaisons that often polarize, rather than enhance, cohesion or mutuality within the team (Hayward, DeMarco, & Lynch, 2000). The Team Assessment Tool could be used to assess current team functioning (Dienemann, 1998). While the beginning registered nurse will not be expected to take a leadership role in conflict negotiation, it is helpful to acknowledge some of the underlying dynamics.

Kritek (2002) refers to the site of conflict negotiation as "the table," and points out that many of these tables are uneven because the power is not evenly distributed among the members at the table. Nurses may assume that the expressed purpose of a team is its actual purpose. However, that assumption may not be valid. Teams often are created because regulatory bodies mandate them, or because those in power think they are a good idea. However, such teams often have little decisionmaking power and authority. Kritek offers strategies for constructive ways of being at an uneven table, including the decision to leave the table if continued involvement compromises personal integrity.

In addition to case management teams, nurses need to participate on shared governance teams, such as policymaking teams or committees, and to effectively communicate their unique perspectives. These skills need to be taught and practiced in relatively safe environments by beginning registered nurses. Advanced practice nurses, such as clinical nurse specialists, can act as role models for leadership behaviors consistent with the goals that support optimal patient outcomes.

CONCLUSION

Trends mandating the use of effective multidisciplinary teams include professional codes of ethics, accrediting bodies, diverse clinical needs of clients receiving health care in a variety of settings, and economics. The results of effective multidisciplinary teamwork will be: a) enhanced patient outcomes; b) reduced redundancy; and c) fewer situations where disciplines interact with patients in isolation. The Team Spirit Model was used as one illustration that emphasizes relationships and recognizes that teams can be at different stages of development, while keeping service as the core purpose of the team. The beginning registered nurse would spend the initial time on a unit-based team as an observer. However, he/she eventually would grow in confidence, contribute professional expertise and provide unique experiences as a relative newcomer to the health field. Since more experienced team members might have grown comfortable with the status quo, the beginning nurse can ask questions that more experienced professionals may not identify. This can be a challenge, since there is much potential for conflict on teams that are related to gender, class, professional discipline, and values. The Team Spirit Model acknowledges these conflicts, but also provides a framework for addressing them.

REFLECTIVE QUESTIONS

1. You have been notified that you will be joining the unit-based multidisciplinary team that meets every Wednesday morning. How would you prepare yourself for the first meeting?
2. During your fourth team meeting, you note that no other nurse team members have verbally contributed during any meetings that you have attended. How would you react with respect to deciding about your verbal contributions during the team meeting?
3. You have cared for Mr. Jones for three days. He says that he knows that his case is being discussed at the team meeting the following day and he wants to attend that meeting. How would you address this request?

RECOMMENDED READINGS

Briefings on JCAHO (2003). *Interdisciplinary Care: Meeting the JCAHO's new requirements and planning for better patient care.* August 28 Audioconference. Available at http://www.hcmarketplace.com/Prod.cfm?id=1810

Crowell, D. (2000). Building spirited multidisciplinary teams. *Journal of PeriAnesthesia Nursing, 15*(2), 108–114.

Hayward, L., DeMarco, R., & Lynch, M. (2000). Interprofessional collaborative alliances: Healthcare educators sharing and learning from each other. *Journal of Allied Health, 29*(4), 220–226.

Stephans, M., Thompson, C., & Buchanan, M., (2002). The role of the nurse on a transdisciplinary early intervention team. *Public Health Nursing, 19*(4), 238–245.

Thompson, E., & Roda, P. (1999). Ensuring competencies of multidisciplinary staff in patient-focused care. *Dimensions of Critical Care Nursing 18*(4), 36–44.

REFERENCES

American Nurses Association (2001). Code of ethics for nurses—Provisions. Available at http://nursingworld.org/ethics/chcode.htm

Annis, T. (2002). The synergy model in practice. *Critical Care Nurse, 22*(5), 76–79.

Blais, K., Hayes, J., Kozier, B., & Erb, G. (2002). *Professional nursing practice: Concepts and perspectives.* Upper Saddle River, NJ: Prentice Hall.

Briefings on JCAHO (2003). *Interdisciplinary Care: Meeting the JCAHO's new requirements and planning for better patient care.* August 28 Audioconference. Available at http://www.hcmarketplace.com/Prod.cfm?id=1810

Brunt, B., Gifford, L., Hart, D., McQueen-Goss, S., Siddall, D., Smith, R., & Weakland, R., (1999). Designing interdisciplinary documentation for the continuum of care. *Journal of Nursing Care Quality, 14*(1), 1–10.

Costello-Nickitas, D. (1997). *Quick reference to nursing leadership.* Albany, NY: Delmar Publishers.

Crowell, D. (2000). Building spirited multidisciplinary teams. *Journal of PeriAnesthesia Nursing, 15*(2), 108–114.

Dienemann, J. (1998). *Nursing administration: Managing patient care.* Stamford, CT: Appleton & Lange.

Griffiths, R., & Crookes, P. (2000). Becoming part of a multidisciplinary healthcare team. In J. Daly, S. Speedy, & D. Jackson (Eds.), *Contexts of nursing.* Sydney: MacLennan & Petty.

Hayward, L., DeMarco, R., & Lynch, M. (2000). Interprofessional collaborative alliances: Healthcare educators sharing and learning from each other. *Journal of Allied Health, 29*(4), 220–226.

Hetherington, L. (1998). Becoming involved: The nurse leader's role in encouraging teamwork. *Nursing Administration Quarterly, 23*(1), 29–40.

Irson, C., & McGillis, G. (1998). A multidisciplinary-shared governance model. *Nursing Management, 29*(2), 37–39.

Kritek, P. (2002). *Negotiating at an uneven table: Developing moral courage in resolving our conflicts.* San Francisco, CA: Jossey-Bass.

Lake, M., Keeling, P., Weber, G., & Olade, R. (1999). Collaborative care: A professional practice model. *Journal of Nursing Administration, 29*(9), 51–56.

Newhouse, R., & Mills, M. (2002). *Nursing leadership in the organized delivery system for the acute care setting: Strategies, structures, and processes for fiscal and clinical integration of care.* Washington, DC: American Nurses Publishing.

Smedley, B., Stith, A., & Nelson, A. (Eds.) (2003). *Unequal treatment: Confronting racial and ethnic disparities in healthcare.* Committee on Understanding and Eliminating Racial and Ethnic Disparities in Healthcare, Board on Health Sciences Policy, Institute of Medicine. Washington, DC: National Academies Press.

Stepans, M., Thompson, C., & Buchanan, M. (2002). The role of the nurse on a transdisciplinary early intervention team. *Public Health Nursing, 19*(4), 238–245.

Thompson, E., & Roda, P. (1999). Ensuring competencies of multidisciplinary staff in patient-focused care. *Dimensions of Critical Care Nursing, 18*(4), 36–44.

Umiker, W. (1998). *Management skills for the new healthcare supervisory.* Gaithersburg, MD: Aspen Publications.

Welch, R. (2003). Decision-making and problem solving. In P. Yoder-Wise (Ed.), *Leading and managing in nursing.* St. Louis, MO: Mosby.

13

Professionalism: The Role of Regulatory Bodies and Nursing Organizations

Vickie A. Lambert and
Clinton E. Lambert

LEARNING OBJECTIVES

After completing this chapter, the reader should be able to:

- Describe regulatory authority
- Discuss the role regulatory authority plays in the protection of the public
- Discuss the role and mission of select major professional nursing organizations
- Delineate the benefits of membership in professional nursing organizations

KEY WORDS

Regulatory authority, licensure, boards of nursing, nurse practice act, professional nursing organizations, accrediting agencies

INTRODUCTION

Regulatory bodies and professional organizations play a vital role in the maintenance and enhancement of professionalism in nursing. It is imperative that mechanisms be in place for a profession such as nursing to provide the public with adequate protection from unsafe actions carried out by nurses. In addition, it is equally important that nursing utilize professional organizations for its advancement and enhancement. The purposes of this chapter are to present, within the 50 states, the District of Columbia, and the five U.S. territories, an overview of the regulatory process of nursing practice and the role played by some of the major professional nursing organizations.

REGULATION OF NURSING PRACTICE

Nursing is a health profession that can pose risk or harm to the public if practiced by people who are unprepared or incompetent. As early as the end of the nineteenth century, nursing recognized the need to implement a mechanism whereby the actions of nurses could be appropriately monitored (i.e., regulated). In 1903, North Carolina became the first state to pass a nurse registration law and issue a license to practice nursing. To further the call for regulation of nursing practice, in 1944, a State Board Test Pool to examine qualified nurse applicants was established by the National League of Nursing Education. Indicating the belief in safe nursing practice, the growth and participation of states in the Test Pool grew rapidly, from 6 in 1944, to 41 by 1949 (Kalisch & Kalisch, 1995). During the 1950s, the remaining states joined the State Board Test Pool, making nursing the first profession to implement the same licensing examination throughout the nation.

Nursing regulation is defined as governmental oversight of nursing practice carried out by each of the 50 states, the District of Columbia, and five U.S. territories, namely Guam, the Virgin Islands, Puerto Rico, American Samoa, and the Northern Mariana Islands. Since members of the public may not have sufficient knowledge or experience in identifying an unqualified health care provider, they are vulnerable to unsafe and incompetent practitioners. It is through the regulatory process that only individuals meeting predetermined qualifications are allowed to engage in nursing practice. Boards of Nursing are the governmental bodies responsible for carrying out the regulation of nursing practice.

Boards of Nursing are authorized to enforce the Nurse Practice Act, and to develop administrative rules and regulations and any other responsibility delineated within the Nurse Practice Act, such as monitoring the quality of nursing programs (National Council of State Boards of Nursing, 2003). A Nurse Practice Act is a state or territorial governmental document that regulates the practice of nursing, creates the Board of Nursing, and empowers the Board to regulate the practice of nursing and enforce the provisions of the Act. A model for a Nurse Practice Act can be found on the Web site: http://www.ncsbn.org/public/regulation/nursing_practice_model_practice_act.htm.

Boards of Nursing achieve the mission of regulation by creating standards for safe nursing care and by issuing licenses to practice nursing. Once a license is issued, it is the responsibility of the Board of Nursing to continually monitor the licensees' compliance with state laws and to take action against any nurse who exhibits unsafe nursing practice. Individuals who serve on Boards of Nursing are appointed to their position. The law in each jurisdiction dictate who may serve on a Board of Nursing. Board membership usually consists of a mix of registered nurses, licensed practical/vocational nurses, advanced practice registered nurses, and consumers. However, five states (California, Georgia, Louisiana, Texas, and West Virginia) have two Boards of Nursing, one for registered nurses and one for licensed practical/vocational nurses (National Council of State Boards of Nursing, 2003). These states generally do not appoint licensed practical/vocational nurses to the registered nurse board. The members of a Board of Nursing meet on a regular basis to oversee the activities of the Board and to take disciplinary action as needed.

Today, all Boards of Nursing are members of the National Council of State Boards of Nursing (NCSBN). The NCSBN is an organization through which Boards of Nursing work together on issues of common interest and concern affecting public safety and welfare, including the development of the licensing examinations for both registered nurses and practical/vocational nurses (NCLEX-RN and NCLEX-PN). In addition to the development of the licensing examinations, the NCSBN performs policy analyses, promotes uniformity in the relationship to regulation of nursing practice, disseminates data related to nursing licensure, conducts research pertinent to the organization's purpose, and serves as a forum for information exchange for its members (National Council of State Boards of Nursing, 2003).

In an attempt to facilitate nurses' ability to provide safe nursing care across state lines, in 1998 the NCSBN approved a policy to remove certain regulatory barriers. As a result, Nurse Licensure Compacts were created (National Council of State Boards of Nursing, 2003). Nurse Licensure Compacts are mutual recognition models of nursing licensure that allow a nurse to: 1) have one license (in his/her state of residency); 2) practice in other states (both physically and electronically); and 3) be subject to each state's practice law and regulations. Under this system of mutual recognition, a nurse may practice across state lines, unless otherwise restricted. However, in order for such mutual recognition to take place, each state must enact appropriate legislation authorizing the creation of the Nurse Licensure Compact. Not all states have adopted a Nurse Licensure Compact agreement. To obtain up-to-date information on which states have implemented, or have pending, implementation of a Nurse Licensure Compact agreement, refer to the Web site at the National Council of State Boards of Nursing: http://www.ncsbn.org/public/nurselicensurecompact/mutual_recognit ion_state.htm.

Another form of nursing regulation, other than licensure, is certification. This is a credential that provides for title protection and recognition of accomplishment. However, it does not include a legal scope of practice. The U.S. government uses the term *certification* to define the credentialing process by which a nongovernmental agency or association such as the American Nurses' Credentialing Center recognizes persons who have met specific requirements (National Council of State Boards of Nursing, 2003). A number of State Boards of Nursing use professional certification as a requirement for granting the authority of registered nurses to practice as Advanced Practice Registered Nurses (APRNs). However, the regulation of APRNs varies widely among Boards of Nursing. It is the advanced practice nurse's responsibility to be knowledgeable about the regulations related to APRNs in the state in which he/she is engaged in practice.

PROFESSIONAL ORGANIZATIONS

Numerous professional nursing organizations exist in the United States. However, many of these organizations address special professional interests of nurses, including the American Association of Critical-Care Nurses, the American Association of Nurse Attorneys, the American Nephrology Nurses' Association, the American Psychiatric Nurses Association, the American Association of Nurse Anesthetists, the Association of Pediatric Oncology Nurses, the American Academy of Nurse Practitioners, the Academy of Medical-Surgical Nurses, the International Association of Forensic Nurses, and the American College of Nurse Midwives. For a sample of the variety of professional nursing organizations in existence, the reader is encouraged to peruse the Web sites: http://dir.yahoo.com/Health/Nursing/Organizations/ and www.nurs. org/orgs.shtml.

With so many special interest nursing organizations, only a few of the major organizations will be discussed. These organizations include the American Nurses' Association, the American Association of Colleges of Nursing, Sigma Theta Tau International, the American Organization of Nurse Executives, and the National League for Nursing.

American Nurses' Association

A full service professional organization, the American Nurses' Association (ANA) represents the nation's 2.7 million registered nurses through its 54 constituent state associations and 13 organizational affiliate members. For a list of these associations and affiliate members, please review the Web site: http://nursingworld.org/SNAweb.htm.

The purpose of the ANA is to advance the profession of nursing by fostering high standards of practice, promoting the economic and general welfare of nurses, projecting a positive and realistic view of nursing, and lobbying the U.S. Congress and regulatory agencies on issues affecting nurses and the public (American Nurses Association, 2003).

The ANA provides leadership in policy initiatives for health care reform. Through its political actions, the ANA has taken positions on a range of issues that include, but are not limited to, Medicare reform, patients' rights, the importance of safer needle devices, whistleblower protections for health care workers, access to health care, funding of nursing education programs, and appropriate reimbursement for health care services. In addition, the ANA continues to work for the collective bargaining rights of nurses, better compensation, improved working conditions, and the implementation of ways in which nursing services can be delivered to meet the current demands in health care. The official professional journal of the ANA is the *American Journal of Nursing.* For additional information the ANA, please refer to the Web site: http://www.ana.org.

The ANA also has three related entities which include the American Nurses' Credentialing Center, the American Nurses' Foundation, and the American Academy of Nursing. The American Nurses' Credentialing Center (ANCC) works to protect nursing and the public by formalizing appropriate standards for nursing credentials. It is the largest and most well-known nursing credentialing organization in the U.S. In addition, the ANCC provides various educational resources, such as credentialing continuing education programs, providing grants and scholarships, awarding funds to support research, and offering review courses for certification examination.

The American Nurses' Foundation (ANF), a charitable affiliate of the ANA, was created for the purpose of raising funds and developing grants to support advances in research, education, and clinical practice. The ANF supports its mission of promoting the health of the public and advancement of nursing through four major activities: provision of nursing research grants, fundraising, provision of extramural projects/ grants, and publishing activities of American Nurses' Publishing. In order to continue meeting its mission, the ANF relies heavily on financial support from individuals, corporations, foundations, and government agencies.

The American Academy of Nursing (AAN) exists for the purpose of enhancing nurse leaders' contributions in transforming the health care system so that the public's well-being is optimized. The approximate 1500+ Fellows of the American Academy of Nursing are nurses who have been recognized as making significant and substantial contributions to the advancement of the profession of nursing. The organization provides educational programs, workshops, publications and conferences for the purposes of enhancing health care knowledge and initiating appropriate changes in the health care system. The official professional journal of the AAN is *Nursing Outlook.*

American Association of Colleges of Nursing

The national voice for America's baccalaureate and other nursing education degree programs, the American Association of Colleges of Nursing (AACN), serves the public interest by providing standards, assisting deans and directors to implement those standards, influencing the nursing profession to improve health care, and promoting public support of baccalaureate and graduate nursing education, research, and practice. Membership in the organization includes over 550 schools of nursing from public and private universities and senior colleges nationwide. These academic institutions are a mix of baccalaureate, graduate, and postgraduate nursing programs. The dean or director of the nursing program of each institution serves as representative to the AACN (American Association of Colleges of Nursing, 2003).

The AACN works in governmental relations and other advocacy activities to advance public policy on nursing education, research, and practice. The organization provides leadership in sustaining federal support for nursing education and research, in shaping legislative and regulatory policy affecting nursing programs, and in ensuring continuing financial support for nursing students. In addition, the AACN operates a national databank reporting statistics on student enrollments and graduation, faculty salaries, budgets, institutional resources, and other trends in baccalaureate and graduate nursing programs. The official professional journal of AACN is the *Journal of Professional Nursing*. For additional information on the AACN please refer to the Web site: http://www.aacn.nche.edu.

An autonomous affiliate of the AACN, the Commission on Collegiate Nursing Education (CCNE) is the only national agency that is dedicated exclusively to the accreditation of baccalaureate and graduate degree nursing education programs. Accreditation by the CCNE is granted through a nongovernmental peer review process that holds nursing education programs accountable to the nursing profession, evaluates the success of nursing programs in achieving their mission, goals and outcomes, assesses the extent to which nursing education programs meet accreditation standards, informs the public of the values of accreditation of a nursing educational program, and fosters continuing improvement in nursing education programs. For additional information on the CCNE, please refer to the Web site: http://www.aacn.nche.edu/Accreditation/index.htm.

Sigma Theta Tau International

The international honor society, Sigma Theta Tau International (STTI), has active members from over 90 countries and territories. As of 2003, STTI sponsored chapters on university and college campuses in the U.S., Canada, Hong Kong, Pakistan, South Korea, Australia, Taiwan, The Netherlands, and Brazil. Membership is by invitation to baccalaureate and graduate nursing students who demonstrate excellent scholarship, and to nurse leaders who exhibit exceptional achievements in nursing. Of the membership, approximately 61% hold a master's or doctoral degree, 48% are clinicians, 21% are administrators or supervisors, and 20% are educators or researchers (Sigma Theta Tau International, 2003).

The purpose of the organization is to create a global community of nurses who lead through the use of scholarship, knowledge, and technology, with the goal of improving the health of people worldwide (Sigma Theta Tau International, 2003). From its inception in 1922, STTI has valued scholarship and excellence in nursing practice. In support of this belief, STTI contributes financially to nursing research, offers educational and research conferences around the world, conducts a biennial convention, offers online continuing education activities, provides career development services, offers an online library, and conducts leadership programs and global health care think-tanks. In addition, the organization produces a variety of publications along with their official professional journal, the *Journal of Nursing Scholarship*. For additional information on Sigma Theta Tau International, please refer to the Web site: http://www.nursingsociety.org.

American Organization of Nursing Executives

A subsidiary of the American Hospital Association, the American Organization of Nurse Executives (AONE) is the national organization for nurses who design, facilitate, and manage care. AONE is considered the leading professional organization for nurses in leadership roles. The purpose of AONE is to represent nurse leaders, approximately 4,000 in number, who improve health care. To accomplish this purpose, AONE provides leadership, professional development, advocacy, and research to advance nursing practice and patient care, promote excellence in nursing leadership, and shape public policy in the health care arena (American Organization of Nurse Executives, 2003).

The services offered by the AONE to its members include providing vision and actions for nursing leadership to meet the health care needs of society, influencing legislative and public policy related to health care, offering services that support management, leadership, education, and development of nurse leaders, and facilitating research and development efforts related to nursing administration and patient care. Several publications are offered by AONE, along with the official professional journal, *Nurse Leader*. To obtain additional information on the AONE, please refer to the Web site: http://www.aone.org.

National League for Nursing

Created in 1893 as the American Society of Superintendents of Training Schools for Nurses and renamed, in 1952, as the National League for

Nursing (NLN), the NLN is considered to be the oldest organization for nursing in the U.S. The purpose of the organization is to advance quality nursing education that prepares the workforce to address the needs of diverse populations in a constantly changing health care environment (National League for Nursing, 2003). To accomplish this purpose, the NLN provides measurement and teaching tools that aid in the evaluation of student and teacher competencies, faculty development activities in the form of workshops, institutes and, online programs, an annual education summit that creates a forum for nurse educators, data related to nursing schools, such as program enrollments and graduation, curriculum innovations, and research activities, and a variety of professional publications that include the organization's official professional journal, *Nursing Education Perspectives.*

Membership in NLN is in the form of two categories, agency and individual. Agency membership includes educational institutions, health care agencies, and allied/public agencies. Individual membership is classified as full, retired, or graduate student nurses. Unlike the American Association of Colleges of Nursing, NLN membership includes nursing programs at all educational levels, nurses and other interested individuals, and agencies other than nursing programs. For additional information on the NLN, please refer to the Web site: http://www.nln.org.

As an independent subsidiary of the NLN, the National League for Nursing Accrediting Commission (NLNAC) is responsible for all accrediting activities of member schools of nursing. Unlike the Commission on Collegiate Nursing Education, the accrediting affiliate of the American Association of Colleges of Nursing, the NLNAC accredits schools of nursing at all levels (practical/vocational, diploma, associate degree, baccalaureate degree, and master's degree). The 15-member Board of Commissioners that governs the NLNAC consists of nine nurse educators, three public representatives, and three nursing service representatives (National League for Nursing Accrediting Commission, 2003). The members of the Board of Commissioners set accreditation policy, make accreditation decisions based on the review of program materials, reports, and recommendations, serve as chairpersons of the program specific evaluation review panels, and decide on corporate matters, such as budget, planning, and administrative policies. For more information on NLNAC please refer to the web site: http://www.nlnac.org.

BENEFITS OF MEMBERSHIP IN PROFESSIONAL NURSING ORGANIZATIONS

Belonging to a professional nursing organization is a vital part of professionalism. With so many credible nursing organizations, it is important for nurses to examine which professional organizations meet their personal needs, fit best with job requirements, and assist in reaching short- and long-term professional goals. Professional organizations offer opportunities that often are not available through other avenues. In addition, professional organizations offer a host of benefits, such as access to:

1. Up-to-date information about the profession by way of journals, publications, newsletters, and Web sites
2. Educational programs through conferences, online programs, workshops, special lectures, and continuing education offerings
3. An avenue for having a voice, by way of state and federal policy changes, for the enhancement of nursing practice and health care delivery
4. Scholarships, research funds, and special project support
5. Agenda setting for the future of nursing education, practice, and research
6. Fellowship with other professional colleagues
7. Standards of excellence for nursing education, practice, and research

To maximize these benefits, nurses must be involved in the activities of the organization selected for membership. Active participation in any nursing organization can provide experiences that positively contribute to nurses' professional growth and development.

SUMMARY

Regulatory bodies and professional nursing organizations play a vital role in sustaining professionalism within nursing. Nursing regulatory bodies and accrediting agencies (independent subsidiaries of select professional nursing organizations) provide standards for safe practice and for quality educational nursing programs. It is only through standards of excellence that nursing will be able to maintain a high level of professionalism throughout the twenty-first century.

The numerous nursing organizations that exist provide avenues for nurses to engage in collegial dialogue and professional activities with individuals with similar interests. Nursing organizations also provide active participants with educational programs and opportunities that can foster professional growth and development. Nurses who take advantage of these opportunities will find that they play a major role in shaping the future of nursing practice, education, and research.

REFLECTIVE QUESTIONS

1. Review the Nurse Practice Act for your respective state or territory. What provisions of the act serve to protect the public from incompetent nurses? For a model of a Nurse Practice Act refer to: http://www.ncsbn.org/regulation/nursingpractice_nursing _practicemodel_act_and_rules.asp.
2. Does your state or territory have a Nurse Compact Agreement? Is so, with which other states or territories? Refer to: http://ncsbn.org.
3. If an accreditation process for nursing educational programs did not exist, what effect would this have on schools of nursing?
4. Review the Web sites for several professional nursing organizations. Based upon your interests, which organizations would serve you best and why? Refer to: http://nursingsociety.org/career/nursing_orgs.html.

RECOMMENDED READINGS

Deleskey, K. (2003). Factors affecting nurses' decision to join and maintain membership in professional associations. *Journal of Perianesthesia Nursing, 18*(1), 8–17.
Flook, D. (2003). The professional nurse and regulation. *Journal of Perianesthesia Nursing, 18*(3), 160–167.
Lewallen, L., & McMullan, K. (2001). Returning to competence after discipline. *JONA's Healthcare, Law, Ethics & Regulation, 3*(3), 88–91.
Reiger, P., & Moore, P. (2002). Professional organizations and their role in advocacy. *Seminars in Oncology Nursing, 18*(4), 276–289.

REFERENCES

American Association of Colleges of Nursing (2003). About AACN. Retrieved November 29, 2003, from http://www.aacn.nche.edu

American Nurses Association (2003). About ANA. Retrieved November 29, 2003 from http://www.nursingworld.org

American Organization of Nurse Executives (2003). Organizational information. Retrieved November 29, 2003 from http://www.aone.org

Kalisch, P., & Kalisch, B. (1995). *The advance of American nursing.* Philadelphia: Lippincott.

National Council of State Boards of Nursing (2003). Nursing regulation. Retrieved November 29, 2003 from http://www.ncsbn.org

National League for Nursing (2003). About NLN. Retrieved November 29, 2003 from http://www.nln.org

National League for Nursing Accrediting Commission (2003). About NLNAC. Retrieved November 29, 2003 from http://www.nlnac.org

Sigma Theta Tau International (2003). About STTI. Retrieved November 29, 2003 from http://www.nursingsociety.org

14

Public Health Nursing:
An Exercise in Citizenship

M. Katherine Maeve

LEARNING OBJECTIVES

After reading this chapter, the reader should be able to:

- Identify six unique characteristics of public health in the United States
- Describe how political affiliations and political processes affect problem identification and goal setting within public health
- Describe how the interdisciplinary nature of public health broadens and expands nursing roles and responsibilities
- Identify three distinct knowledge bases used by public health nurses
- Describe how public health nurses uniquely enact citizenship in their practice

KEY WORDS

Social justice, politics, population health, communities, criminal justice system

INTRODUCTION

Public health is best when nothing happens—when there are no outbreaks of infectious diseases, when our food and water are safe to consume, when the air is safe to breathe, when children are immunized, and when everyone has equal access to quality health care (Garrett, 2000). Public health nurses have a long history of advancing the public's health, although their contributions have not been widely recognized outside the nursing community. A recent editorial in the *American Journal of Public Health* (Stover & Bassett, 2003) drew attention to the notion that while public health advocates, research institutes, private foundations, and the government have all contributed to the advancement of public health, the actual endeavors of public health practitioners (including nurses) often are overlooked. The purpose of this chapter is to acquaint the reader with historical issues associated with both public health and public health nursing. An exemplar of how a public health nursing perspective drives nursing practice and research will be presented. It will be argued that, unlike any other nursing specialty, public health nursing is an exercise in citizenship.

WHAT IS PUBLIC HEALTH?

At the turn of the last century, public health leaders began to consider strategies to mitigate constant epidemics of infectious diseases. In the late 1800s and early 1900s, the industrial revolution led to large numbers of poor (often immigrant) workers moving into cities that were wholly unprepared to accommodate their burgeoning populations, especially when they were of different cultural traditions (Garrett, 2000; Sidel, Drucker, & Martin, 1993). The mixing of dense populations, living in unsanitary conditions and working long hours in unsafe and exploitative industries with wave after wave of cholera, smallpox, typhoid, tuberculosis (TB), yellow fever, malaria, and other diseases, was a formula for disaster (Turnock, 2001). Women commonly died during childbirth, and even if they lived, it was just as likely the baby they gave birth to would not.

However, it was the success of the industrial revolution that provided the capital to begin funding public health projects. As municipalities were better funded, sanitation improved, safe water supplies were developed and protected, and animal and pest control strategies were put into place. In addition, since individuals earned more money, they could buy better food, making for a population with healthier immune systems. People were able to afford better and safer housing, so that actual spaces between individuals and families increased. As a result, dramatic reductions in infectious diseases were realized (Sidel, Drucker, & Martin, 1993).

The decline of TB during this period demonstrates how social conditions intersect with public health efforts in a way that affects the incidence of disease. In 1900, for every 100,000 U.S. residents, 194 died from tuberculosis (TB). By 1940, the death rate from TB had dropped to 46 per 100,000 (Turnock, 2001). This dramatic drop occurred before antibiotics were developed to treat tuberculosis. While improved social conditions did not eliminate TB, they did have a dramatic effect on how entire communities suffered from tuberculosis (Sidel, Drucker, & Martin, 1993; Turnock, 2001).

By the beginning of this century, the field of public health had grown exponentially, and continues to evolve. Turnock (2001) identified six unique features of contemporary public health practice in the U.S.: a social justice foundation; an inherently political nature; a link with government; an ever-expanding public health agenda; a grounding in science; and an uncommon culture/bond.

Social Justice Foundation

Since 1848, social justice has been acknowledged as fundamental to sound public health practices (Anderson & McFarlane, 2000; Krieger, 1998, 2000; Turnock, 2001). In this view, public health is a social matter. To public health advocates, all persons are entitled to live in safe environments, with access to enough resources to sustain themselves and their children. These basic human entitlements include the right to adequate health care services.

Inherently Political Nature

It will be obvious to most that social justice is also a political issue. Social justice issues embedded within the public health agenda, however, are often the cause of conflict and confrontation (Turnock, 2001). The numerous issues surrounding HIV/AIDS in the U.S. and worldwide reflect how this public health threat has been politicized, with both good results as well as some less desirable consequences. Ultimately, public health is negotiated, just as any other political issue is negotiated (Garrett, 2000).

Link with Government

Federal, state and local governments play a large part in enforcing provisions of public health policies, such as monitoring water and sewer safety, product safety, workplace safety standards and the like (Anderson & McFarlane, 2000; Garrett, 2000; Turnock, 2001). These same government agencies, with their associated bureaucracies, are also involved in deciding which public health problems will be prioritized and supported with government money. Obviously, priorities will change between governmental administrations. Generally, in the U.S., we have come to expect that Republican administrations will favor some issues, and Democratic administrations will favor others. Further, there are many levels of governmental bureaucracies (local, state, and federal) that must be negotiated, and they might be of any political persuasions at any given time with very diverse, perhaps opposing, objectives. In the end, the necessary link with government means that public health organizations have the authority to enforce policies, but developing those policies within government bureaucracies can be challenging.

Public health districts also provide direct health care services, primarily to the indigent. For instance, it is common for public health departments to provide child immunizations, blood pressure clinics, clinics that specialize in sexually transmitted diseases, and the like.

Ever-Expanding Public Health Agenda

Traditional domains of public health interest include biology, environment, lifestyle, and health service organization. Though public health initially focused on infectious diseases and related environmental risks, public health approaches now are used widely for a variety of problems (Anderson & McFarlane, 2000; Garrett, 2000; IOM, 1988; Krieger, 1998, 2000; Levy & Sidel, 1997; Maeve, 2003; Marquart, Brewer, & Mullings, 1999; Mundt, 1998; Stanhope & Lancaster, 2000; Storlie, 1970; Turnock, 2001).

For instance, when statistics indicated that an alarming number of motor vehicle accidents and related deaths were caused by drunk drivers, it became apparent that legal sanctions against those drivers were imperative, as was the notion of educating the public not to drive drunk. Today, the number of deaths associated with drunk driving accidents is reported widely, and law enforcement officials are often held accountable when rates are overly high for any given area. As a result, penalties are harsher. Most days, Americans see some evidence of the public health campaign advertisement "Friends don't let friends drive drunk." Improving traffic light systems and safety devices, such as seat belts and air bags, were also public health strategies that dramatically reduced the mortality and morbidity associated with accidents.

Grounding in Science

According to Turnock (2001), public health consists of five basic sciences: epidemiology, biostatistics, environmental science, management sciences, and behavioral sciences. Each of these sciences is included in the core curriculum of public health professionals. Nursing curricula also contain each of these sciences, in addition to our own substantive contributions to the science of public health (Anderson & McFarlane, 2000; Stanhope & Lancaster, 2000).

Focus on Prevention

The concept of prevention is central to all public health practice (Anderson & McFarlane, 2000; Garrett, 2000; IOM, 1988; Krieger, 1998, 2000; Levy & Sidel, 1997; Maeve, 2003; Marquart, Brewer, & Mullings, 1999; Mundt, 1998; Stanhope & Lancaster, 2000; Storlie, 1970; Turnock, 2001). Three levels of prevention are widely acknowledged and used for policy and planning purposes: primary, secondary, and tertiary. Primary prevention is about the true avoidance of disease through health promotion activities and protective actions. For example, educating people about necessary levels of nutrition to maintain health is a classic primary prevention strategy. Secondary prevention concerns early detection, intervention, and treatment for adverse health conditions, with the goal of early detection of diseases. Screening at-risk children for lead contamination is an example of secondary prevention. If a child is found to have lead levels, interventions can be implemented to remove lead from the child's environment and provide appropriate treatment before toxic lead levels are reached. Tertiary prevention is employed after adverse health conditions have already developed and caused damage to the individual. The goals of tertiary prevention are to limit disability, and rehabilitate or restore people to their maximum capabilities. If a child who has ingested lead manifests the kind of symptoms that suggest brain damage, a tertiary prevention approach would utilize medical services as appropriate, as well as ensure that the child received special education to help him keep on track with growth and development tasks and be successful in school.

Uncommon Culture

One of the most unique features of public health, in the U.S., is the diverse number of professions involved (Anderson & McFarlane, 2000;

Stanhope & Lancaster, 2000; Turnock, 2001). Professionals who practice in public health may include nurses, physicians, anthropologists, engineers, epidemiologists, biostatisticians, lawyers, nutritionists, social workers, and many more examples too numerous to name. This creates a very different culture than any one of those professions might develop within another context. Most nurses are comfortable when their dayto-day work occurs in an environment where there are other nurses. However, when working on public health projects, there may be many types of people with competing priorities, different beliefs, and different approaches. Because of this, public health nurses become very knowledgeable about a much broader spectrum of subjects than they would ever be exposed to in a hospital setting. For instance, a nurse whose second career choice would have been geology, might be happy working with environmental clean-up committees. Public health nursing gives nurses the opportunity to do nursing, but with a much broader scope of practice and expanded opportunities.

As we can see in the above descriptions, public health acknowledges and assumes responsibility for a wide scope of issues that influence the health and wellness of individuals, families, and communities. The Institute of Medicine (IOM) (1988) provided a useful definition of public health as "fulfilling society's interest in assuring conditions in which people can be healthy" (p. 7). This view acknowledges the premise that society has an interest in the health of its members—we all live in the same world. Garrett (2001) noted early American public pioneers understood "that preventing disease in the weakest elements of society ensured protection for the strongest (and richest) in the larger community" (p. 11).

WHAT IS PUBLIC HEALTH NURSING?

In 1996, the Public Health Nursing Section (PHNS) of the American Public Health Association (APHA) issued a position statement regarding the definition and role responsibilities of a public health nurse:

> Public health nursing is the practice of promoting and protecting the health of populations using knowledge from nursing, social, and public health sciences. (p. 1)

The PHNS states that the title "Public Health Nurse" designates a nursing professional with educational preparation in public health and nursing science, with goals focused on population-level outcomes. The primary focus then is to promote health and prevent disease for entire population groups, as they are found in neighborhoods, communities, states, and countries. In addition, the notion of population groups also consists of collections of individuals who have similar characteristics or share common phenomena.

For example, if a community has a large number of low-birth-weight babies, public health nurses may target those babies after their release from the hospital to ensure that babies are adequately nourished and are growing and developing appropriately. Nurses also may recognize the need to provide education to the community's pregnant women about the causes and consequences of low birth weight. For the purposes of planning, new mothers with low-birth-weight babies form an aggregate of women who might live in various geographic areas across the community, but provide the focus for care. Individual mothers and babies will receive care, but that care is planned for in terms of the aggregate. The success of this program would then be measured in terms of how it affects the incidence of low-birth-weight babies in the target population.

The process of public health nursing practice is similar to the nursing process described in many foundational nursing texts. This systematic process is:

1. Health and health care needs of a population are assessed, especially those at particular risk for illness, injury, disability or premature death.
2. Based on current scientific knowledge, an intervention plan is developed that takes into account available resources, community culture and expectations, accepted practice standards, and goals of the program.
3. Plan is implemented.
4. Formative and summative evaluations are developed throughout the program to determine the extent of the intervention, and what effect it has on individuals and the population.
5. The results of the process are developed and disseminated to influence and direct care services and health resources, influence and inform public policy, and inform future research directions. (PHNS/APHA, 1996, pp. 1–2)

PUBLIC HEALTH NURSING PIONEERS

In the United States, nursing has a long and rich history of attending to the health of vulnerable population groups, communities, and neighborhoods. Two nursing pioneers from the turn of the century, Lillian Wald and Margaret Sanger, changed forever the image of nurses as handmaidens to physicians, or women who "take orders" from anyone! These remarkable women had a clear vision of what they wanted and were willing to do whatever it took to make it happen.

In 1893, Lillian Wald, who became known as the "mother of public health nursing," established a district nurse service that became known as the House on Henry Street (Swanson, 1997). Wald was outraged at the squalor and disease she found among immigrants living on the lower east side of New York at the turn of the century. Wald and her colleagues began to live in the neighborhood, identified themselves socially within the neighborhood, and fought for improved living conditions. While much of Wald's efforts were related to providing direct health care (indeed, she employed several physicians to *assist her*), she also understood the effect of social conditions upon health and recognized that only through social justice advocacy could these conditions change. And change they did! Wald and her colleagues entered the democratic process on behalf of their community and *with* their community to effect change. Wald recognized that entering into the democratic process as a nursing practice issue was an exercise of citizenship.

Margaret Sanger was another pioneer public health nurse. Sanger was one of eleven children. Her mother always was pregnant and sick. She died at a relatively young age from TB, which Margaret attributed to her mother's multiple pregnancies. Because of this, Margaret decided to become a nurse and help pregnant women. Ultimately, she found that helping women have safer births was a noble effort, but almost as many women were dying of botched abortions as from actual births. She was determined to get to the root of the problem itself—unwanted and back-to-back pregnancies. Despite considerable opposition by churches and government, Margaret developed classes and gave lectures to women and girls living in New York's ghettos about how their bodies worked and how to prevent conception. She was harassed, arrested, and had her office and equipment confiscated and destroyed by thugs and police. Sanger's contribution of citizenship was outside the democratic process that was available to her at the time, but she was clear in her vision. Despite these obstacles, Sanger ran a crusade for women's biological and reproductive rights that challenged the traditional way of thought, and introduced concepts that shifted the course of American society.

Lillian Wald and Margaret Sanger represent an ideal of what public health nursing can be. Obviously, these were extraordinary nurses with extraordinary amounts of energy and dedication. They also were extraordinary citizens.

Described below is one example of a program developed for a particularly vulnerable group of women. Though the program is not fully implemented, it represents the trajectory of how public health nursing practice can evolve into a research program, and, ultimately, inform an intervention program.

A NURSING PARTNERSHIP WITH CRIMINAL JUSTICE

Nationally, health care and criminal justice professionals are increasingly exploring the intersection between health behaviors and outcomes, and criminal behaviors and outcomes. Recognizing the intersection between these professional interests is the belief that social problems (including health disparities, crime, and recidivism) are not solved when there is intellectual isolation between disciplines (Maeve, 1999, 2001, 2003; Marquart, Brewer, & Mullings, 1999).

Traditionally, law enforcement's approach to the crime problems has been "investigation, prosecution, and incarceration." Now, criminal justice professionals are exploring collaborations with other disciplines that include "prevention, intervention, and treatment" as a way to address the high rates of crime and incarceration (Drake, personal communication, December 6, 2002). As discussed earlier, prevention, intervention and treatment are synonymous with the levels of prevention used in public health practice.

One important intersection between criminal justice interests and health interests concerns the large numbers of inmates released from jails and prisons every year. Though the numbers of persons released from prisons each year is substantial (600,000), a staggering *15 million individuals* go in and out of county jails annually (Bureau of Justice Statistics, 2002; Maeve, 2003; Travis, Solomon, & Waul, 2001). Because of the increased incidences of chronic and acute physical, dental, mental, and social illnesses present in all incarcerated populations, the release and reintegration of individuals back into the community, without adequate treatment or mechanisms to ensure continuity of care, has been referred to as a public health crisis (Hammett, Roberts, & Kennedy, 2001; Maeve, 2001, 2003; Marquart, Brewer, & Mullings, 1999).

Of the 15 million individuals released from county jails every year in the U.S., three million are women (Bureau of Justice Statistics, 2002). In the vast majority of cases, women's crimes are directly or indirectly related to substance use and abuse. Though the possession or use of drugs may not be the proximate cause of arrest, crimes such as disorderly conduct, prostitution, shoplifting, and check and/or check-card fraud most often are committed in order to get money to buy drugs.

The majority of women entering jail are young, single mothers of dependent children who largely come from economically disadvantaged neighborhoods; are poorly educated; have increased incidence of chronic physical illness; often have recent injuries occurring prior to or during their arrests; have experienced limited and inconsistent health care prior to incarceration; have longstanding emotional and mental health problems; have poor dentition; have experienced both physical and sexual abuse, usually beginning in their childhoods; and have longstanding drug and alcohol problems (Hammett, Roberts, & Kennedy, 2001; Maeve, 1999, 2000, 2001, 2003; Marquart, Brewer, & Mullings, 1999). Additionally, 10% of incarcerated women are pregnant (Bureau of Justice Statistics, 2002). Therefore, incarcerated women have been identified as one of the most vulnerable groups of women in American society.

Providing health care to incarcerated women (and men) is difficult at best, but particularly difficult within jails (Maeve, 2001). Jail populations tend to be somewhat fluid as a result of the rapid cycle of arrests and releases. Because of constant changes within the jail population, chronically underfunded county jail systems often are only able to care for acute illnesses and injuries. Incarceration, in and of itself, places women (and men) in largely overcrowded, risky environments where inmates are easily exposed to infectious diseases (particularly TB, HIV, and hepatitis) and violence (Hammett, Roberts, & Kennedy, 2001; NCCHC, 2002; Travis, Solomon, & Waul, 2001). Furthermore, these health problems do not remain behind jail or prison walls.

A recent study noted that, on a national level, approximately 90% of jails and prisons have screening structures in place that reflect CDC guidelines. However, few actually adhere to the guidelines for screening and treatment of infectious diseases (NCCHC, 2002). Therefore, it is not altogether unexpected that inmates will become infected with a disease such as TB, HIV, or Hepatitis, and will carry those infections back to their families and neighborhoods (Hammett, Roberts, & Kennedy, 2001, Maeve, 2001, 2003).

Previous research indicates that the constant cycling of women (and men) in and out of jail, without adequate treatment or follow-up, leads to a number of unfortunate collateral consequences, including child abuse, family violence, the spread of infectious diseases, homelessness, and community disorder (Maeve, 2001, 2003). Within the neighborhoods where the women in Maeve's study lived, there were higher incidences of accidents; higher incidences of premature and low-weight babies; higher incidences of deaths from chronic illnesses (e.g., heart disease, hypertension, diabetes, HIV/AIDS); higher incidences of infectious diseases such as TB, HIV/AIDS; higher incidences of mental health illnesses; poorer educational outcomes; higher incidences of violent crimes; and higher arrests of both women and men. These neighborhoods also were saturated, seemingly, with crackcocaine and alcohol.

In 1978, the World Health Organization (WHO) defined health as "a state of enough physical, mental and social well-being to enable people to work productively and participate actively in the social and economic life of the community in which they live" (p. 5). Clearly, this vision of health cannot be actualized in communities where poverty, crime, substance abuse, and violence are everyday occurrences. Nor can health flourish in families and neighborhoods where a substantial percentage of fathers and mothers are either in prison, or in and out of jail on a regular basis, with their children living in a constant state of flux (Maeve, 2001, 2003; Wallace & Wallace, 1997).

It was clear from the study that incarcerated women, and women at risk for incarceration, needed more than mere medical care. Medical care would satisfy only one piece of their complex health needs. This group of women needs what Mundt (1998) called "true healthcare" (p. 7) that is not dependent upon a medical referral, but is born of proactive nursing care encompassing all aspects of health—physical, mental, and social. Mundt (1998) has called for nurses to develop health care systems for the underserved that are comprehensive, grounded in advocacy, feature interdisciplinary collaboration, and are developed in ways that can document and demonstrate how interventions have a direct impact on health outcomes.

Collaborations between traditional health care providers and systems, and the criminal justice system, could have meaningful outcomes on health at the individual, family, and community levels. Such collaborations could reduce crime and recidivism, and serve the overall goals of the community and various disciplines.

NURSING CARE PARTNERSHIP PROGRAM

The Nursing Care Partnership Program was developed with local criminal justice professionals in an attempt to break the cycle of repeated incarcerations for women (Maeve, 2003). The explicit goals of the program are to help women become healthier and stay out of jail. It is believed that attending to women's health issues and needs *before* their release from jail, and helping them address those issues *after* their release, will provide a more seamless transition from jail back into the community and will positively influence health issues embedded within criminal activity. The Nursing Care Partnership Program partners women being released from jail with nurses who work with women intensively to accomplish the goals of the program. Nursing interventions are directed towards helping women make health-promoting choices within life contexts less likely to include reoffending and rearrest, thus increasing women's desistance from further criminal behaviors. In brief, the Nursing Care Partners are integrally involved in:

1. Identifying individual needs and priorities with women prior to their release
2. Connecting with women immediately upon release
3. Linking women with the resources they needed after release to stabilize their lives
4. Providing quality comprehensive accessible health care services specific for this particular group of women
5. Helping women learn how to make health-promoting choices over time
6. Recognize desistance from crime as a "work in progress"

Women are recruited for the program prior to their release from jail. In partnership with nurses, release plans are developed according to individual needs. Primary health care, including dental and mental health care, is provided by the program for the first year after each woman's release, giving the women support and time to develop their own resources. Other features and services through the program include

TABLE 14.1   Health Achievement Markers

1. Routine & appropriate primary health care with treatment, as indicated
2. Psychiatric evaluation with treatment, as indicated
3. Abstinence from drugs and/or alcohol
4. Dental evaluation and treatment, as indicated
5. Practicing safe sex
6. No unplanned pregnancies
7. Maintenance of all prescribed drug regimens
8. No emergency room visits for nonemergency conditions
9. Participation in individual and/or group counseling, as individually indicated
10. Health care insurance coverage (Medicare, Medicaid, and/or private source)
11. Appropriately caring for (or appropriately participating in care of) dependent children
12. Permanent housing arrangement
13. Regular and legitimate source of income
14. Basic high school diploma and/or GED certificate
15. Adherence to probation requirements

educational offerings, parenting support, and employment counseling. Though direct health care services are available to women only for the first year after their release, women will have access to their nursing care partner, and any classes/support groups associated with the program after their first year.

Interventions have been designed to address local practices and services, including local practices within the criminal justice system. Helping women become healthier and stay out of jail is the goal shared by nurses and criminal justice professionals. However, the women's participation in the program is not courtmandated. To develop trusting and successful relationships with these women, nurses cannot function as agents for the police or courts. Nursing's commitment to caring cannot be accomplished from the disciplinary standpoint necessary for police and corrections officers.

Findings of previous research (Maeve, 2001) have led to the identification of health achievement markers for newly released women that are reflective of making health-promoting choices. Further, these markers are also consistent with the kinds of life contexts less likely to include reoffending, rearrest, and reincarceration (Maeve, 2003).

Funding for the program is pending and will include specific documentation to evaluate its effectiveness in terms of health outcomes, and in correlation with numbers and patterns of arrests. Specific research aims for the program are to:

1. Determine which health achievement markers are significant predictors of rates of offending among women who participate in the Nursing Care Partnership Program and women who do not
2. Compare rates of offending, and times, with offenses (hazard rates) among women newly released from jail who participate in a Nursing Care Partnership Program and women who do not
3. Engage women before and after release from jail in participative action research to generate knowledge about issues of health, about events, circumstances and/or structures affecting women's reintegration, and about how these phenomena relate to desistance from crime
4. Identify how the Nursing Care Partnership Program affects women's reintegration and desistance from crime

Crime is a significant and complex social issue, with enormous human and economic costs (Hammett, Roberts, & Kennedy, 2001; Maeve, 2001, 2003; Marquart, Brewer, & Mullings, 1999; Travis, Solomon, & Waul, 2001). Incarcerated women who are engaged in persistent cycles of imprisonment often related to substance abuse represent one of the most vulnerable groups of women in our society. Their complicated health status, in and out of jail, has tremendous implications for their own, their family's, and their community's immediate and long-term well being. The human and economic consequences of repeated incarcerations are substantial, often overwhelming individuals, families, and communities forever. To interrupt these cycles of repeated incarceration, innovative interdisciplinary interventions must be developed, particularly interventions that address issues of social health.

CONCLUSION

Nursing is uniquely positioned to intervene with many socially significant health issues, including crime, incarceration, and release. But it is not enough to just *think* about our obligations to the social health of our communities. As a practice discipline, nursing must *do something* about social health. The gap between the *haves* and the *have nots* in our society grows wider every day, every year. In the U.S., *this differential always translates into health disparities.* Therefore, nurses need to join Drevdahl (1995) when she notes that "it is imperative that community nurses stop simply recounting the injustices present in their communities and start employing interventions that breach usual social structures" (p. 22). Doing so will not only fulfill nursing's most obvious professional obligations, it also will contribute our citizenship in this much neglected but growing area of human experience (Maeve, 2001). Today, we need more Lillian Walds and more Margaret Sangers.

REFLECTIVE QUESTIONS

1. What are the three levels of prevention used in planning by public health nurses?
2. Compare and contrast the basic nursing process with the public health nursing process.
3. Identify nurse(s) who sit on your local Board of Health, or provide leadership within local public health departments, and find out how they take part in the political processes in your community. Does nursing have a voice in your community?
4. What are the strengths and weaknesses of interdisciplinary teams in public health?
5. What interests do you have outside nursing that could be incorporated into your nursing practice in a public health setting?

RECOMMENDED READINGS

Drevdahl, D. (1995). Coming to voice: The power of emancipatory community interventions. *ANS, 18*(2), 13–24.

Krieger, N. (1998). A vision of social justice as the foundation of public health: Commemorating 150 years of the spirit of 1848. *AJPH, 88*(11), 1603–1606.

Mundt, M. (1998). Exploring the meaning of "underserved": A call to action. *Nursing Forum, 33*(1), 5–10.

Swanson, J. (1997). Historical factors: Community health nursing in context. In J. Swanson & M. Nies, *Community health nursing: Promoting the health of aggregates* (2nd ed.). Philadelphia: W. B. Saunders.

Wallace, R., & Wallace, D. (1997). Socioeconomic determinants of health: Community marginalisation and the diffusion of disease and disorder in the United States. *British Medical Journal, 314*(7090), 1341–1345.

REFERENCES

American Public Health Association, Public Health Nursing Section (1996). *The definition and role of public health nursing.* Washington, DC: Author.

Anderson, E. T., & McFarlane, J. (2000). *Community as partner: Theory and practice in nursing* (3rd ed.). Philadelphia: Lippincott.

Bureau of Justice Statistics (2002). *Prisoners in 2001.* Washington DC: U.S. Dept. of Justice.

Drevdahl, D. (1995). Coming to voice: The power of emancipatory community interventions. *Advances in Nursing Science, 18*(2), 13–24.

Garrett, L. (2000). *Betrayal of trust: The collapse of global public health.* New York: Hyperion.

Hammett, T., Roberts, C., & Kennedy, S. (2001). Health-related issues in prisoner reentry. *Crime & Delinquency, 47*(3), 390–409.

Institute of Medicine, National Academy of Sciences (1988). *The future of public health.* Washington, DC: National Academy Press.

Krieger, N. (1998). A vision of social justice as the foundation of public health: Commemorating 150 years of the spirit of 1848. *American Journal of Public Health, 88*(11), 1603–1606.

Krieger, N. (2000). Passionate epistemology, critical advocacy, and public health: Doing our profession proud. *Critical Public Health, 10*(3), 287–294.

Levy, B. S., & Sidel, V. W. (1997). *War and public health.* New York: Oxford University Press.

Maeve, M. K. (1999). Adjudicated health: Incarcerated women and the social construction of health. *Crime, Law & Social Change, 31,* 49–71.

Maeve, M. K. (2000). Speaking unavoidable truths: Understanding early childhood sexual and physical violence among women in prison. *Issues in Mental Health Nursing, 21,* 473–498.

Maeve, M. K. (2001). Waiting to be caught: The devolution of health for women newly released from jail. *Criminal Justice Review, 26*(2), 143–169.

Maeve, M. K. (2003). Nursing care partnerships with women leaving jail: Effects on health and crime. *Journal of Psychosocial Nursing and Mental Health Services, 41*(9), 30–40.

Marquart, J., Brewer, V., & Mullings, J. (1999). Health risk as an emerging field within the new penology. *Journal of Criminal Justice, 27*(2), 143–154.

Mundt, M. (1998). Exploring the meaning of "underserved:" A call to action. *Nursing Forum, 33*(1), 5–10.

National Commission on Correctional Healthcare (2002). *The health status of soon-to-be released inmates* (Vol. I). Chicago: Author.

Sidel, V., Drucker, E., & Martin, S. (1993). The resurgence of tuberculosis in the United States: Societal origins and societal responses. *Journal of Law, Medicine & Ethics, 21*(3–4), 303–316.

Stanhope, M., & Lancaster, J. (2000). *Community & public health nursing* (5th ed.). Philadelphia: Mosby.

Storlie, F. (1970). *Nursing and the social conscience.* New York: Appleton-Century-Crofts.

Stover, G., & Bassett, M. T. (2003). Practice is the purpose of public health. *American Journal of Public Health, 93*(11), 1799–1801.

Swanson, J. (1997). Historical factors: Community health nursing in context. In J. Swanson & M. Nies, *Community health nursing: Promoting the health of aggregate* (2nd ed.). Philadelphia: W. B. Saunders.

Travis, J., Solomon, A., & Waul, M. (2001). *From prison to home: The dimensions and consequences of prisoner reentry.* Washington, DC: Urban Institute.

Turnock, B. (2001). *Public health: What it is and how it works* (2nd ed.). Gaithersburg, MD: Aspen.

Wallace, R., & Wallace, D. (1997). Socioeconomic determinants of health: Community marginalisation and the diffusion of disease and disorder in the United States. *British Medical Journal, 314*(7090), 1341–1345.

World Health Organization (WHO) (1978, September). Report of the International Conference on Primary Healthcare. Geneva, Switzerland: Author.

15

Rural Health in America: Challenges and Opportunities

Catherine Reavis

LEARNING OBJECTIVES

The learning objectives and related activities of this chapter will:

- Define rurality as applied to delivery of health care services throughout rural America
- Identify the complexities of American demographics that influence rural health and health care delivery
- Describe the general state of American health and pertinent rural health issues
- Discuss many available services providing health care to rural Americans
- Present an overview of nursing education and preparation that enable nurses to provide rural health care in a variety of settings
- Match rural health care challenges with nursing opportunities in order to meet rural health care needs

KEY WORDS

Isolation, disadvantage, poverty, health status, diversity

INTRODUCTION

The United States is a complex blend of peoples of different ethnicity and rich culture, living in a vast array of environments. Health issues are as complex as the country's inhabitants, where demographics and geographical conditions dictate the challenges and opportunities. As health and health care are inextricably linked to economy and demography, rural health care offers a unique profile and related opportunities. For example, where the rural economy is stagnant or losing population, health status suffers. Rural ageing populations require more health care. In areas suffering the loss of industry, the rural population dependent on this industry for economic viability suffers mental anguish and related mental health conditions. The loss also affects the family and institutions such as schools and churches. These patterns of change occur in urban areas of America as well, but services to assist with the process of change and meet the health care needs of the community often are not available to rural and remote Americans (Ricketts, 1999). This chapter will attempt to provide a definition of rurality, describe the demographics contributing to rurality, give the reader a sense of the state of the nation's health and special needs of rural peoples, discuss services and resources to meet health care challenges, illuminate health care gaps, and discuss the role of nursing in addressing rural health concerns.

DEFINING RURALITY

The two most common designations of rurality are defined by the U.S. Bureau of the Census and the U.S. Office of Management and Budget (OMB). The Census Bureau classes populations according to the density of persons. Periodic counts of inhabitants in America by Bureau of Census personnel provide the numbers of inhabitants and use the figures to define urban as "all territory, population and housing units in urbanized areas and in places of 2,500 or more persons outside urbanized areas" (Ricketts, 1999, p. 7). Rural areas are all "territory, population and housing units not classified as urban" (Ricketts, 1999, p. 7). The OMB designation identifies counties as metropolitan or nonmetropolitan based more on economics and integration of metropolitan areas with peripheral counties. OMB designation takes into account not only the census data, but commuting patterns and business activity. Since the OMB definition of rurality is a constant process, for purposes of this text, the definition of rurality will be understood as that defined by the U.S. Bureau of the Census, as described above. Both designations are useful in setting policy and planning programs of support for urban and rural populations at both the federal and state levels.

DEMOGRAPHICS

Selected demographic data about America and influencing economics should precede a discussion of rural health needs and proffer a foundation for discourse about resources and services to meet those needs. Urban flight in the last decade has caused significant and uneven shifts in rural populations. While rural counties experienced an increase of growth (70%), this growth was concentrated in only 40% of the rural counties (Ricketts, 1999). The number of rural counties experiencing a decrease in population rose from 600 to 855 between 1995–1999 (Ricketts, 1999). Mining- and farming-dependent counties had the greatest relative decrease in population growth as economics influenced demands for goods and services from other industries.

As employment opportunities for immigrants, especially Hispanics and Asians, increased, shifts in the ethnicity of rural populations were stimulated, thereby reconstructing existing demographics. In the rural South, African Americans comprise 18% of the population. In the west, American Indians, and Alaskan natives make up 9% of rural counties. Overall, Hispanics constitute 11% of rural America (Eberhardt, Ingram, & Makuc, 2001). These ethnic dispersions make rural settings uniquely different regarding health issues and access to health care services.

At the extreme of rurality are the frontier areas of the United States. These vast territories are sparsely populated, with 2–20 persons per square mile. Almost all frontier counties lie between the Pacific Coast Mountains and the 98th meridian, running from approximately the middle of North Dakota through mid-Texas. These frontier areas comprise Native American populations living on or near reservations with others that have common tribal heritage. Native Americans exist as independent, autonomous nations within the United States and contract for many services including health care. Contracted health care providers may deliver services that are administered by members of the Indian Nation. While Native Americans are recognized as members of a nation within the American nation, and health care regulation and financing are viewed as separate from the rest of America, health care delivery and considerations may also be integrated into existing systems. For example, Native Americans may use drugs manufactured in America and, thereby, benefit from drug regulation by the Federal Drug Administration, an agency protecting the health of all Americans. The United States Department of Health and Human Services (DHHS) has programs that are concerned with the health of all Americans, including Native Americans. Native Americans have many of the same health concerns as other rural peoples in America, but have a high incidence of diabetes mellitus, substance abuse, and depression when compared with the American population as a whole (Hartley, Bird, & Dempsey, 1999). Since Native Americans populate the extremely rural frontier counties, they offer special health care challenges specific to their ethnicity as well as challenges related to access to health care.

Economic changes in rural America have had a profound effect on health care. American rural counties have shifted from being primarily agrarian to employing only 7.6% of their populations in agriculture and related industries. Rural communities suffer challenges to economic viability by not being competitive in attracting new business, suffering significant poverty, and compromising educational and social opportunities (the "rural digital divide," for example). Much of America is still undeveloped and gaps in technology prohibit rural residents from being in touch with the rest of the nation and the world (DHHS, 2002). Effective, accessible health and social services for rural populations are essential to the health and well-being of Americans and also serve as economic opportunities for people working in the health care industry. In rural communities, health care services may provide and generate up to 20% of jobs.

STATE OF THE NATION'S HEALTH

Estimates of the health concerns of the American public give a generalized view of the health of the nation (National Health Interview Survey, 1998). Noninstitutionalized adults were the source of data in the 2002 study conducted by the Centers for Disease Control and Prevention (CDC), National Center for Health Statistics. Sixty-five percent of adults reported excellent or very good health, in spite of the fact that 17% had no health insurance and 14% had no usual source of medical care. Prevalent disease states reported were cardiovascular (12%), hypertension (19%), respiratory (2%), emphysema/asthma (9%), cancer in ages 18–64 (6%) and ages greater than 65 (18%), diabetes mellitus (5%), ulcer disease (9%), kidney disease (2%), and mental health, especially depression, (12%). Americans have set the stage for many of the nation's health issues by smoking (25%), not engaging in regular physical activity (60%), and being overweight (35%) or obese (20%) (DHHS, 2002). These data suggest Americans have spent more health care dollars on interventions for acute and chronic diseases instead of engaging in active health promotion campaigns. This unwise use of resources especially affects rural Americans where the following statistics describe the disproportionate lack of health care resources and services.

RURAL HEALTH IN AMERICA

According to Ricketts (1999), factors contrasting urban and rural health that nurses, desiring to work in rural or remote area, must consider are:

1) Rural areas have approximately 50% fewer physicians than urban areas, with 90% of the specialty physicians practicing in urban areas.
2) Rural residents are less likely to have health insurance from employers, and the rural poor are less likely to receive Medicaid benefits than the urban poor.
3) Rural residents suffer more poverty. On the average, per capita income is $7,417 less in rural areas than in urban areas. Nearly 24% of rural children live in poverty.
4) Rural residents are twice as likely as urban residents to die in motor-vehicle accidents and from unintentional injuries.
5) Alcohol abuse and use of smokeless tobacco are significant health concerns for rural youth.
6) Rural residents are less likely to receive routine dental care.
7) Rural men are committing suicide at a significantly higher rate than men in urban areas, with fewer mental health professionals per capita to provide care.
8) Lack of transportation in rural areas is a significant barrier to access to health care services.
9) A larger proportion of rural residents are elderly compared with national norms.

RURAL HEALTH RISK FACTORS

Many health problems place Americans at risk for disease and emphasize the need for health promotion in the delivery of health care services. However, difficult and different health challenges face most rural counties. According to the Centers for Disease Control and Prevention (Eberhardt, M. S., Ingram, D. D., Makuc, D. M., 2001), health risks unique to America's rural populations are:

1) Adolescents and adults living in the most rural counties are the most likely to smoke.
2) Adults 18–49 years of age in the rural Western counties are more likely to consume five or more drinks in one day than adults in urban counties.
3) Women living in the most rural counties have the highest rates of obesity.
4) The population physically inactive during leisure time was highest in rural counties in the South.
5) Rural counties in the South and West have the highest infant mortality rates.
6) Death rates of children and young adults (ages 1–24) are highest in the most rural counties.
7) Death rates of working-age adults (ages 25–64) are highest in the rural South.
8) Death rates from ischemic heart disease were highest in the rural South.
9) Death rates from chronic obstructive pulmonary diseases are highest in rural counties.
10) Deaths from unintentional injuries are 80% higher in the most rural counties than in fringe counties of large metropolitan counties.
11) Suicide rates for males age 15 years or over are lowest in large metropolitan counties, and increase steadily as counties become less urban.
12) Birth rates for adolescents are more than 30% higher in rural counties than in large metro counties.
13) Limitation in activity due to chronic health conditions among adults is more common in rural counties.
14) Total tooth loss among seniors increases as urbanization declines.

Nurses working in rural areas of America would be advised to consider the list of special health risks to vulnerable rural populations. Attention needs to be focused on health promotion, since many health risks lead to increases in morbidity and mortality. Significant change to higher levels of healthier rural populations can be attained if health care providers focus on "health care" rather than "illness care."

SERVICES

Strong rural social networks have both positive and negative effects on the delivery of health care services. Positive forces occur from the general sense of familiarity in rural communities that allow providers access to knowledge of persons in need of services. In rural areas where most people know each other, health care needs may be part of the overall community consciousness. An individual's health care needs may be identified by neighbors and/or close contacts who feel compelled to assist the individual in accessing health care services through a sense of community and neighborliness. This tradition seems to be carried over from early pioneer days in America when people lived in rural communities and shared resources in order to survive. Conversely, this familiarity may exert a negative effect on delivery of services to those rural people feeling an invasion of privacy and stigmatization from certain services. For example, families using health care services provided by Medicaid may feel stigmatized, as only people in a lower income bracket can qualify for those services. In addition, only certain health care providers accept Medicaid patients, since the government reimbursement for Medicaid services may be less than other managed-care organizations. Therefore, patients covered by Medicaid are limited in the number of health care providers who can t treat them. In general, rural populations lack access to health care services, and have poorer health and greater poverty (DHHS, 2002).

Directly related to poor access to health care services are the high cost of healthcare, the number of uninsured, and the lack of qualified providers. American health care is paid for by a variety of methods including, but not limited to, fee for service, insurance premiums, or federal assistance. The cost of the service is set by the provider, and for uninsured patients the service is paid for by the patient at the time of service. In the past, and often in the present, poor patients in rural America have been unable to afford the health care provided, and have paid the physician with goods and services, such as trading farm produce for an office visit or for medicine.

An alternate method of paying for health care services is through insurance. Persons who make periodic payments to private insurance companies are thereby insured, and the insurance company may pay for selected health care services as provided for in the health care agreement or policy. These periodic payments may vary from reasonable to very expensive and unaffordable by many Americans, especially those in lower income brackets. In selected populations of Americans who qualify for federal and/or state government health care insurance programs such as Medicare or Medicaid, the individual may pay a small amount of the service called a co-pay, and the governmental program reimburses the provider for the remainder of the service costs.

Not all Americans can qualify for governmental insurance programs, and only twenty percent of rural Americans are insured through private companies. Not just people in lower income brackets may qualify for health care through funds from federal health insurance programs (Ricketts, 1999). Elderly and disabled Americans may also receive health care services via federal programs. Medicare, a federally funded health care program, is the primary source of health care reimbursement in rural areas (Ricketts, 1999). Americans over 65 years of age, or who have been declared disabled, may qualify for Medicare health insurance. It provides health insurance coverage for over 38 million Americans. As a greater percentage of rural Americans become elderly, Medicare reimbursement will play an even more significant role in the delivery of health care to rural populations (Mueller, Schoenman, & Dorosh, 1999). However, Medicare only pays for certain services, and at present, it does not pay for medications, although legislation is pending to change this policy. Many elders have more than one disease or medical condition, and medication to manage their illnesses may cost hundreds of dollars per month. As persons over 65 are more likely to be retired and living on a fixed income, assisted by Social Security benefits, the cost of medications may be so high that rent and food may be sacrificed to purchase medicines.

Children and mothers of children may receive health care benefits through federal and state health care programs such as Medicaid and State Children's Heath Insurance (CHIP) programs. Children qualify for Medicaid if their parents are determined to meet certain criteria, which primarily means living below the poverty level. Since the health of the child is directly related to the health of the mother, Medicaid also provides health care dollars for mothers who qualify. Generally, Medicaid pays for clinical preventive services, such as immunizations and well check-ups, clinic visits for illness, hospitalizations, medications, and procedures. Enrollment in these federal health care programs varies from state to state. It is related to economic factors such as the poverty level of the respective state, access to providers, and provision of Rural Health Clinics or Federally Qualified Health Clinics in underserved areas. Without insurance, rural persons are caught in a double bind; they come from rural areas that have high levels of poverty, and the cost of health care services often prohibits the uninsured from paying a fee for service.

Sixty-five million Americans living in rural areas benefit from 225 United States Department of Health and Human Services (DHHS) programs. Despite widespread support from the government, the availability of health care services for Americans is lacking due to poor coordination between various legislative and administrative departments. The DHHS issued a Task Force Report in July 2002 addressing the following goals:

1) Improve rural communities' access to quality health and human services.
2) Strengthen rural families.
3) Strengthen rural communities and support economic development.
4) Partner with state, local, and tribal governments to support rural communities.

Important influences on the access to quality health care in rural areas include the lack of providers and limited facilities in which to receive care. As of 2001, only 9% of U.S. physicians practice in rural areas where 20% of the nation's population lives. Only one primary care physician is available for every 2,857 individuals in rural America, compared with one physician for every 614 citizens nationally (Sinay, 2001).

Currently, 22 million Americans live in Health Professions Shortage Areas (HPSAs) or Medically Underserved Areas (MUAs). Both MUAs and HPSAs are defined by criteria designating underserved populations. Where state regulations are favorable, bridging of this health care gap is accomplished through mid-level providers, such as Physician Assistants (PAs) (nonnursing personnel), and Advanced Practice Nurses (APNs).

Both physicians and Advanced Practice Nurses (APNs) may have received federal assistance toward their educational preparation expenses in exchange for payback services in rural health upon completion of their respective degrees (Pathman, Konrad, & King, 2002).

Rural hospitals across America are closing at an alarming rate due to multiple factors, chief among them being the disproportional reimbursement for services from federal health care programs such as Medicare. Hospitals experiencing financial difficulty may qualify for assistance through several federal programs that help equalize hospital cost burdens while providing access to care for rural Americans. A rural hospital with a given number of patient encounters may qualify as a Critical Access Hospital. If volume warrants, a rural hospital also may qualify for fixed-cost assistance through a Prospective Payment System. However, guidelines regarding qualifications for federal assistance are very stringent and hospitals may treat too many patients to qualify, but not enough to remain financially solvent without federal assistance. Hospitals that depend solely upon federal reimbursement (i.e., Medicare), soon acquire negative balances and become too deeply in debt to remain viable.

Rural health care across America most often is provided in one of 3,500 existing rural health clinics. A clinic is designated as a rural health clinic if a mid-level practitioner (i.e., a Physician Assistant [PA] or Advanced Practice Nurse [APN]) is available 50% or more of the time the clinic is open, and if the PA or APN provides more than 2,100 office visits annually) (Sinay, 2001). PAs or APNs provide health care services within the scope of practice regulations of each individual state. Nationally, APNs have proved to provide quality, cost-effective health care with high patient satisfaction ratings (Murphy, 2001). Such rural health clinics have increased services and decreased emergency room usage through delivery of quality health care.

With the dearth of physicians in rural America, PAs and APNs have become legally authorized to receive reimbursement for services they have provided to underserved populations. Thus, it is not unusual for a PA or APN to be the only provider in a specified geographic area. The federal guidelines for rural health clinics vary according to the type of clinic, and may be served solely by a PA or APN with medical oversight, or have a physician on site for a specified amount of time. These clinics remain viable as they receive cost-based Medicare and Medicaid reimbursements. In many remote areas, these clinics are the only health care for rural residents, and offer an excellent and challenging practice arena for APNs. An APN is prepared through an accredited Masters of Nursing program and has an authorized scope of practice in patient care by the state of licensure. In addition to a standard Masters in Nursing core curriculum, specialty coursework and a national certification exam qualify these APNs to be competent, caring providers of health services. The skills of an APN are based on the concepts associated with assessment, diagnosis, treatment (including prescriptive authority), health promotion, and anticipatory guidance for patients within their specialty areas. APNs may serve patients as Family Nurse Practitioners, Certified Nurse Midwives, Certified Registered Nurse Anaesthetists, Pediatric Nurse Practitioners, Acute Care Nurse Practitioners, Adult Nurse Practitioners, Psychiatric/Mental Health Nurse Practitioners, Geriatric Nurse Practitioners, and Women's Health Nurse Practitioners. The APN curricula and national certification examinations are regarded as the gold standard for international advanced practice. Information on credentialing internationally may be obtained through the American Nurses Credentialing Center Web site at http:// www.nursingworld.org/ancc/inside/about/aboutCl.html. Canada and the United Kingdom work collaboratively with American nurse educators to advance the concepts of APNs and address access to health care all over the world.

Preparation beyond a Bachelor's degree in Nursing prepares nurses in America to assume additional responsibilities in practice. One such Advanced Practice Nurse authorization in America is certification as a Clinical Nurse Specialist (CNS). Many clinical specialists work outside hospitals in rural areas to provide public health services and manage public health clinics. These services are valued especially in economic downturns (i.e., the first years of the twenty-first century). While public health clinics in America are another way to deliver health care services, the scope of services offered varies widely from state to state due to legislative priorities. Some states offer a full complement of services in multisite facilities serving both rural and urban patients. More often, states have limited state public health departments providing a few specialty services such as immunizations for children or women's reproductive health care. CNSs are prepared to manage such clinics and offer cost-effective services.

Many health care services and policies in America are coordinated through the Department of Health and Human Services (DHHS) (see http://www.hhs.gov/). The DHHS administers some 12 agencies concerned with all populations, including Native Americans. DHHS programs (300+) are concerned with protecting the health of Americans. Within the DHHS, the Office of Rural Health Policy (ORHP) promotes better health care service in rural America, supports rural policy and decision-making, and ensures a rural voice in the consultative process. Established in August 1987 by federal administrators, the ORHP subsequently was approved by the U.S. Congress in December of that year. It now is located within the structure of the Health Resources and Services Administration (HRSA). Congress charged the ORHP with informing and advising the DHHS on matters affecting rural hospitals and health care services, coordinating activities within the department that relate to rural health care, and maintaining a national information clearinghouse.

American health professionals utilize a variety of publications to keep abreast of current and emerging issues and solutions. Two publications that help connect rural health professionals to the national health perspective are *The Nation's Health,* the official newspaper of the American Public Health Association (see http://www.apha.org/thenations-health), and *The Journal of Rural Health* published by the National Rural Health Association (see http://www.NRHArural.org/). Although many rural areas do not have Internet connections, those that do have Internet access are able to enjoy recent updates from the Centers for Disease Control and Prevention (see http://www.cdc.gov/), the Department of Health and Human Services (see http://www.os.dhhs.gov/), and the Office of Rural Health (see http://ruralhealth.hrsa.gov/).

CHALLENGES

In July 2000, the Secretary of Health and Human Services, in collaboration with the DHHS, issued a national plan for health entitled *Healthy People 2010: Understanding and Improving Health.* This plan was the result of a consultation process that included health experts, the public, and the Healthy People Consortium, a public/private alliance of over 350 national organizations and 270 state agencies. Since its inception in 1979, *Healthy People 2010* has served as a national health planning process and established prevention priorities that have been adopted and adapted throughout the country. This is the third time that DHHS developed 10-year health objectives for the nation. Currently, most states and many localities use the *Healthy People 2010* framework to guide local health policies and programs.

Healthy People 2010 contains broad-reaching national health goals for the new decade. It focuses on two major themes: 1) increasing the quality and years of healthy life; and 2) eliminating racial and ethnic disparities in health status. Also unveiled were the first-ever leading health indicators, comprising ten areas of health status, based upon *Healthy People 2010* objectives. These measures give Americans a guide to perceiving and attaining health and will allow for easy assessment of the overall health of the nation, as well as that of specific communities. Individuals will be able to make comparisons between the national goals and plan for health improvements over time. The nation's progress in achieving these health goals over the course of the decade will be monitored through 467 objectives grouped into 28 focus areas. The focus areas are devoted to a comprehensive array of diseases, conditions, and public health challenges.

Many of the *Healthy People 2010* objectives target interventions designed to reduce or eliminate illness, disability, and premature death among individuals and communities. Other objectives target broader issues, such as improving access to quality health care, strengthening public health services, and improving the availability and dissemination of health-related information. Each of the objectives is targeted for specific improvements to be achieved by 2010 (DHHS, 2000). The ten leading health indicators cover physical activity, overweight and obesity, tobacco use, substance abuse, mental health, injury and violence, environmental quality, immunization, responsible sexual behavior, and access to health care. Since rural populations have both limited access to health care and a higher incidence of diseases related to many of the targeted health indicators, individuals, communities, and health care providers could improve overall health by attending to the objectives. Rural health care providers and patients can access information, teaching tools, and plans for behavior change on the *Healthy People 2010* Web site, http://www.healthypeople.gov/BeHealthy/. The leading health indicators are supported by 21 specific measurable objectives that reflect the influence of behavioral and environmental factors and community health interventions. Rural health care providers and the communities they serve can engage in collaborative initiatives to support the *Healthy People 2010* objectives. By monitoring these 21 measures, rural communities will be able to assess their current health status and monitor it over time.

NURSING EDUCATION TO MEET HEALTHCARE CHALLENGES

Meeting the challenges of health care in the present century requires a level of preparation by the American nurse that was not required or envisioned in the past century. As nursing has evolved from the system established by Florence Nightingale in the late 1800s, the preparation of American nurses has diversified and will continue to develop to meet health care demands through the twenty-first century. Programs to prepare nurses have origins in the community, hospital, and academic settings. Nurses may be prepared at a prelicensure level and function in a limited scope as nurse aids and technicians. Nurses may be licensed by state Boards of Nursing to function as Licensed Professional (also Vocational) Nurses, Registered Nurses, and Advanced Practice Nurses. Educational preparation for these levels span a continuum, from hospital Certificate and Associate Degrees from community colleges, to Bachelors, Masters, and Doctoral preparation in accredited colleges and universities. The role and scope of practice also vary from state to state, and within states according to clinical settings. In both urban and rural settings, the need for services may force nurses to push the extremes of the scope of their practice.

Generally, in the last century and across all educational settings, preparation of nurses has lagged behind the needs for services and assisting Americans in accessing health care. Nursing has not been the only profession failing to meet the demands in a new century of health care. A host of professional organizations and governmental agencies has been guiding nursing education for future health care needs. Of the many federal agencies and independent nongovernmental agencies tracking the nation's health status and making related recommendations, the Pew Health Professions Commission is notable. The commission issued a series of reports with the purpose of guiding the education of the nation's health professions workforce. According to the fourth report of the Pew Health Professions Commission (1998), most of the nation's health education institutions are preparing professionals to deal with yesterday's health care system. In an attempt to focus on future needs, four recommendations made by the Pew commission to address America's health care challenges in the upcoming decades are: 1) reconsider the nature of health care work including preparing upcoming professionals with new skills and staffing in new configurations; 2) restructure the regulation of health care professionals, 3) increase the level of health care professionals with alignment of the demands of the system, and 4) realign training and education to meet the changing needs of the care delivery system (Pew, 1998). Five recommendations of the commission followed the identification of delivery system needs. The commission recommended for all health professional groups the following: 1) change professional training to meet the demands of the health care system; 2) ensure the workforce reflects the nation's population diversity; 3) require interdisciplinary competence in all health professionals; 4) continue to move education into ambulatory practice; and 5) encourage public service of all health professional students and graduates. Particular recommendations that affect the educational opportunities of rural populations are recommendations 2 and 5. Recommendation 2 ensures that the workforce reflects the nation's population diversity and targets students from medically underserved areas (MUAs). The commission reports that students from MUAs demonstrate a greater willingness to return to serve these communities and provide culturally sensitive health care that is best understood by a workforce from the MUA. Educating nurses and APNs from MUAs will improve access to health care in these rural areas. Recommendation 5 encourages public service for all health professional students and graduates. This recommendation can only enhance the opportunities for nurses to work in public health service areas that are disappearing from America's rural service area. Among 21 competencies for health professionals listed by the commission are many to improve rural underserved populations. Pertinent recommendations to improve rural health are: 1) rigorously practice preventive health care; 2) improve access to health care for those with unmet health needs; and 3) provide culturally sensitive care to a diverse society. The recommendations of the commission have the potential to address health care issues of both urban and rural populations, and many nursing educational institutions are incorporating the suggestions in the redesign of curricula and practice.

NURSING OPPORTUNITIES

Nursing is in a unique position to adapt education to meet America's health care needs, especially those of rural populations. New roles and adaptations are already meeting the needs of rural vulnerable populations. The role model that has its origins in serving the underserved was historically the community health nurse. These nurses broke from the traditional nursing setting of the hospital to offer care to people in their homes. Called *visiting nurses* in the early part of the twentieth century, these nurses assisted patients and their families holistically, from basic hygiene needs to nutritional support. Social services such as food banks and unemployment assistance were nonexistent at this time, and the visiting nurse adapted her skills to address other needs and assist families in achieving a higher standard of living. The visiting nurse evolved into the community nurse or home health nurse over time, and into a role that delivered primary health care services to many vulnerable populations, especially rural ones. The community health nurse is concerned with the biophysical, psychological, physical, social, and behavioral dimension of patients. The community health nurse assists patients and their families to interact with the health care system to achieve desired health care goals (Clark, 2002). Most professional nursing program curricula contain elements to prepare the graduate for the community-health nursing role in a variety of settings within rural populations. Community-oriented nursing practice encompasses the following nursing interventions (Stanhope & Lancaster, 2000):

1) disease prevention
2) health promotion
3) health protection
4) health maintenance
5) health restoration
6) health surveillance

The education of a professional nurse is especially suited to holistic care in rural underserved areas. The concepts of community health nursing in rural populations can be applied in clinics, provider offices, acute care facilities, and outreach services such as hospice or home health. The prior list of settings is by no means comprehensive, and innovative nurses in rural areas need only identify population needs in order to stimulate a role expansion of the community health nurse. An example of an expanded role in response to community need is the parish nurse. Based on the role and scope of community nursing, parish nursing is a blend of nursing concepts that meet both the health and spiritual needs of a designated population. The support is usually anchored in a religious institution and the community of parishioners tied to that religious institution constitute the practice setting for the nurse. Nurses working in parish settings report a high degree of job satisfaction, since the holistic approach of nursing care is embodied in the fullest sense (Cagle, 2002).

SUMMARY

Rural health care in America encompasses a diverse and complex set of issues in settings as multidimensional as the unique populations within. Each rural community can only respond positively to competent, caring nurses who are sensitive to the transcultural issues inherent in the populations they serve. Nurses in America have the education and training to meet these needs if, in turn, they have the spirit of caring and love for underserved populations. Nurses who embody the principles of their profession have the opportunity to become part of the fabric of the rural community and work together to meet the health care needs of all.

APPLICATION EXERCISE

Choose a special rural population with a health issue of interest to you. An example might be farm equipment accidents in migrant populations or suicide in rural adolescents. Access the Web sites listed in this chapter to find answers to your questions and help you understand the scope of the problem and possible solutions. Write a short report about the nature of the health concern and what you as a nurse might suggest as interventions to help resolve the health care issue. Plan to share your findings with your class.

REFLECTIVE QUESTIONS

- Think about the social disadvantage that is experienced by many rural-dwelling people. How do you think this social disadvantage affects health?
- What special skills do nurses working in rural areas need? When you answer this, consider isolation as an issue.
- What cultural diversity issues present particular challenges to rural nurses?

RECOMMENDED READINGS

Department of Health and Human Services (2000). *Healthy People 2010: Understanding and Improving Health.* Retrieved June 16, 2003, from http://www.health.gov/healthypeople

Department of Health and Human Services (2002). *HHS Rural Task Force Report to the Secretary. Department of Health and Human Services, Health Resources and Services Administration.* Retrieved June 16, 2003, from http://ruralhealth.hrsa.gov/PublicReport.htm

Eberhardt, M. S., Ingram, D. D., Makuc, D. M., et al. (2001). *Urban and Rural Health Chartbook. Health, United States, 2001.* Hyattsville, MD: National Center for Health Statistics.

Ricketts, T. C. (1999). *Rural Health in the United States.* New York: Oxford University Press.

Sinay, T. (2001). Productive efficiency of rural health clinics: The Midwest experience. *The Journal of Rural Health, 17,* 239–249.

REFERENCES

Cagle, K. (2002). Parish nursing: Faith and healing, hand in hand. *Pulse/ The Atlanta Journal-Constitution,* July, 15–16.

Clark, M. J. (2002). *Community health nursing: Caring for populations* (4th ed.). Englewood Cliffs, NJ: Prentice Hall.

Department of Health and Human Services (2000). *Healthy People 2010: Understanding and Improving Health.* Retrieved June 16, 2003, from http://www.health.gov/healthypeople

Department of Health and Human Services (2002). *HHS Rural Task Force Report to the Secretary. Department of Health and Human Services, Health Resources and Services Administration.* Retrieved June 16, 2003, from http://ruralhealth.hrsa.gov/PublicReport.htm

Department of Health and Human Services, Centers for Disease Control and Prevention (2002). *Summary Health Statistics for U.S. Adults: National Health Interview Survey. Vital and Health Statistics.* Series 10, Number 209. SHHS. Hyattsville, MD: National Center for Health Statistics.

Eberhardt, M. S., Ingram, D. D., Makuc, D. M., et al. (2001). *Urban and Rural Health Chartbook. Health, United States, 2001.* Hyattsville, MD: National Center for Health Statistics.

Hartley, D., Bird, D., & Dempsey, P. (1999). Rural mental health and substance abuse. In T. C. Ricketts (Ed.), *Rural health in the United States.* New York: Oxford University Press.

Mueller, C., Schoenman, J., & Dorosh, E. (1999). The Medicare program in rural areas. In T. C. Ricketts (Ed.), *Rural health in the United States.* New York: Oxford University Press.

Murphy, C. E. (2001). Practice identity, collaboration, and optimal access to effective healthcare. *Journal of Pediatric Healthcare, 15,* 98–100.

National Health Interview Survey (1998). Centers for Disease Control and Injury. National Center for Health Statistics. Retrieved December 2003, from: http://www.cdc.gov/nchs/nhis.htm

Pathman, D., Konrad, R., & King, T. (2002) Medical training debt and service commitments: The rural consequences. *Journal of Rural Health, 16,* 264–272.

Pew Health Professions Commission (1998). Recreating health professional practice for a new century. The Fourth Report of the Pew Health Professions Commission. Retrieved November 11, 2004 from http://futurehealth.ucsf.edu/compubs.html.

Ricketts, T. C. (1999). *Rural health in the United States.* New York: Oxford University Press.

Sinay, T. (2001). Productive efficiency of rural health clinics: The Midwest experience. *The Journal of Rural Health, 17,* 239–249.

Stanhope, M., & Lancaster, J. (2000). *Community & public health nursing* (5th ed.). St. Louis: Mosby.

16

Meeting the Health Care Needs of a Diverse Society

Akram Omeri and Margaret M. Andrews

LEARNING OBJECTIVES

Upon completion of this chapter, the student should be able to:

- Discuss the nature of the diversity of U.S. society, including social, economic, and cultural variations
- Analyze racial and ethnic disparities that influence health access and outcomes for the people of the U.S.
- Examine the major components of *Healthy People 2010*, the national prevention agenda that identifies the leading indicators used to measure the health of the nation
- Understand the importance of minimizing inequities in the provision of health care services in the U.S., and in contemporary nursing practice
- Examine and discuss the impact of evidenced-based transcultural nursing knowledge in promotion of health and well-being of people from culturally and linguistically different backgrounds in the U.S.

KEY WORDS

Cultural diversity, multiculturalism, ethnic health policy, transcultural nursing, making a difference

INTRODUCTION

As in many nations, people in the United States who come from various ethnic, cultural, and socioeconomic backgrounds often experience marked *disparities* in health care. The occurrence of many diseases, injuries, and other public health problems is disproportionately higher in some groups, access to the health care delivery system is more restricted, and the overall quality of health care is deemed to be inferior for people from certain racial, ethnic, and cultural populations. These disparities have become the focus of federal, state, and local government studies over the past two decades. The *Healthy People 2010* initiative has been the nation's disease prevention and health promotion agenda for the past two decades. This initiative began in 1979 with a report by the Surgeon General, which established the precedent for setting national health objectives and monitoring their progress over time.

This chapter explores the diversity in U.S. society in an attempt to provide an understanding of the social and cultural milieu, the role of social policy and direction in health initiatives, and the potential impact of research-based, transcultural nursing knowledge in minimizing inequalities in nursing and health care.

IMPACT OF POPULATION TRENDS ON HEALTH CARE IN THE U.S.

Important changes in the U.S. population will shape future efforts to improve health and health care. Two major changes in the demographic characteristics of the U.S. population are the growth in the population of elderly, and the increasing racial and ethnic diversity of the nation. From 1950 to 2000, the proportion of the population that was elderly rose from 8 to 12 percent. By 2050, it is projected that one in five Americans will be 65 years of age or older. The racial and ethnic composition of the country also has changed over time. The Hispanic and Asian/Pacific Islander populations have grown more rapidly than other groups in recent decades. In 2000, more than 12% of the U.S. population identified themselves as Hispanic, and 4% as Asian or Pacific Islander (Department of Health and Human Resources, DHHR, 2000, 2002).

Improvements in health care delivery have contributed to a marked increase in the overall health and longevity of people in the U.S., with average life expectancy increasing from 50 in 1900 to 77 in 2003. Unfortunately, not all racial and ethnic groups have experienced these gains to the same degree. Despite notable progress in the overall health of the U.S. population, there are continuing disparities in the burden of illness and death experienced by African Americans, Hispanics, Native Americans, Alaska Natives, and Asian Pacific Islanders. In general, African Americans have shorter lives than any other group, and American Indians, Alaska Natives, and Hispanics are often disadvantaged when compared with the white population.

African Americans, Asian Americans, and Hispanics are more likely than Whites to experience difficulty communicating with their health care providers, to perceive that they are treated disrespectfully when receiving health care services, and to experience barriers to care, including lack of insurance or a regular physician or nurse practitioner. A substantial proportion of people from diverse racial and ethnic backgrounds indicate that they would receive better care if they were of a different race or ethnicity (Collins et al., 2002).

To understand the changes occurring in U.S. health care, it is necessary to examine the changing demographics of the nation. While the White majority is aging and their numbers are decreasing, the Black, Hispanic, Asian, Native Hawaiian and Other Pacific Islander, and American Indian/Alaska Native populations are young and growing in numbers.

Racial, ethnic, cultural, and socioeconomic backgrounds influence the degree to which each person's health care needs are met. Substantial disparities exist in income and education, especially among Whites, African Americans, and Hispanics. Although most are employed in the workforce, African Americans and Hispanics have lower rates of health insurance coverage than their White counterparts, and they are more likely to have a poorer health status and higher rates of chronic disease. Findings from the Commonwealth Fund indicate that the availability of affordable, comprehensive health insurance is fundamental to ensuring quality health care for individuals from diverse cultures. Policy makers must continue to develop creative and practical options for expanding health coverage and assess them for their potential to reduce the number of uninsured minorities (Collins et al., 2002).

In a study by the Commonwealth Fund (Collins et al., 2002), Hispanics and Asian Americans are the least well served by the U.S. health care system. The study reveals that three factors ensure that minority populations receive optimal health care:

1. effective patient-physician communication
2. overcoming cultural and linguistic barriers
3. access to affordable health insurance

Meeting the health care needs of the diverse U.S. society requires knowledge of the cultural and socioeconomic factors that affect each person's health and that influence the amount, frequency, and quality of health care.

ETHNIC DIVERSITY IN THE U.S. POPULATION

Every decade, the U.S. federal government conducts a national census of the population—the most recent being in 2000. In the U.S. the following panethnic population groups have been federally defined and recognized for census purposes: White, Black, Hispanic, Asian, Native Hawaiian or Other Pacific Islander, and American Indian/Alaska Native. To reflect the nation's growing diversity, the Census 2000 considered race and Hispanic origin to be two separate concepts, and provided citizens with the option of choosing one or more racial identities, or of choosing the category, *Some Other Race.* The following is a brief description of the major population categories:

- *White* refers to a person having origins in Europe, the Middle East, Australia, New Zealand, or North Africa. Those who self-identify as White include people of German, Italian, Irish, Polish, Australian, or Arab heritage. This group comprises 75.1% of the total population and has a median age of 37.7 years (U.S. Census Bureau, 2000).
- *Black* or *African American* refers to persons having origins in any of the original black racial groups of Africa, some of whom migrated in more recent years from the Caribbean or South America. The Black or African American population comprises 12.3% of the total population, and the median age is 30.2 years (U.S. Census Bureau, 2000).
- *Hispanic* or *Latino* refers to people whose heritage is from Spanish-speaking countries such as Spain and Central or South American nations. People who identify their origin as Hispanic or Latino can be of any race. This group comprises 12.5% of the total population, and has a median age of 25.8 years (U.S. Census Bureau, 2000).
- *Asian* refers to people having origins in any of the original peoples of the Far East, Southeast Asia, or the Indian subcontinent (e.g., China, India, Japan, Korea, or the Philippines). *Native Hawaiian*

or *Other Pacific Islander* refers to people who have their origins in Hawaii, Guam, Samoa, or other Pacific Islands. These two groups comprise 4.4 % of the total population, and have a median age of 32.7 years.

- *American Indian/Alaska Native* refers to people having origins in any of the original peoples of North America, and who maintain cultural identification through tribal affiliation or community recognition. Included in this category are those from the 550 federally recognized nations, or those who self-identify as members of Native American nations. These groups comprise 0.9% of the total population, and have a median age of 28 years.

- *Some Other Race* was added to the 2000 census because millions of people failed to respond to the other categories in previous censuses. In 2000, approximately 2% of the U.S. population identified as being of "two or more races."

CRITIQUE OF THE PANETHNIC POPULATION CLASSIFICATION SYSTEM

Historically, the federal panethnic population classification was formulated so that demographic data about traditionally under-represented populations could be gathered in a systematic manner. Among the rationales for establishing the panethnic population classification was that group-specific statistical information could be systematically gathered and used to help government officials make equitable decisions about public policies and allocation of resources for specific groups of people. The use of panethnic population groups has gained widespread acceptance and has been embraced by many people as a convenient way to refer to the hundreds of cultures and subcultures in the U.S.

The creation of the panethnic groups has had a tremendous influence on the way in which people think about ethnic groups, and has affected the health care services people from diverse backgrounds receive. In addition to establishing specific ethnic minority groups, the unique characteristics of each group's culture and subculture have become hopelessly enmeshed with others in the same category.

One disadvantage to the use of panethnic groups is that each group is treated homogeneously and consideration is seldom given to the myriad health-related beliefs and practices that exist within each group. For example, there are hundreds of cultures and subcultures subsumed under the broad category known as Whites. Those of Italian, Irish, Australian, Polish, or German ancestry are categorized in the same group despite vast differences. Similarly, there may be no recognition given to the differences among the dozens of cultures representing those who identify themselves as Hispanic *or* Latino, a group that includes Spanish-speaking individuals from Spain, Central America and South America.

Second, in some instances, people placed in a particular category might not agree that this is where they belong or might object to the nomenclature given. For example, some people who trace their ancestry to Africa prefer to be called Black, whereas others call themselves African American. Using an incorrect label to describe people in certain categories might foster a sense of marginalization and being unwelcome in the company of other groups.

Lastly, there are numerous other nonethnic cultures and subcultures that nurses interact with besides those included in the federal panethnic categories, for example, the gay/lesbian/transgender culture, the deaf culture, the cultures of professions such as nursing or medicine, and other nonethnic cultures.

POLICY INITIATIVES TO IMPROVE HEALTH: *HEALTHY PEOPLE 2010*

Since the original report, *Healthy People 2000* (U.S. Department of Health & Human Services, 1993) was released *Healthy People 2010* (U.S. Department of Health and Human Services, 2001) also has been released. Both of these reports address specific health conditions disproportionately affecting racial and ethnic communities. *Healthy People 2010* is the third generation of this health initiative. It is intended to address the health problems of the nation as it enters the twenty-first century using the knowledge and skills of national, state, and local government agencies, individual and group participants in communities, members of health care delivery systems, voluntary groups, and public and private sector organizations and agencies. The focus of the initiative is to close the gaps in health outcomes, particularly racial and ethnic disparities as they relate to diabetes, AIDS, heart disease, infant mortality, cancer screening and management, and immunizations. Other groups being targeted include women, youth, the elderly, people of low income and education, and people with disabilities.

Healthy People 2010 has two major goals:

1) Increase quality and years of healthy life
2) Eliminate health disparities among different segments of the population

Healthy People 2010 aims to promote healthy behaviors, promote healthy and safe communities, improve systems for personal and public health, and prevent or reduce diseases and disorders. The initiative provides a tool for monitoring and tracking health status, health risks, and the use of health services.

Derived from *Healthy People 2010* objectives, the *Leading Health Indicators* reflect the major public health concerns in the U.S. and were chosen based on their ability to motivate action, the availability of data to measure their progress, and their relevance as broad public health issues. These indicators are physical activity, overweight and obesity, tobacco use, substance use, responsible sexual behavior, mental health, injury and violence, environmental quality, immunization, and access to health care.

The U.S. Department of Health and Human Services also seeks to promote more diversity in the health care professions, including nursing. The diversity in nursing is monitored by the federal Division of Nursing, which is housed within the Bureau of Health Professions, Health Resources and Services Administration, U.S. Department of Health and Human Services. According to the latest *National Sample Survey of Registered Nurses* (2000), only 12.3% of registered nurses in the U.S. represent racial or ethnic minority groups and only 5.4% are men. There is widespread recognition that a culturally diverse nursing workforce is essential to meeting the health care needs of the nation's population. Although nursing schools enroll more diverse students than medical colleges (10.5%) or dental colleges (11%), the overwhelming majority of students in baccalaureate nursing programs are females (91%) from nonminority backgrounds (73.5%) (American Association of Colleges of Nursing, 2001).

In addition to the federal initiatives, programs and research on health disparities and diversity in the nursing profession have been conducted by several of the most prestigious private foundations and agencies in the United States (e.g., Henry J. Kaiser Family Foundation, Commonwealth Fund, Pew Charitable Trust, Robert Wood Johnson Foundation, Kellogg Foundation, and others).

INFLUENCE OF INCOME ON HEALTH

The relationship between health and socioeconomic status is significant in that there is a correlation between income and access to health care delivery systems and to the quality of health care (Agency for Health Research and Quality, 2002).There is also a higher probability that people will be exposed to environmental health hazards when they reside in low-income housing and neighborhoods, which in turn tend to have higher levels of pollution and exposure to toxic substances than middle and upper income neighborhoods (U.S. Department of Health & Human Services, 2003).

The concept of *poverty* is subject to multiple definitions and interpretations.

National poverty data are calculated using the official U.S. Census Bureau definition of poverty, which has remained standard since it was introduced in the mid-1960s and is useful for measuring progress against poverty. Under this definition, *poverty* is determined by comparing pre-tax cash income with the *poverty threshold*, which adjusts for family size and composition (U.S. Bureau of the Census, 2002). In 2003, the poverty threshold for a family of four living in one of the 48 contiguous states or Washington, D.C. was $18,400 (compared with $23,000 for Alaska and $21,169 for Hawaii). The *poverty guidelines* are another version of the federal poverty measure. They are issued each year in the *Federal Register* by the Department of Health and Human Services. The guidelines are a simplification of the poverty thresholds for administrative purposes, for example, determining financial eligibility for federal programs such as Head Start, National School Lunch, Low-Income Energy, Medicaid, Aid to Families with Dependent Children, and so forth (U.S. Department of Health & Human Services, 2003).

Nearly 33 million people (11.7% of the U.S. population) live in poverty. The percentage of people living in poverty according to ethnicity is as follows: non-Hispanic Whites, 7.8%; Blacks, 22.7%; Asian/ Pacific Islanders, 10.2%; Hispanics, 21.4%; and American Indian/Alaska Native, 25.9%. Of all family groups, poverty is highest among those headed by single women, especially if they are Black or Hispanic, in which case the poverty rates exceed 35%. Twenty-six percent of all female-headed families are poor, compared with 4.9% of families in which males are present. Children under six years of age are particularly vulnerable to poverty. An appalling 18.2% of all U.S. children under age six are poor. If these children live in families with a single female as head of household (and no spouse present), the poverty rate skyrockets to 48.9% (U.S. Bureau of the Census, 2002).

Poverty levels also differ depending on where people live. The metropolitan poverty rate is 16.5% which is twice the rate found in suburbs (8.2%). For rural areas—the countryside and small towns—the poverty rate is 14.2%. The poverty rate also varies by region and within regions. The greatest poverty in the United States is found in the South (13.5%), whereas the lowest poverty is found in the Midwest (9.4%) (U.S. Bureau of the Census, 2002).

Less income means less nutritious food; less heat in winter and fresh air in summer; more crowded living conditions and, thus, more likelihood of contracting communicable diseases; less knowledge about illness or health; fewer visits to primary care providers such as physicians or nurse practitioners; fewer dental visits; less preventive care; and lower quality of health care. In addition, people from lower socioeconomic groups tend to live and work in more polluted, hazardous, and strenuous environments (Agency for Health Research and Quality, 2002).

States with the highest levels of income inequality also have the highest morbidity and mortality rates. The reason why poverty matters is because health care costs often prevent the poor from having access to the highest technology and best health care providers. In the words of former Surgeon General C. Everett Koop, "When I look back on my years in office, the things I banged my head against were all poverty" (Coontz, 1992, p. 270).

Health insurance is the means by which individuals and families seek to ensure that health care costs can be met. However, health insurance is not accessible to all, as will be made evident in the following discussion of health insurance in the U.S.

HEALTH INSURANCE IN THE U.S.

Most U.S. citizens are covered by some type of health insurance, and many people are covered by more than one provider. Some segments of the population, however, are particularly likely to lack health insurance, for example, minorities. The degree to which some members of society are not covered by health insurance is an important measure of the country's overall well-being.

Medicare is a federal health insurance program that covers 41 million elderly and disabled Americans under the age of 65. Currently, minorities account for nearly 20% of Medicare beneficiaries. In 2030, racial and ethnic minorities are projected to account for 26% of Medicare beneficiaries 65 years of age or older. This trend has particular implications for the Medicare program, as racial and ethnic minority beneficiaries tend to have poorer health than White beneficiaries. While 43% of African American beneficiaries and 42% of Latino beneficiaries assess their own health as fair or poor, only 25% of White beneficiaries do so (CMS, 2000).

Among the low-income population (with incomes below 200% of the federal poverty level), the federal *Medicaid* program rivals employer-based insurance as the source of coverage. For example, more than one-third of low-income African Americans (41%) and American Indian/Alaska Natives (43%) have Medicaid coverage (CMS, 2000). Medicaid eligibility is limited to individuals who fall into specified categories. The federal statute identifies over 25 different eligibility categories for which federal funds are available. These categories can be classified into five broad coverage groups:

- Children
- Pregnant women
- Adults in families with dependent children
- Individuals with disabilities
- Individuals 65 or over

Medicaid is a state-administered program and each state sets its own guidelines regarding eligibility and services.

Employment-based private health insurance plans cover 64% of the people in the U.S. Twenty-four percent are covered by a government health plan, including Medicare (13%), Medicaid (10%), and military health insurance (3%). Given that many people are covered by more than one plan, the total exceeds 100% (Kaiser Commission on Medicaid and the Uninsured, 2003).

Fourteen percent of the U.S. population (39 million people) lack health insurance coverage. Ten percent of Whites, 19% of Blacks, 32% of Hispanics, 18% of Asian/Pacific Islanders, and 12% of American Indian/Alaska Natives have no health insurance coverage. With 27% uninsured, young adults (age 18 to 24) were more likely than any other age group to lack health insurance coverage. Because of Medicare, the elderly are at the other extreme, with only about 1% lacking coverage. Children age 12-17 are slightly more likely than younger children to lack health insurance, 12% compared with 11%. Among poor children, 22% have no health insurance coverage. Of the 11 million uninsured children, one out of six Black children and one out of four Hispanic children are uninsured, compared with 1 out of 11 White children (U.S. Census Bureau, 2003). Uninsured population in the U.S. was reported as 44 million in a News Release statement by the U.S. House of Representatives (2003).

The cost of health insurance for a typical group family insurance policy costs $7,954 (single is $3,060). This represents 15% of the median family income ($52,000). Only about 35% of families today earn a sufficient income to prevent more than 10% of their gross income from going toward the purchase of health insurance for the family (Nichols, 2003). For the many who are self-insured, the cost of insurance, and the percentage of income, is much higher. An explanation for the paradox of high tax and expenditure on health without improvements in the nation's overall health is presented in the next section.

HEALTHCARE EXPENDITURES

In 2000, national health care expenditures in the United States totaled $1.3 trillion, and health expenditures as a percentage of the gross domestic product (GDP) was 13%. The United States continues to spend more on health care than any other industrialized nation in the world. While U.S. health care utilizes some of the world's most highly advanced equipment and procedures, Americans pay for this through high taxes and insurance premiums.

Despite the large health care expenditures, the U.S. *does not have the best health care system in the world.* Rather, it has one of the best emergency care systems. By and large, advanced U.S. health care technology has not translated into better health statistics for its citizens. For example, the U.S. ranks near the bottom in international comparisons related to various health indicators such as life expectancy, infant mortality, and related categories.

The lack of emphasis on primary prevention has adversely affected the overall health and well-being of Americans. In Europe during the last century, for example, life expectancy nearly doubled after nations purified their drinking water and created sanitation systems. In the U.S. during this century, by contrast, the highest breast cancer rates are found in neighborhoods around the chemical industry. Some of the disparities in the health status of differing ethnic groups are discussed in the next section.

DISPARITIES IN HEALTHCARE

Disparities in health care have been well documented in recent decades across a broad range of health conditions and for a wide range of populations. Disparities have been identified for racial and ethnic minorities, women, children, elderly, low-income populations, people with special needs (such as chronic illness, disabilities, and end-of-life issues), and those living in rural areas or in the inner city.

Health inequalities inflict various injustices upon ethnic minorities in the United States of America (Jarrett, 2000a). The impact of policies on macro social systems contain and suppress ethnic minorities and propagate inequalities in the social, physical, mental, economic, legal, political, religious, cultural, and educational systems. Jarrett (2000b) discussed the finding that the impact of such policies promotes inequality in ethnic minorities in the U.S.

Aguilar highlights the unresponsiveness of the health care system towards ethnic minorities (cited in Jarrett, 2000). She describes the health system as plagued with multiple deficiencies in service delivery, resulting in a lack of access to appropriate health care services. She notes inequalities in the distribution of funds to support the appropriate design and implementation of health services for specific groups. Aguilar highlights lack of cultural education and information about different cultural groups as a major contributor to inequalities, inefficiencies, and inaccessibility of health services.

The outcomes related to the deficiencies in the health care system are evident in the following examples, which illustrate the unequal incidence of disease and of access to health services for ethnic minority groups:

- Cancer mortality rates are 35% higher in Blacks than Whites, though much can be done to eliminate this disparity by administering population- and community-based prevention programs and improving the effective delivery of both preventive and treatment services.
- Cervical cancer is five times higher in Vietnamese women in the United States than in White women.
- African American diabetics are seven times more likely to have amputations and develop kidney failure than White diabetics.
- 15% of African Americans, 13% of Hispanics, and 11% of Asian Americans feel that they would have received better care if they were of a different race or ethnicity.

- Hispanic children are nearly three times as likely as White children to have no usual source of health care.
- African Americans are 13% less likely to undergo coronary angioplasty and one-third less likely to undergo coronary bypass surgery than their White counterparts.

ETHNIC HEALTH POLICY IN THE U.S.: ROOTS AND DIRECTIONS

Approaches to the Provision of Culturally Competent Nursing and Health Care

Implications of providing culturally meaningful health care are numerous. It is evidenced from research that when care is culturally congruent with the values and beliefs of people, health and healing will improve in quality and cost-effective ways. Evidenced-based transcultural nursing knowledge discoveries will enable nurses to:

- Provide quality and culturally congruent and competent care that meets the cultural care needs of the diverse populations in the U.S.
- Promote transcultural nursing and cross-cultural education as core areas of study in the health care professions, in an attempt to inform health practices with research-based transcultural knowledge and to address discrimination, alienation, marginalization, stereotyping, and racism
- Encourage commitment to "health for all," that is, a belief that good health is a right for all, rather than a privilege. This requires improvement in access and care to diverse populations in the U.S.

Application of Leininger's three modes of actions and decisions as portrayed in the Sun-rise Enabler (Leininger & McFarland, 2002), based on the theory of Culture Care Diversity and Universality, could prove beneficial. These action modes are described briefly below as a guide to the provision of culture specific nursing care to diverse populations.

Cultural Care Preservation/Maintenance

Evidenced-based transcultural knowledge will inform practitioners as to what culture care modes could be/need to be maintained and preserved without clashing with treatment modalities that need to be applied for example, for Afghan refugees in New South Wales, Australia, understanding of Islam and its code of practice is extremely important. Their religiosity and their practices need to be understood and preserved by nurses and other health service providers to promote culturally meaningful care and respect for their beliefs, in order to achieve the best health care outcomes for this group of people (Omeri, Lennings, & Raymond, 2003).

Cultural Care Accommodation/Negotiation

Accommodating culture in healthcare in culturally meaningful ways is the provision of health related information in the language of specific cultural groups. Knowledge of cultural and religious festivities relating to significant life events such as birth or death is also important transcultural knowledge that needs to be known and understood by nurses and other health care professions and accommodated when appropriate.

Cultural Care Repatterning/Restructuring

Repatterning a cultural lifeway is a process of change, which involves giving up the old, and perhaps culturally meaningful ways, and adopting new and different care patterns. This process of change is often a three-way process involving the clients as receivers of care, and the nurse or other health care professionals as providers of care along with as the health care system. In some aspects, this change is very slow and at times may not be possible. It involves a great deal of negotiation and involvement of the clients.

Madeleine Leininger wrote that "Transcultural nursing is a growing and highly relevant area of study and practice today that has great relevance for nurses living and functioning in a multicultural world" (Leininger, 1995; Leininger & McFarland, 2002). This area of study and practice often requires different ways of knowing and helping people of diverse cultural backgrounds. Transcultural nursing allows nurses to think about what may be different or similar among people with regard to their special care needs and concerns. As nurses discover the client's particular cultural beliefs and values, through research, they learn ways to provide culturally sensitive, compassionate, and competent care that is satisfying and meaningful to the client and congruent with their lifeway practices (Leininger & McFarland, 2002). This process of discovery of cultural knowledge, in addition to enabling nurses to develop deep understanding and appreciation for cultures, will allow nurses to develop insights about their own cultural background (self awareness) and how to use such knowledge appropriately with clients, families, communities, and health care services.

In 1991 Leininger explicated her *Theory of Culture Care Diversity and Universality* with two major constructs of culture and care: describing, explaining, and predicting nursing similarities and differences focused primarily on human care and caring in human cultures. Leininger used world view, social structure, language, ethnohistory, environmental context, and the generic (folk) and professional systems to provide a comprehensive and holistic view of influences in culture care and wellbeing. The three modes of nursing decisions and actions—culture care preservation and/or maintenance, culture care accommodation and/or negotiation, and culture care repatterning and/or restructuring—are ways to provide *culturally congruent* or *culturally competent* nursing care (Leininger, 1991, 1995; Leininger & McFarland, 2002).

Transcultural nursing concepts address an essential domain of knowledge to guide transcultural nursing practice. *Cultural imposition* is one transcultural nursing concept that often leads to cultural clash, dissatisfaction, intolerance, anger, prejudice, discrimination, noncompliance, and a host of other behaviors. Cultural imposition practices, which often stem from cultural ignorance, cultural blindness, ethnocentrism, and biases, remain a major and unrecognized problem in nursing. Cultural imposition is defined as "the tendency of an individual or group to impose their beliefs, values, and patterns of behaviour upon another culture for varied reasons" (Leininger 1990, 1991, 1995; Leininger & McFarland, 2002). Leininger and others state that cultural imposition practices between nurses and clients can be observed in situations in which the nurse believes her/his views are the right, best, and most therapeutic professional ways, and that the client's views are strange, bizarre, and not desirable for their health.

Health and illness are largely culturally defined, constructed, and maintained, and therefore local health systems tend to fit their values and practices (Kleinman, 1980; Haviland, 1993; Helman, 1994). Additionally, Western scientific theories based on high technologies may be of limited benefit to some cultures because of cultural differences. The phenomenon of cultural imposition can be described as harking back to the colonial historical past, when dominant cultures took over less dominant cultures in an oppressive way. Western health service practitioners, including nurses and other health practitioners, with their new technological knowledge, may not realize that indigenous health care values and norms are culturally determined and often do not change readily (Leininger & McFarland, 2002).

Underpinning transcultural nursing are values of equity, justice, fairness, understanding, and tolerance for differences. Leininger's theory has been used to identify underserved ethnic populations within a community, which is described as the first step in eliminating inequalities in health care among racial and ethnic minorities and providing culturally congruent health care (Zust & Moline, 2003). Transcultural nursing concepts provide ways to identify ethnocentric practices that come about through cultural blindness. Culturally sensitive and aware transcultural nurses, as primary health and nursing care providers, can advocate on behalf of clients, families, and communities for health care that is equitable because it is culturally congruent, culturally competent, and accessible.

MODELS OF CULTURALLY COMPETENT NURSING CARE

Cultural competence, according to Campinha-Bacote (2002), "is a process, not an event" that consists of five integrated constructs: cultural awareness, cultural knowledge, cultural skills, cultural encounters, and cultural desire. She defines it as an "ongoing process in which the healthcare provider continuously strives to achieve the ability to effectively work within the cultural context of the client" (individual, family, community) (p. 181). Her model assumes that "there is a direct relationship between the level of competence of health care provider and their ability to provide culturally responsive healthcare service" (p. 181). Another model focuses on a combination of cultural assessment skills and the nurse's critical thinking skills to provide the necessary knowledge on which to base culturally competent and contextually meaningful care for clients—individuals, families, groups, communities, and institutions (Andrews & Boyle, 2003).

In an attempt to foster excellence in transcultural nursing practice, Leuning, Swiggum, Barmore Wiegert, and McCollough-Zander (2002) proposed a set of standards for transcultural nursing. The standards, based on Leininger's culture care theory and Campinha-Bacote's model of cultural competence, are intended to provide criteria for the evaluation of nursing care, a tool for teaching and learning, as well as increasing public confidence in the nursing profession.

In order for faculties of nursing to be able to guide student nurses to develop competence in caring for the growing multicultural populations, there is an urgent need for faculties to have the opportunity and the choice to undertake core studies in transcultural nursing. Faculties of nursing have an ethical and moral responsibility to inform their teaching and research with essential transcultural nursing knowledge. This knowledge is essential to guide students toward safe, responsive, meaningful, and culturally competent care, congruent with the lifeway practices of the culturally diverse groups in U.S. and elsewhere in the world.

STRATEGIES FOR ELIMINATING HEALTH DISPARITIES

The United States government has implemented several programs aimed at eliminating health disparities and promoting health for all citizens. The following section is a summary of the major programs:

- *Healthy People 2010* is a set of health objectives put forth by the U.S. Department of Health and Human Services for the purpose of improving the health of the nation. *Healthy People 2010* is intended to be used by many different people, states, communities, and professional organizations, including groups such as the American Nurses Association, the Transcultural Nursing Society, and related groups, to help in the development of programs to improve health.
- *Healthy People 2010* builds on initiatives pursued over the past two decades. The 1979 *Surgeon General's Report, Healthy People, and Healthy People 2000: National Health Promotion and Disease Prevention Objectives* established national health objectives and served as the basis for the development of state and community plans. Like its predecessors, *Healthy People 2010* was developed through a broad consultation process, built on prevailing scientific knowledge, and designed to measure programs over time (U.S. Department of Health & Human Services, 2002).
- According to the Agency for Health Research and Quality (2002), the goal of eliminating health disparities will be met through commitment to:

- Understanding why disparities in health care exist by continuing to incorporate research on disparities in health care into other research efforts
- Uncovering the root causes for the differences
- Identifying and implementing effective strategies to eliminate disparities
- Continuing to gather data related to disparities
- Working more closely with communities to assure that research is relevant to the populations in them and implemented quickly
- Evaluating the importance of cultural competence to health care disparities
- Building capacity for health services research among minority institutions and minority investigators

- The National Center for Cultural Competence seeks to address disparities in health care through:

  - Training, technical assistance and consultation
  - Networking, linkages and information exchange
  - Knowledge and product development and dissemination

Major emphasis is placed on policy development, assistance in conducting organizational cultural competence self-assessments, and strategic approaches to the systematic incorporation of culturally competent values, policy, structures, and practices within organizations (National Center for Cultural Competence, 2003).

The way is open for nurses to contribute to achieving these practical and policy objectives through the application of research-based transcultural knowledge.

CONCLUSION

Meeting the health care needs of diverse populations in the U.S. is one of the greatest challenges faced by nurses and health care professionals. This chapter provides an overview of population trends relating to cultural diversity and the ways it affects the roles of nurses and health care professionals. It highlights a critique of panethnic classifications, the disadvantages experienced by ethnic populations, and the influence of such classifications on the attitudes and behavior of Americans toward ethnic groups. The chapter also highlights policy initiatives, health insurance, and disparities in health care. Culturally competent nursing and health care, including several current models of practice, are presented. The chapter also highlights the importance of transcultural nursing knowledge and its application to practice in an attempt to improve the health and well-being of the diverse populations in the U.S.

ACKNOWLEDGMENT

Special acknowledgment to Helen Hamilton, consulting editor and coeditor of the publication: Clare, J., & Hamilton, H. (Eds.). (2002). *Writing research: Transforming data into text.* Edinburgh: Churchill Livingstone.

REFLECTIVE QUESTIONS

1. How does transcultural nursing knowledge contribute to the reduction of health disparities?
2. What other transcultural nursing knowledge would be helpful to understand and reduce health disparities?
3. How does evidenced-based-transcultural nursing knowledge foster promotion of health and well-being of the diverse U.S. populations?

RECOMMENDED READINGS

Andrews, M. M., & Boyle, J. S. (2003). *Transcultural concepts in nursing care* (4th ed.). Philadelphia: Lippincott.
Omeri, A., Malcolm, P., Ahern, M., & Wellington, B. (2003). Meeting the challenges of cultural diversity in the academic settings. *Nurse Education in Practice, 3,* 5–22.

REFERENCES

Agency for Healthcare Research and Quality (2002). *AHRQ focus on research: Disparities in healthcare.* AHRQ Publication No. 02-M027, March 2002. Rockville, MD: Author. http://www.ahrq.gov/news/focus/disparhc.htm.

Aguilar, M. A. (2000). Health. In A. A. Jarrett (Ed.), *The impact of macro social systems on ethnic minorities in the United States.* London: Praeger.

American Association of Colleges of Nursing (2001). *Effective strategies for increasing diversity in nursing programs.* Washington, DC: Author.

Anderson, L. M., Scrimshaw, S. C., Fullilove, M. T., Fielding, J. E., & Normand, J. (2003). Culturally competent healthcare systems: A systematic review. *American Journal of Preventative Medicine, 24*(3S), 68–79.

Andrews, M. M., & Boyle, J. S. (2003). *Transcultural concepts in nursing care* (4th ed.). Philadelphia: Lippincott.

Campinha-Bacote, J. (2002). The process of cultural competence in the delivery of healthcare services: A model of care. *Journal of Transcultural Nursing, 13*(3), 181.

CMS (2000). Medicare Current Beneficiary Survey. U.S. Census Bureau, Current Population Statistics, 2000.

Collins, K. S., Hughes, D. L., Doty, M. M., Ives, B. L., Edwards, J. N., & Tenney, K. (2002). Diverse communities, common concerns: Assessing healthcare quality for minority Americans. The Commonwealth Fund 2001 Healthcare Quality Survey. Retrieved July 10, 2003 from http://www.cmwf.org

Coontz, S. (1992). *The way we never were: American families and the nostalgia trap.* New York: HarperCollins.

Haviland, W. (1993). *Cultural anthropology* (7th ed.). Orlando: Harcourt Brace Jovanovich College Publishers.

Helman, C. (1994). *Culture, health & illness* (3rd ed.). Oxford, UK: Butterworth Heinemann.

Jarrett, A. A. (2000a). Introduction. In A. A. Jarrett (Ed.), *The impact of macro social systems on ethnic minorities in the United States.* London: Praeger.

Jarrett, A. A. (Ed.) (2000b). *The impact of macro social systems on ethnic minorities in the United States.* London: Praeger.

Kaiser Commission on Medicaid and the Uninsured (2003). Health insurance coverage in America: 2001. Data update, 2003.

Kleinman, A. (1980). *Patients and healers in the context of culture.* Berkeley: University of California Press.

Leininger, M. M. (1990). The significance of cultural concepts in nursing. *Journal of Transcultural Nursing, 2*(1), 52–59.

Leininger, M. M. (1991). *Culture care diversity and universality: A theory of nursing.* New York: National League for Nursing Press.

Leininger, M. M. (1995). *Transcultural nursing: Concepts, theories, research, and practices.* New York: McGraw-Hill.

Leininger, M. M., & McFarland, M. R. (2002). *Transcultural nursing: Concepts, theories, research, and practices.* New York: McGraw-Hill.

Leuning, C., Swiggum, P. D., Barmore Wiegert, H. M., & McCullough-Zander, K. (2002). Proposed standards for transcultural nursing. *Journal of Transcultural Nursing, 13*(2), 40–53.

Mays, R. M., De Leon Siantz, M. L., & Wehweg, S. A. (2002). Assessing cultural competence of policy organisations. *Journal of Transcultural Nursing, 13*(2), 129–144.

National Center for Cultural Competence (2003). *Addressing disparities in healthcare delivery.* Retrieved July 17, 2003 from www.Georgetown.edu/research/ gucdc/nccc

News Release, U.S. House of Representatives (2003). Bush administration ignores 44 million uninsured in U.S. as it awards contracts for universal health care in Iraq. Retrieved November 12, 2004 from http://www.house.gov/commerce_democrats/press/108nr17.htm (personal communication with Dr. M. Andrews, co-author).

Nichols, L. M. (2003). Increasing stress on the U.S. healthcare system: Structural crisis or temporary? Special Committee on Ageing. U.S. Senate. Hearing to Examine the State of the Nation's Healthcare System, March 10, 2003.

Omeri, A. (2003). Assuring culturally competent nursing care: Whose responsibility? *Nursing Review,* September, 7.

Omeri, A., Lennings, C., & Raymond, L. (2003). *Report of a research study investigating access to and appropriateness of healthcare services for the Afghan refugee community in NSW, Australia.* Department of Family & Community Health, Faculty of Nursing, Sydney University. Sydney, Australia.

Omeri, A., Malcolm, P., Ahern, M., & Wellington, B. (2003). Meeting the challenges of cultural diversity in the academic settings. *Nurse Education in Practice, 3,* 5–22.

U.S. Bureau of the Census (2000). *2000 census of population and housing.* Washington, DC: U.S. Government Printing Office.

U.S. Bureau of the Census (2001). *Population profile of the United States: 2000.* Available at http://www.census.gov

U.S. Bureau of the Census (2002). *Poverty in the United States: 2001,* Series P-60, No. 219. Washington, DC: U.S. Government Printing Office.

U.S. Bureau of the Census (2003). Health Insurance Coverage: Highlights: 2003. Retrieved November 12, 2004 from http://www.census.gov/hhes/hlthins/hlthin03/hlth03asc.html.

U.S. Department of Health & Human Services (1993). *Healthy people 2000: National health promotion and disease prevention objectives.* (DHHS Publication No. PHS 91-50212) Washington, DC: U.S. Government Printing Office.

U.S. Department of Health & Human Services (2001). *Healthy people 2010: Understanding and improving health.* (Superintendent of Documents

Stock No. 017-0550-9). Washington, DC: U.S. Government Printing Office.

U.S. Department of Health & Human Services (2002). *Projected supply, demand and shortages of registered nurses: 2000–2002.* Retrieved from http://bhpr.hrsa.gove/healthworkforce/reports/rnproject.report.htm

U.S. Department of Health & Human Services (2003). *National healthcare quality report.* Rockville, MD: Agency for Healthcare Research and Quality.

Wenger, A. F. (1999). Cultural openness: Intrinsic to human care. *Journal of Transcultural Nursing, 10*(1), 10.

Zust, B. L., & Moline, K. (2003). Identifying underserved ethnic populations community: The first step in eliminating health disparities among racial and ethnic minorities. *Journal of Transcultural Nursing, 14*(1), 66–74.

17

Critical Thinking in Nursing: Beyond Clinical Judgment to Perspective, Context, and Meaning

William K. Cody

LEARNING OBJECTIVES

At the completion of this chapter, the student will be able to:

- Describe the relevance of critical thinking to nursing
- Describe the main characteristics of critical thinking
- Apply basic concepts of critical thinking to various areas of nursing practice
- Identify resources for further reading and study of critical thinking

KEY WORDS

Conclusion, context, evidence, logical analysis, meaning, nursing frameworks, perspective, premise, reason, reflection, relevance, soundness

INTRODUCTION

Critical thinking has been much written about and talked about within the discipline of nursing over the past decade (see Alfaro-LeFevre, 2004;

Gray, 2003; Hicks, 2003; LeMone & Burke, 2004; Seymour, 2003). In the United States, accrediting agencies mandate nursing education programs to include in their curricula content and processes to prepare nurses to exercise critical thinking in practice. At times the treatment of critical thinking in the literature may seem to imply that critical thinking is merely a circumscribed set of skills, no more challenging or broad-ranging in its complexities than, for example, physical assessment or medication administration. However, the American Association of Colleges of Nursing (AACN, 1998) states that the faculty of critical thinking includes "*questioning, analysis, synthesis, interpretation, inference, inductive and deductive reasoning, intuition, application, and creativity*" (p. 9, emphasis added). The same cannot be said for *any* single, circumscribed content area in nursing. Rather, critical thinking refers to a broad intellectual approach to the whole of nursing science and nursing practice.

WHY CRITICAL THINKING?

More than a mere skill set, critical thinking can be considered *the application of reason and reflection to* any *situation or discourse,* and the capacity to *identify evidence for one's beliefs, evaluate its significance* and *change one's thinking* accordingly. This broad range of thought processes encompasses virtually all of professional nursing practice and has relevance to all aspects of life, health, and health care. Since critical thinking infiltrates all aspects of nursing practice, one may wonder why it is necessary to consider it separately. Is critical thinking not subsumed within the learning processes engaged in the traditional areas studied in nursing curricula, such as interpersonal relations, pathophysiology, psychology, pharmacology, management, teaching-learning, and bioethics? The answer is both *yes* and *no.* Although it is true that critical thinking processes are necessary and expected in most aspects of professional practice, it is highly advisable also to consider the process of thinking critically separately, so as to identify and better understand the rational and intuitive grounding of one's reflections, understandings, and beliefs, and to be more aware of the processes involved in one's decision making.

The fact that the process of thinking critically has been so often emphasized and examined in nursing bears witness to the importance of sustained and careful attention to the nature of the *knowledge base* we use in the day-to-day and hour-to-hour practice of nursing. Indeed, it is incumbent upon every professional nurse to reflect upon the knowledge used for understanding people and making decisions, the philosophical and theoretical frameworks that guide us to questions, the questions to which they then guide us, what counts as knowledge or evidence for decision-making, and why we come to believe that we know what we know. Professionalism mandates continuous education beyond entry level to maintain currency. By exercising one's capacity for critical thinking in the study and practice of nursing, the nurse can come to a deeper understanding of the human condition, better identify the crucial questions arising in nursing practice situations, and better identify justifications for action or inaction in a given nursing care situation.

THE CRITICAL THINKING MOVEMENT: EDUCATION FOR LIFE

The full breadth of the critical thinking movement is not often addressed in nursing texts. Scholars have delineated diverse modes of critical thinking for millennia, as exemplified in the European tradition by Plato and Aristotle, but the contemporary movement can be traced to publications by Ennis (1962) and Glaser (1941), from which many branches grew in the second half of the twentieth century (Ennis, 1962; Paul, 1993; Thayer-Bacon, 2000). The movement was initially conceived as an extension, or blossoming, of the democratization of education (Paul, 1993). The ideal was to cultivate formidable intellectual abilities in all youth, not only among those who graduated from private colleges and universities. Critical thinking was tied to a progressive vision of greater democracy. Knowledge, discernment, logic, critical analysis of the views of others, and dialogue with persons holding different views were considered vital to this project. These dimensions of the critical thinking movement have strong implications for nursing.

Although various critical thinking theorists define the process differently, all are strong advocates for an increased emphasis on critical thinking in *all* education broadly. Ennis (1987) is a proponent of reasoned reflection as the basis for decision-making and action. McPeck (1981) advocates reflective skepticism as the basis for engaging in specific activities. Paul (1989) promotes "disciplined, self-directed thinking" that is dialogical and morally grounded as a process leading to the "perfection" of thinking in a particular domain (p. 214). Lipman (1988) specifically advocates "skillful, responsible thinking that facilitates good judgment because it (1) relies upon criteria, (2) is self-correcting, and (3) is sensitive to context" (p. 39). Siegel (1988) proposes that critical thinking means that a persistent rationality is the preeminent basis for one's beliefs and actions. Critical thinking as a component of professionalism cannot be considered alone but rather, in the context of a broad liberal education in arts and sciences and a commitment to life-long learning.

SELECTED CONCEPTS OF CRITICAL THINKING

All health care professionals, including nurses, are continually faced with situations in which careful thinking about specific elements of the situation is necessary for the discharge of their duties in caring for people. Reasoning must be applied to such situations, and conclusions drawn so that actions can be taken or withheld. The very value of *rationality* (reasoning) is the primary assumption underlying the discourse about critical thinking. If we do not agree that rationality indeed informs our thinking about human affairs in a unique way, then the relevance of critical thinking as a process for decision-making becomes questionable. This is not to say that rationality underpins all human affairs. It is often clear in the realm of personal values, interests, and passions, that rationality has a marginal or even oppositional role vis-à-vis individual beliefs and values in actual living.

The centrality of rationality in critical thinking relates to the scientific dimensions of nursing, since rationality is an inherent quality of science, but not necessarily of all dimensions of life or art. Reasoning and logical analysis are necessary components of critical thinking. However, if these are applied only to what may seem to be the salient, objective factors in a given situation without *also* giving deep consideration to perspective, context, relevance, and meaning, the resulting analysis will likely be hollow and mechanistic, and of little value for decision-making in the significant life situations where nursing care takes place.

A few fundamental concepts are useful in improving the exercise of critical thinking in health care situations and in reflecting on such situations. In health assessments, interviews, triage, and other ways of coming to know the person(s) to be cared for, information is gathered that may or may not allow for a conclusion to be drawn about the person and her/his situation and health. Knowledge and information from other sources (education, experience, tradition, workplace routines, research, anecdotes, and other sources) are *applied* to the available data *about* the situation at hand. Together, these bits of information and knowledge, stated as assertions, comprise the *reasons*, or *premises*, for whatever *conclusions* may be drawn.

Case Example

In differentiating a common cold from influenza, the information to be taken into consideration includes the time of year in which the illness occurs, whether or not the person received an annual influenza vaccination, whether or not the person had a known exposure to influenza, whether or not high fevers and body aches are present, and whether or not the person states something to the effect of "I know this is the flu." From medical science we know that influenza is the more serious illness, far more prone to complications, with a significant number of fatalities annually. So, from a medical perspective, if the information available leads to the reasoned conclusion that the person has influenza, the care will be different than it would if the conclusion were that the person had a common cold.

In considering the reasons or premises for a particular conclusion, the critical thinker considers the *validity* of the evidence and the *logical connections* between and among the various pieces of information. Validity refers to the *soundness, relevance,* and *meaningfulness* of the premises given for a particular conclusion. Soundness is the degree to which an assertion can be said to be free of error, fallacy, or misapprehension. Relevance is the extent to which an assertion pertains to the immediate and actual situation at hand. Meaningfulness relates to the understandings of the situation by those who are living it. The strongest premises for drawing conclusions (to state the obvious) are those that are sound, relevant, and meaningful. The critical thinker must reflect on the evidence with *openness* (or *skepticism*), with *self-discipline,* and *within its historico-cultural and ethical context.* The critical thinker must focus on the strength of the premises in drawing a conclusion, be sensitive to the life context of the situation, and be self-correcting, by thinking about the quality of her/his own thinking *while* she/he is thinking (Ennis, 1987; Lipman, 1988; McPeck, 1981; Paul, 1989; Siegel, 1988).

Thinking critically in this manner is necessary in order to justify taking action in the realm of health care, where the actions of practitioners can be life-saving or life-threatening, where seemingly small actions can lead to very significant consequences, and where the autonomy of the person cared for must always be respected in decision-making. Moreover, the full life context of the situation and the various perspectives of all the individuals directly involved in the situation should be taken into account. Critical thinking requires time for data gathering, reflection, and discussion. Improving your critical thinking skills is not likely to make you a faster working nurse. For this very reason, there are elements of the health care establishment (bureaucrats, administrators, and payer sources) that do not always support the continued development of critical thinking among nurses (Weinberg, 2001).

As we move from the level of making relatively obvious differentiations in the presentation of various illnesses to the level of seriously considering the full complexity of life situations in the context of diverse families and communities, the challenges of applying critical thinking in practice, and the real complexity and depth of thought required to do so, become more apparent. Ultimately, in any given health care situation, there are endless interpretations of reality among the parties involved and infinite possibilities as to how the situation will eventually unfold. Critical thinking is needed in nursing *not* to simplify the processes of thinking about the deep complexities of life, health, and health care, but rather *to ensure that the complexities of life are recognized, appreciated, and respected* by nurses, with the realization that ultimately, it is not possible for the health care provider, whether physician, nurse, or other professional, to resolve all the problems and ease all the pain an individual may have.

CRITICAL THINKING WITH AND ABOUT NURSING FRAMEWORKS

As the centerpiece of an educational reform movement, critical thinking has been regarded widely as a process that is generalizable across subjects and disciplines. An emphasis on the processes of inquiry, logical reasoning, and reflection, as opposed to rote memorization of facts or theories, has been its hallmark. Through the years, a number of works have been produced exploring and illustrating views on critical thinking *within* specific disciplines. McPeck (1981) and Resnick (1987), along with a number of others, claim that critical thinking actually is not learned in the abstract, but precisely in the detailed subject matter of a specific discipline.

Critical thinking in nursing should not be construed to refer simply to tidy linear processes of judging according to predefined criteria, choosing diagnostic labels from menus, problem-solving in a context of cause-effect thinking, implementing interventions grounded in the notion of an objective reality, and evaluating outcomes based on predefined norms. To consider critical thinking only a biomedical concept without explicating a perspective specific to nursing is to ignore nursing's distinctive place in the multidisciplinary health care team and the unique role of the nurse in society. Just as the lawyer has an obligation to apply critical thinking to the practice of law, and the physician has an obligation to apply critical thinking to the practice of medicine, the nurse has a professional obligation to exercise and apply critical thinking specifically to the practice of nursing *as* nursing.

Thinking is unavoidably shaped and colored by the historico-cultural context of the thinker. The multidimensional influences of history, culture, environment, language, economics, and education are always with us. The critical thinking movement promotes engagement with other cultures and multiple perspectives. It is, however, even more fundamental to the development of critical thinking abilities *to know oneself as a person and a nurse, to be able to articulate one's basic beliefs about human beings, health, and health care, and to understand where one's beliefs and values come from.* What beliefs, values, and assumptions about human beings and health drive your practice? How do you connect these with your everyday practice, and how do you know if your actions and intentions in practice are consistent with your belief system or not? What does your belief system drive you to attend to in practice (from the vast panoply of possible aspects of human beings and their health), and why?

NURSING FRAMEWORKS AS AIDS TO UNDERSTANDING

Nursing frameworks can be useful in coming to know self as person and nurse (Cody, 2000). A crucial move to promote deeper and more authentically critical thinking in nursing is the use of nursing theoretical frameworks to guide practice. The use of nursing theoretical frameworks adds depth to nursing practice that cannot be attained any other way. This is because nursing frameworks are the only theoretical frameworks rooted in philosophies of nursing and intended solely to guide nursing practice and research. For example, the nurse who uses Watson's (1999) framework concerned with human caring places the philosophy, science, and act of caring in the forefront of her or his performance as a nurse. She or he would attempt, by forming a transpersonal relationship with the person and seeking to participate in transcendence within actual caring occasions, to facilitate the wholeness and growth of the person, conceived as body-mind-spirit. Familiarity with the literature on Watson's framework and the thoughts of Watson scholars around the world is necessary to think critically about one's practice in this context.

The nurse who uses Parse's (1998) framework concerned with human becoming places the philosophy and science of unitary becoming in the forefront of her or his performance as a nurse, in which she or he offers true presence to the other in the context of the nurse-person relationship, and seeks to cocreate the quality of life desired by the person. Familiarity with the relevant literature is again necessary in this context. Using a nursing framework that resonates with one's values provides a philosophically and logically sound and consistent guide to practice across a range of settings and situations, and is thus an indispensable aid to the effective use of critical thinking.

Nursing frameworks embrace the discipline's unique societal and professional mission. Each one offers a structure of beliefs, values, concepts, and principles to guide nursing practice. As a professional, the nurse should be well versed in the frameworks of the discipline and have advanced knowledge in at least one framework to guide her or his practice. This aspect of ongoing professional education requires critical thinking, and a number of aids to analysis and evaluation of nursing frameworks exist (for example, see Fawcett, 2000). The nurse should also be well aware of alternative frameworks and conceptualizations in a way that connects one's own reflections with the varieties of possibilities envisioned by frameworks from nursing and other disciplines.

The use of nursing frameworks enables us to engage in critical thinking in many ways, such as the following:

- Exploring alternative visions of reality and seeking to understand how others experience their humanity and their relation to the universe
- Differentiating nursing science and nursing service from those of other professions, thereby offering a unique service to humankind
- Creatively designing innovative ways to be with clients and to offer assistance to them in ways they value

- Critiquing the status quo in relation to injustice and fundamentally unfair societal policies
- Doing all these things in a community of similar-thinking colleagues who speak the same language, share one's understandings about people, health, and health care, and wish to be genuinely engaged toward a common purpose in bettering humankind

Case Example

The nurses on a busy nursing unit within a large health care organization decide to use a nursing framework as an overall guide for their practice. Thus, they are better able to agree upon the goals of nursing care, to share a common definition of health and well-being, to be consistent in the ways in which different nurses offer care, to communicate with one another about the salient particulars of each case, to contribute more demonstrably a unique component to the multidisciplinary team's overall care of the person and family, and to document the care given more consistently. These capacities, in turn, support the use of critical thinking by the nurses around the central shared goal of improving care, health outcomes, and quality of life.

CRITICAL THINKING: MORE THAN CLINICAL PROBLEM SOLVING

Contemporary health care in the developed world includes state-of-the-art equipment and pharmaceuticals, practitioners with highly specialized knowledge, and systems, policies, and codes of ethics that are in place to promote the safety and dignity of persons, and fairness in the delivery of health care services. Unfortunately, in addition to the elements listed above, other less desirable elements of society also shape and color contemporary health care to some extent, as undeniable dimensions of contemporary life. Beliefs, systems, and behavior patterns that can be identified through critical thinking as white supremacist, sexist, ethnocentric, classist, and homophobic persist among powerbrokers and practitioners. Many health care workers labor with too little education beyond biomedical technology to offer competent care consistently to whole persons or to demonstrate profound respect for human dignity in all health care situations. Overuse and misuse of technology are common, as are egregious pricegouging, profiteering, and monumental waste of resources. Critical thinking in nursing means having the capacity to apprehend, question, and analyze these aspects of health care when they come to light, as well as the capacity to reason critically within the full context of life, community, and society.

DIVERSITY AND POSSIBILITY

It is through critical thinking that the nurse can provide the proper balance of culturally sensitive care and individualized care by being continuously aware that every ethnic group has common patterns of beliefs and activities, but open to the insight that a particular individual within that group does not necessarily follow these. Situations arise in which the routine of the health care agency, the culture of the person, and the person's individual preferences represent three different perspectives on the same situation. It is not uncommon to witness colleagues in health care making snap judgments about persons based on their race or ethnicity, their age, their sex, their class, and so forth. Critical thinking abilities empower the nurse to think through such situations and design care that does not succumb to such faulty thinking, but rather creatively addresses the uniqueness of each situation. Through application of critical thinking, the nurse can uphold nursing values, including the wholeness of persons, the interrelatedness of person and environment, and the inherent dignity of each person. Critical thinking can cut through stereotypes; it can help us to imagine *Why not?* when confronted with a novel life pattern; and it can serve to analyze and critique dimensions of justice and ethics in the delivery of health care.

Questions that we may ask ourselves to stimulate and sustain critical thinking in a variety of situations include the following:

- What is the goal of my practice in this situation, and how can I best keep sight of it amid the complexity?
- How does a nursing perspective on this situation differ from the perspective of medicine or other disciplines?
- Whose perspective is of central importance here? The client's . . . or someone else's?
- What unexamined assumptions underlie the assertions being made in this situation?
- How does the information available in this given situation relate to the scientific knowledge of similar phenomena? How valid is the data I have collected? From where did it come, and can I trust it?

- Is the information I have collected really relevant to the crux of the situation as the client or others may see it?
- What is the meaning of the situation for the client? For the family? For society? For the health care agency for which I work? Whose perspective is central to decision-making here?

It is most important in critical thinking to stay open to new possibilities of understanding. Indeed, the person who is not open to new possibilities of understanding could hardly be said to be thinking critically at all. The critical thinker is willing to and prepared to experience the unexpected while thinking about complex situations—and is perhaps even enthusiastic about it!

Case Example

Among certain populations in the United States in which poverty is severe and persistent over generations (such as the homeless population with whom this author has worked for 10 years), most families comprise single mothers and their children, and the extended family is, for the most part, a matriarchal network of women and children in similar situations, with little consistent adult male presence. Consider the unemployed mother of three children with three different fathers who is now homeless with her children. She left her last boyfriend because he was using illegal drugs and she found no options other than the street and the shelter.

If you were asked to analyze this family's situation, what would you list among the factors contributing to their becoming homeless? What would you point to as evidence? Some might say that poor choices in sex partners, lack of birth control, and drug use contributed to the homelessness, while others might say that unemployment and lack of needed government programs were the decisive factors. The nurse must be capable of thinking incisively about these situations while maintaining a profound respect for the woman and her children to be able to care for this woman and her children as whole persons. The nurse should also be self-aware enough to identify the underlying values that color and shape her/his perceptions.

THE CENTRALITY OF ATTENTIVE LISTENING

Much of health care is practiced as objective science and taught as objective science. In chemistry, biology, pathophysiology, and pharmacology, objectivity functions as a tool that helps us to understand the form and function of physical phenomena, and to predict how these may react under certain conditions. Where this approach to science, experimentation, knowledge, and prediction is appropriate, objectivity serves its purposes very well. Many of the phenomena that confront nurses in day-to-day practice, however, are experiential, unique to the person living the experience, or in the common parlance, *subjective*. In recent years, it has become more widely accepted to treat pain as clients describe it subjectively, and it is not too hard to see that phenomena such as grieving or loneliness are essentially subjective; they are uniquely experienced by the person living the experience.

Critical thinking can be put to best use in nursing if it is applied in a context of *listening to clients*. Despite advances in democracy, consumerism, and bioethics, much of health care remains extremely paternalistic. Among practitioners, programs, and systems, it is not difficult to find examples of paternalism—a diminution in the effective autonomy of the person, ostensibly for her/his own good—throughout health care and human services (Cody, 2003). Paternalistic attitudes and interventions are commonly associated with what the purveyors consider to be objective facts about the situation. However, the actual factors that are truly relevant to the situation can only by known by listening to the person who is living the experience. It is only by listening to clients that one can obtain the most crucial bits of information to which one can even apply critical thinking!

For example, the ability to listen attentively and engage authentically with persons is crucial if the nurse is to understand who the most important family members are for the person—not always the spouse, offspring, or parent, as one might assume. Many persons have concerns about the illnesses they are living with that make it difficult for them to absorb any new information. Listening for these concerns and addressing these as the first step in a teaching plan paves the way for more meaningful learning. Further, in today's high-tech, acute-care environments, where many persons are living with multiple system problems and technology dependence, the need for persons, families, and health care professionals to make life-changing (or even life-ending) decisions on painfully short notice has become quite common. The connection between the ability to listen attentively and the ability to critically think through complex nursing care situations cannot be overemphasized.

DIFFERENT INFORMATION AND EVIDENCE
TO ADDRESS DIFFERENT QUESTIONS

In a scientific field that also encompasses human care, it is sometimes necessary for clinicians to remind themselves that traditional scientific evidence is not the only kind of information or knowledge that is needed for competent practice. As Fawcett, Watson, Neuman, Walker, and Fitzpatrick (2001) amply demonstrate, it is necessary for the nurse to seek different kinds of information to address different questions that arise in nursing practice, research, education, and administration. According to Fawcett and colleagues, the evidence sought to address *empirical* questions is scientific data—information systematically collected from people experiencing the phenomenon under study, analyzed through rigorous processes. The evidence sought to address *ethical* questions is found in standards of practice, codes of ethics, and philosophies of nursing—representations that are fundamentally different in kind from empirical evidence. The validity of such evidence is derived from public discourse subject to philosophical analysis and interpretation, leading to some form of public assertions of basic ethical principles. The evidence needed to address *personal* questions in nursing practice is found in each person's own experience and is that which is reflected on in reflective practice. The evidence sought to address *aesthetic* questions in nursing is found in works of art (nursing or non-nursing) and criticism. Thus, a novel, play, film, painting, or song may in some sense inform one's practice, in that it can characterize or portray an experience in such a way as to broaden our understandings of it.

A Case Example of Varieties of Evidence

Hector is a 30-year-old man living with human immunodeficiency disease (HIV). Jen is a 28-year-old registered nurse caring for Hector on his first hospital admission for complications of HIV, specifically, pneumocystic carinii pneumonia. Upon their initial meeting, Hector tells Jen of several concerns he has regarding his care. His life partner, who has health care power of attorney, is male, and Hector wants his partner to room in as much as possible, but he does not want his parents to know about his partner. His family background includes a deep devotion to a certain religious tradition, which Hector respects in his interactions with his family, but in his own personal life he is not religious and not a practicing member of the church. Hector has certain concerns about the details of his care. He says that he has had "pneumonia" before and "got over it very quickly" by doing a lot of breathing exercises and coughing, and he is looking forward to doing that again in this instance. He says he is very troubled whenever he has to hear details about his diagnostic tests, cell counts, and such, and he would prefer not to have to hear any more than is absolutely necessary for his care. Hector also tells Jen that he is deeply saddened by this first significant opportunistic infection, although he has anticipated that it would come sooner or later, and he needs lots of quiet time to reflect on what it means to his life, his career, and his family, to be dealing with a potentially fatal illness at this time of his life.

Jen, Hector's nurse, has cared for a number of persons living with HIV and has kept current with the scientific literature on HIV-related care. She has taken a keen interest in HIV as represented in the arts. She also has developed the attentive listening skills and critical thinking skills to care for Hector both effectively and meaningfully. Jen has reflected on her own mortality, her feelings about persons close to her living with potentially fatal illnesses, and her experiences caring for persons who died, and is comfortable with her memories, beliefs, and values about these experiences. Jen is very cognizant of the various issues involved in juggling the relationships and interactions of the partner and the family of origin. She is aware of her ethical obligations regarding the person's decision-making or those of his designee, should he become incapacitated; and she is aware of the aesthetic considerations in maintaining a supportive, comfortable environment in Hector's room despite the potential for turmoil. Jen understands the likely misapprehension that Hector has right now regarding this pneumonia (which is interstitial and cannot be significantly helped by coughing), but she also understands that Hector may not be ready to hear this at the time of his admission. Jen is also aware of the difficulties that Hector may have in finding adequate quiet time for reflection in the midst of an acute-care hospital setting, but she takes note of his desire for such reflection to be supported and shares this information with the next nurse coming on shift. Clearly, all of these considerations offer unlimited opportunities for Jen to exercise critical thinking in caring for Hector.

CONCLUSION

Critical thinking is a crucial component of all professional nursing practice. It relates not only to biomedically oriented clinical judgment, but also to the whole context of life as it is humanly lived, and all that the nurse brings to her/his practice. Enhancing one's critical thinking is about *education for life*. Fundamental concepts of critical thinking are rationality, logic, premises, soundness, validity, relevance, meaning, perspective, and context. As a profession, nursing has an obligation to apply critical thinking to the practice of nursing *as* nursing. In this regard, nursing frameworks offer means of enhancing knowledge of self, clarity in one's perspective of the discipline, and critical thinking. Using nursing frameworks with enhanced critical thinking offers increased possibilities for improving care and the quality of life.

REFLECTIVE QUESTIONS

1. What does it mean to consider the whole life situation of persons to whom you offer care?
2. Think of a situation in which critical thinking about multiple kinds of evidence is necessary for understanding. What is most important for you personally to know to make a decision?

RECOMMENDED READINGS

Alfaro-Lefevre, R. (2004). *Critical thinking in nursing: A practical approach* (3rd ed.). Philadelphia: Saunders.

Fawcett, J., Watson, J., Neuman, B., Walker, P. H., & Fitzpatrick, J. J. (2001). On nursing theories and evidence. *Journal of Nursing Scholarship, 33*(2), 115–119.

hooks, bell (1997). *Cultural criticism and transformation* (videotape). Northampton, MA: Media Education Foundation.

Paul, R. (1993). *Critical thinking: What every person needs to survive in a rapidly changing world.* Santa Rosa, CA: Foundation for Critical Thinking.

Thayer-Bacon, B. J. (2000). *Transforming critical thinking: Thinking constructively.* New York: Teachers College Press.

REFERENCES

Alfaro-Lefevre, R. (2004). *Critical thinking in nursing: A practical approach* (3rd ed.). Philadelphia: Saunders.

American Association of Colleges of Nursing (1998). *The essentials of bacca-laureate education for professional nursing practice*. Washington, DC: Author.

Cody, W. K. (2000). Theoretical concerns: Nursing science frameworks as means of knowing self. *Nursing Science Quarterly, 13*, 188–195.

Cody, W. K. (2003). Paternalism in nursing and healthcare: Central issues and their relation to theory. *Nursing Science Quarterly, 16* (4), 288–296.

Ennis, R. H. (1987). A taxonomy of critical thinking dispositions and abilities. In J. B. Baron & R. J. Sternberg (Eds.), *Teaching thinking skills: Theory and practice*. New York: W. H. Freeman and Company.

Ennis, R. H. (1962). A concept of critical thinking. *Harvard Educational Review, 32*(1), 81–111.

Fawcett, J. (2000). *Analysis and evaluation of contemporary nursing knowledge: Nursing frameworks and theories*. Philadelphia: F. A. Davis.

Fawcett, J., Watson, J., Neuman, B., Walker, P. H., & Fitzpatrick, J. J. (2001). On nursing theories and evidence. *Journal of Nursing Scholarship, 33*(2), 115–119.

Glaser, E. (1941). *An experiment in the development of critical thinking*. New York: Teachers College Press.

Gray, M. T. (2003). Beyond content: Generating critical thinking in the classroom. *Nurse Educator, 28*(3), 136–140.

Hicks, F. D. (2003). Critical thinking and clinical decision-making in critical care nursing: A pilot study. *Heart & Lung, 32*(3), 169–180.

LeMone, P., & Burke, K. M. (2004). *Medical-surgical nursing: Critical thinking in client care* (3rd ed.). Upper Saddle River, NJ: Prentice Hall Health.

Lipman, M. (1988). *Philosophy goes to school*. Philadelphia: Temple University Press.

McPeck, J. (1981). *Critical thinking and education*. New York: St. Martin's.

Parse, R. R. (1998). *The human becoming school of thought*. Thousand Oaks, CA: Sage.

Paul, R. (1989). Critical thinking in North America: A new theory of knowledge, learning and literacy. *Argumentation, 3*, 197–235.

Paul, R. (1993). *Critical thinking: What every person needs to survive in a rapidly changing world*. Santa Rosa, CA: Foundation for Critical Thinking.

Resnick, L. B. (1987). *Education and learning to think*. Washington, DC: National Academy Press.

Seymour, B. (2003). Valuing both critical and creative thinking in clinical practice: Narrowing the research-practice gap? *Journal of Advanced Nursing, 41*(3), 288–296.

Siegel, H. (1988). *Educating reason: Rationality, critical thinking, and education*. New York and London: Routledge.

Thayer-Bacon, B. J. (2000). *Transforming critical thinking: Thinking constructively*. New York: Teachers College Press.

Watson, J. (1999). *Postmodern nursing and beyond*. Edinburgh, New York: Churchill Livingstone.

Weinberg, D. B. (2001). *Code green: Money-driven hospitals and the dismantling of nursing*. Ithaca, NY: Cornell University Press.

18

Making the Transition to Professional Nursing: Becoming a Lifelong Learner

Jane Conway and Margaret McMillan

LEARNING OBJECTIVES

Those who have read this chapter should be able to:

- Consider strategies which maximize learning opportunities in a range of contexts
- View themselves as autonomous, action-oriented learners
- Appreciate the interaction between lifelong learning and professional development
- Develop strategies to address self-development
- Appreciate the interaction between classroom-based learning activities and clinical practice

KEY WORDS

Transition, graduate, accountability, lifelong learning, curriculum, clinical education, facilitator

INTRODUCTION

This chapter is based on the belief that the transition from student to graduate and practitioner requires the development of the ability to critically examine our own and others' practice and be accountable for our own actions. These abilities are often linked to the idea of being a lifelong learner (Buchan, 1998) and are seen as increasingly important to professional nursing practice in the twenty-first century (Clark, Maben, & Jones, 1997). The authors recognize that, for many student nurses, clinical practice is the goal of nursing education. However, as will be demonstrated, the principles that underpin learning in the clinical area are explored in on-campus learning activities and are transferable across contexts.

In writing about the development of registered nurses, Benner (1984) has identified that the ability to integrate theory and practice to the point of being able to generalize is essential to development from novice (newly qualified nurse) to later and more advanced levels of nursing. However, Benner also acknowledges that there are particular challenges in being able to transfer concepts across contexts. Effective clinicians are aware that *context* is the crucial moderator in nursing practice, and have developed mechanisms for managing situations contextually rather than seeking to manage all situations in the same way. Such ability to transfer core concepts across situations and modify actions according to context is an indication of *expert* nursing practice (Benner, 1984). Clinical learning experiences provide nursing students with the opportunity to begin to develop the skills of identifying general principles of practice, transferring them across contexts, and modifying actions based on principles of management.

Dale (1994) argues that experiential knowledge (the knowledge that arises from the integration and subsequent analysis of theory in practice) is not adequately developed in nursing students. Thus, without clinical learning experiences which provide the opportunity to integrate classroom theory into real-life practice situations, nursing students have little opportunity to develop the lifelong learning skills of critical thinking and reflective practice considered important to professional practice (Benner, 1984; Benner, Tanner, & Chesla, 1996), nor to appreciate that how we view the interrelationship between academic and clinical learning is what creates our definition of nursing.

Experiential knowledge is not merely being exposed to an experience. It is that which emerges when the experience is structured to achieve learning as an outcome of the experience. Therefore, students should use the theoretical base developed from university-based activities to frame the clinical experience so that learning, rather than merely experiencing, occurs. Students should ask themselves, "What is it that I want to achieve from this learning experience, and how does this relate to my ability to practice nursing?"

HOW CAN I BEST DEVELOP NEW KNOWLEDGE?

In order to learn, we need to develop the process skills for lifelong learning (Maslin-Prothero, 2001; Griffitts, 2002; Armstrong, Johnston, Bridges, & Gessner, 2003). These process skills are the basis of learning and are transferable across disciplines. In the case of nursing, nursing knowledge provides specific content which, when processed, results in nursing action. That is to say, when we become nurses, we have developed general learning skills and we demonstrate our use of these through being able to "think and act like a nurse." In order to be lifelong learners in relation to nursing practice, we need to become what has been termed *reflective practitioners* (Brookfield, 1993). We need to reflect about what we do as nurses, how we respond as nurses and individuals, and what we would do again in a similar situation. We then need to act when a similar situation occurs. The skills of reflective practice unite theoretical and clinical concepts.

In Figure 18.1 below, Gibbs (1988) provides a useful framework for situation analysis that is both thought- and action-oriented and allows

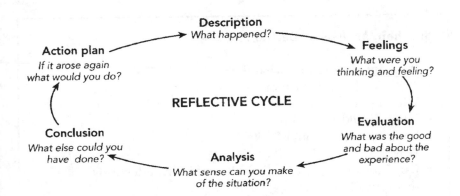

FIGURE 18.1   The reflective cycle.
Gibbs, 1988.

for consideration of the affective aspects of nursing experience and provides opportunity to explore how the learner as a reflective practitioner felt about the experience. Such an approach is particularly useful in nursing as it acknowledges human and emotional as well as intellectual domains of decision making.

Classroom-based learning activity provides us with the opportunity to explore, in a relatively safe environment, what we know, what we do, and who we are as nurses, so that we are more prepared for professional practice situations. Clinical learning activity provides us with the opportunity both to test out what we have learned in practice and to confront new situations from which we can further our learning. However, we can only learn if we are prepared to do so. It is important that we value learning as much as we value what we have learned. It is our ability to question ourselves and our practice that enhances our professional development.

Little (1996) has developed a framework of questions that is applicable in both classroom and clinical learning situations. These questions provide a useful guide to developing lifelong learning skills, yet are equally important questions for clinical decision making. The framework recognizes that learning is inherently a personal experience, and places emphasis on the subjective nature of learning (Griffitts, 2002). In order to be accountable for their practice, nurses need to become subjectively engaged in that practice.

Little's approach consists of the following sets of questions related to a range of areas.

Situation/Analysis or Decision Making

- What information do I have?
- What further information do I need?
- What options/alternatives do I have?
- What should I prioritize?
- What action/s should I take?
- Why?
- Can I justify this action (lawfully, ethically, effectively, theoretically, etc.)?

The Learning Process

- What do I already know?
- How do I know it?
- What do I need to know?
- Where will I find it?
- What resources can I use?
- How will I know that I know?
- Why should I learn it?

Perceptions

- What are my feelings?
- What are my beliefs about the situation?
- What are my assumptions?
- How have I derived these beliefs/assumptions?
- How do my feelings/beliefs
  - affect my interpretation?
  - affect my response?
  - relate to espoused professional values?
- Why do I hold this belief/assumption?
- What are alternative beliefs/assumptions?

Learning Processes

- What is the validity of my source?
  - Legislation
  - Data based on research
  - Opinion
  - Practice
  - Expertise
  - Experience
- What is the currency of the knowledge, skills, behavior?
- What is the support for this view?
  - Political/ideological
  - Cultural
- What other ideas/concepts/skills does it relate to?
- How does it relate to my view of the world (current understanding)?

The Situation Revisited

- How does my learning relate to/apply in this situation?
- How does my learning relate to/affect my original ideas?
- What gaps/misconceptions did my learning identify?
- What ideas/skills did my learning confirm?
- What response would I give now in the situation?

Reflection on

- **Situation analysis**

  - How well did I use the data?
  - How well did I define the situation in need of a response?
  - How comprehensive were my alternatives?
  - How well can I justify my response?

- **The learning process**

  - How valid/relevant were my sources?
  - How comprehensive were my sources?
  - How effective was my learning?

- **The group process**

  - How well did I contribute?
  - Wh9t was my role in the groups?
  - How effective was each member's contribution?
  - Did the group remain on task?
  - Did the group attend to process, that is, how people were feeling/responding/behaving, etc.?

This framework of questions is useful because it encourages us to look at situations in context and to appreciate that, as learners and professionals who make sound clinical judgments, we are required to interact effectively with others, provide reasoning and support for our actions and decisions, and be aware that we are accountable for our own learning and practice actions.

Whilst both Gibbs's and Little's frameworks are relevant to a number of practice disciplines, including nursing, there is potential for nurses selectively to utilise the *learning* components of models such as these and to overlook the critical elements related to action. Ultimately, professional accountability is related to actions, not a capacity to generate ideas. Although theory is important, because it provides a framework for the work nurses do, it is of little consequence unless it results in effective nursing actions. Conversely, practice can become meaningless unless we seek to understand it through conceptualizing the practice of nursing. Such integration of theory and practice leads to our moving beyond *becoming* nurses to *being* nurses who integrate our knowing, doing, and being to produce what is meaningful, client-focused management of situations. Being reflective practitioners means that we are, both personally and professionally, constantly transformed and emancipated from our previous ways of thinking and acting (Brookfield, 1993; Cranton, 1994; Frierc, 1972; Mezirow, 1985).

> We agree that the goal of nursing education is to prepare nurses: to be more responsive to societal needs, more successful in humanizing the highly technological milieus of healthcare, more caring and compassionate, more insightful about ethical and moral issues, more creative, more capable of critical thinking and better able to bring scholarly approaches to client problems and issues and to advocate ethical positions on behalf of clients. (Bevis & Watson, 1989, p. 1)

We are also concerned that the attitude that clinical and classroom learning are separate entities may result in the mistaken perception that there is an insurmountable division between the theoretical and practical aspects of nursing. Students of nursing need to be encouraged to develop skills in reflective practice and situation analysis, not for the purpose of intellectualizing or rationalizing nursing practice, but for the purpose of identifying and maintaining excellence in clinical practice and meeting the goals of nursing identified above by Bevis and Watson. Figure 18.2 represents what we perceive to be the relationships between context and lifelong learning processes and curriculum and improved practice. Achieving improved practice required the process skills of lifelong learning and reflective practice.

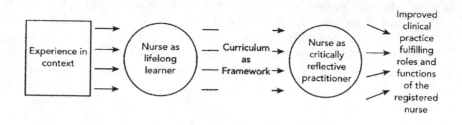

FIGURE 18.2   An educational equation for improved nursing practice.
Conway & McMillan, 2000, p. 273.

USING EDUCATION AS A SPRINGBOARD TO A DIVERSITY OF PRACTICE ROLES

In order to gain the most out of learning experiences, it is important that each experience be approached as a way of linking theory and practice, and as an opportunity for further learning and generation of new perspectives. The role of the registered nurse is increasingly one of health care facilitator/manager as well as direct caregiver. Students of nursing should be encouraged to view the role of the registered nurse as multifaceted, incorporating functions of both health care giver and health care facilitator (Andersen, 1991). Andersen's model identifies a number of nursing roles that students should explore while in the clinical setting. Increasingly, nurses are required to engage in roles beyond that of direct patient care giver and engage in *systems level intervention*, such as contributor in multidisciplinary teams, researcher, and manager, through which they facilitate quality patient care. At the very least, students need to think about how the roles and functions that registered nurses perform have shaped, and been shaped by, the practice situation.

Nursing students should explore roles other than direct care giver. In most nursing programs, the primary emphasis is placed on providing clinical experience in a range of settings (e.g., mental health, acute care and the community). However, it is unclear whether students are encouraged to explore a range of nursing roles and functions while in those settings (Conway & McMillan, 2000). In order to prepare for the diversity of practice, students themselves should analyze each situation and try to determine what nursing roles and competencies are applicable. For example, students should ask themselves:

- What is the role of the registered nurse here? Is the registered nurse in this context a *health care giver* or a *health care facilitator*?
- Does the role require skills as a clinician, researcher, educator, manager, or communicator, or a combination of these?
- What knowledge base is required for sound clinical decision making?

Asking questions such as these encourages us to explore the diverse roles and functions of nurses and to differentiate between the roles of registered nurses and other levels of nurses.

CONCLUSION

Nursing is emerging as a distinct entity (May & Fleming, 1997) with curricula that emphasize nursing as a discipline distinguished from others (Duffy, Foster, Kuiper, Long, & Robison, 1995; Greenwood, 1996). Contemporary nursing curricula include discipline specific knowledge, and integrate knowledge from other disciplines to inform the practice of nursing. This differs from previous practices of modifying knowledge from other disciplines to suit nursing situations. Thus nursing education serves both an epistemological and political purpose, and students should be able to articulate and conceptualize the nature of their discipline and apply their thinking to actual practice. Contemporary nursing education challenges nurses to question and justify practice, and emphasizes the ability to think about nursing, as well as the ability to perform nursing actions to best manage nursing situations. The challenge for students is to develop an integrated approach to practice which values thoughtful, highly skilled and efficient action, and to continue with lifelong learning and professional development.

REFLECTIVE QUESTIONS

1. How can you become more responsible and accountable for your own learning?
2. How can you plan and evaluate your ongoing professional development?
3. Who can assist you with meeting these needs?

RECOMMENDED READINGS

Andersen, B. M. (1991). Mapping the terrain of the discipline. In G. Gray & R. Pratt (Eds.), *Towards a discipline of nursing.* Melbourne: Churchill Livingstone.

Benner, P., Tanner, C., & Chesla, C. (1996). *Expertise in nursing practice: Caring clinical judgement and ethics.* New York: Springer Publishing.

Lipe, S., & Beasley, S. (2003). *Critical thinking in nursing: A cognitive skills workbook.* Philadelphia: Lippincott.

Palmer, A. M., Burns, S., & Bulman, C. (1994). *Reflective practice in nursing: The growth of the professional practitioner.* Oxford: Blackwell.

REFERENCES

Andersen, B. M. (1991). Mapping the terrain of the discipline. In G. Gray & R. Pratt (Eds.), *Towards a discipline of nursing.* Melbourne: Churchill Livingstone.

Armstrong, M. L., Johnston, B. A., Bridges, R. A., & Gessner, B. A. (2003). The impact of graduate education on reading for lifelong learning. *The Journal of Continuing Education in Nursing, 34*(1), 19–27.

Benner, P. (1984). *From novice to expert: Excellence and power in clinical nursing practice.* Menlo Park: Addison Wesley.

Benner, P., Tanner, C. A., & Chesla, C. A. (1996) *Expertise in nursing practice: Caring, clinical judgment, and ethics.* New York: Springer Publishing.

Bevis, E. O., & Watson, J. (1989). *Toward a caring curriculum: A new pedagogy for nursing..* New York: National League for Nursing.

Brookfield, S. (1993). On impostorship, cultural suicide and other dangers: How nurses learn critical thinking. *Journal of Continuing Education in Nursing, 24*(5), 197–205.

Buchan J. (1998). Nurses off the peg. *Nursing Standard. 13*(1), 23–24.

Clark, J., Maben, J., & Jones, K. (1997). Project 2000: Perceptions of the philosophy and practice of nursing: Shifting perceptions—a new practitioner? *Journal of Advanced Nursing, 26*(1), 161–168.

Conway, J., & McMillan, M. (2000). Maximising Learning Opportunities. In J. Daly, S. Speedy, & D. Jackson (Eds.), *Contexts of nursing: An introduction* (1st ed.). Sydney: MacLennan & Petty.

Cranton, P. (1994). *Understanding and promoting transformative learning : A guide for educators of adults.* San Francisco: Jossey-Bass.

Dale, A. (1994). The theory-theory gap: The challenge for nurse teachers. *Journal of Advanced Nursing, 20,* 521–524.

Duffy, N., Foster, C., Kuiper, R., Long, J., & Robison, L. (1995). Planning nurses' education for the 21st century. *Journal of Advanced Nursing, 21,* 772–777.

Friere, P. (1972). *The pedagogy of oppression.* Harmondsworth: Penguin.

Gibbs, G. (1988). *Learning by doing: A guide to teaching and learning methods.* Oxford: Further Education Unit, Oxford Polytechnic.

Greenwood, J. (Ed.) (1996). *Nursing theory in Australia: Development and application.* Sydney: Harper Educational.

Griffitts, L. (2002). Geared to achieve with lifelong learning. *Nursing Management, 33*(11), 22–24.

Howatson-Jones, I. L. (2003). Difficulties in clinical supervision and lifelong learning. *Nursing Standard, 17*(37), 37.

Little, P. (1996). *Questions for learning.* Unpublished workshop material. PROBLARC. University of Newcastle.

Maslin-Prothero, S. (2001). *Bailliere's study skills for nurses.* London: Bailliere Tindall.

May, C., & Fleming, C. (1997). The professional imagination: Narrative and the symbolic boundaries between medicine and nursing. *Journal of Advanced Nursing, 25,* 1094–1100.

Mezirow, J. (1985). A critical theory of self directed learning. *New Directions for Continuing Education, 25,* 17–30.

Townsend, J. (1994). Challenge models for learning and knowing. In M. McMillan & J. Townsend (Eds.), *Reflections on contemporary nursing practice.* Sydney: Butterworth.

Index

𝕊 *Springer Publishing Company*

101 Careers in Nursing

Jeanne M. Novotny, PhD, RN, FAAN
Doris T. Lippman, EdD, APRN, CS
Nicole K. Sanders, BSN, RN
Joyce J. Fitzpatrick, PhD, MBA, RN, FAAN, Editors

Few careers offer the advantages of nursing: flexibility, room for growth, satisfaction from helping others. And there is a desperate need for nurses; demand will exceed supply for some time to come.

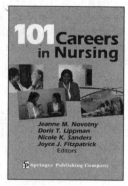

This concise volume provides an overview of what's possible in a nursing career. It profiles 101 different types of nursing careers, including a basic description, education requirements, skills needed, compensation, and related web sites and professional organizations. Personal stories from the practicing nurses highlight the content.

Students, career changers, find a wealth of informati

Contents:

* Introduction, *J.M. Novotny,*
* 101 Career Descriptions, such
  Armed Services Nurse, Cor
  Nurse, Disaster/Bioterrorism
  Care Transport, Forensic Nu
  Disabilities Nurse, Occupatio
  Donation Counselor, Peace C
  Assurance Nurse, Risk/Mana
  Transplant Nurse
* Launching Your Career Search
* Notes from My Interview Exp
  N.K. Sanders
* Guide to Certification in Nursir
* Glossary of Career Acronyms

2003   240p

750.364 LARCENY; FROM LIBRARIES

SEC. 364. LARCENY FROM LIBRARIES - -
ANY PERSON WHO SHALL PROCURE, OR TAKE IN
ANY WAY FROM ANY PUBLIC LIBRARY OR THE
LIBRARY OF ANY LITERARY, SCIENTIFIC,
HISTORICAL OR LIBRARY SOCIETY OR
ASSOCIATION, WHETHER INCORPORATED OR
UNINCORPORATED, ANY BOOK, PAMPHLET, MAP,
CHART, PAINTING, PICTURE, PHOTOGRAPH,
PERIODICAL, NEWSPAPER, MAGAZINE,
MANUSCRIPT OR EXHIBIT OR ANY PART THEREOF,
WITH INTENT TO CONVERT THE SAME TO HIS OWN
USE, OR WITH INTENT TO DEFRAUD THE OWNER
THEREOF, OR WHO HAVING PROCURED OR TAKEN
ANY SUCH BOOK, PAMPHLET, MAP, CHART,
PAINTING, PICTURE, PHOTOGRAPH, PERIODICAL,
NEWSPAPER, MAGAZINE, MANUSCRIPT OR
EXHIBIT OR ANY PART THEREOF, SHALL
THEREAFTER CONVERT THE SAME TO HIS OWN
USE OR FRAUDULENTLY DEPRIVE THE OWNER
THEREOF, SHALL BE QUILTY OF A MISDEMEANOR.

MICHIGAN COMPILED LAWS.

11 West 42nd Street, New York, NY 10036-8002 • Fax: 212-941-7842
Order Toll-Free: 877-687-7476 • Order On-line: www.springerpub.com